World malaria report 2009

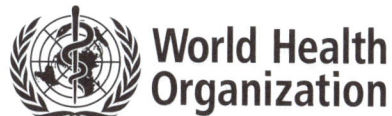

WHO Library Cataloguing-in-Publication Data

World malaria report 2009.

1.Malaria - prevention and control. 2.Malaria - drug therapy. 3.Antimalarials. 4.National health programs. 5.Statistics.
I.World Health Organization.

ISBN 978 92 4 156390 1   (NLM classification: WC 765)

Photos on cover: ©*WHO / Stephanie Hollyman*

Contents

Foreword

Dr Margaret Chan, *Director-General World Health Organization*

The findings in the *2009 World Malaria Report* are cause for cautious optimism. While much remains to be done, the data presented here clearly suggest that the tremendous increase in funding for malaria control is resulting in the rapid scale up of today's control tools. This, in turn, is having a profound effect on health – especially the health of children in sub-Saharan Africa. In a nutshell, development aid for health is working.

The global momentum that has been built to tackle malaria is extraordinary. It has brought together the governments of malaria endemic countries, foundations, bilateral donors, multilateral organizations, private companies, nongovernmental and faith-based organizations, and civil society. In the process, it has sparked the creation of public-private partnerships that are speeding up the development of new tools to fight this terrible scourge.

This report demonstrates that funding has resulted in steady increases in the coverage with malaria control interventions, especially insecticide-treated mosquito nets. It also shows that where these interventions have been fully scaled up, the malaria burden falls dramatically. On recent visits to African countries, I have witnessed the empty beds in the malaria wards and heard what this means for doctors, nurses, and families. This is the human side of the statistics set out in the report. Although still limited, early data suggest that the impacts being observed in health facilities are being mirrored by population level declines in all-cause child mortality. This is the sort of good news we all need.

Yet there are potential threats to our fragile success. The most serious of these is the further spread of resistance to artemisinins, which has been identified in malaria parasites in Asia. Although the extent of the spread of this resistance is still being determined, we need to act quickly to mitigate the threat. The World Health Organization, with support from a variety of donors and partners, has taken a leading role in efforts to characterize and contain artemisinin resistance in South-East Asia. We know, right now, three of the things that we urgently need to do: 1) halt the marketing and use of oral artemisinin monotherapies; 2) provide universal access to diagnostic testing for malaria; and 3) strengthen routine surveillance for malaria and regular monitoring of antimalarial drug efficacy.

We can save millions of lives over the coming years by scaling up the malaria control tools that we already have available. However, we know that the malaria parasite is a formidable opponent, and that if we are to ultimately eradicate malaria, we need new tools. The unprecedented recent spending on the research and development of these tools, including a vaccine against malaria, is a critical component of the long-term strategy against malaria. At the same time, we need to support operational research as an integral part of malaria programming so that we can learn as we implement and continuously refine our delivery strategies.

Ultimately, the power of malaria control interventions must be matched by the capacity to deliver those interventions to all who need them. If we fail to use these unprecedented global health resources to strengthen health systems, then we will have squandered a tremendous opportunity.

Mlehan

Acknowledgements

The following collected and reviewed national data from malaria-endemic countries – *WHO African Region:* Hammadi (Algeria); National Malaria Control Programme (Angola); Laly Roger (Benin); National Malaria Control Programme (Botswana); Laurent Moyenga (Burkina Faso); Hypax Mbanye (Burundi); Kouambeng Celestin (Cameroon); Antonio Lima Moreira (Cape Verde); Moyen Jean Méthode (Central African Republic); National Malaria Control Programme (Chad); Yssouf Amina (Comoros); National Malaria Control Programme (Côte d'Ivoire); Lydie Kalindula Azama (Democratic Republic of the Congo); National Malaria Control Programme (Equatorial Guinea); Tewolde Ghebremeskel (Eritrea); Worku Bekele (Ethiopia); Antimi J. Solange (Gabon); National Malaria Control Programme (Gambia); Constance Bart Plange (Ghana); Felicia Owusu-Antwi (Ghana); Amadou Oury Diallo (Guinea); Evangelino Quade (Guinea-Bissau); National Malaria Control Programme (Kenya); National Malaria Control Programme (Liberia); Benjamin Fanomezana Ramarosanatana (Madagascar); National Malaria Control Programme (Malawi); National Malaria Control Programme (Mali); National Malaria Control Programme (Mauritania); Samuel Mabunda (Mozambique); National Malaria Control Programme (Namibia); Abani Maazou (Niger); Aro Modiu Aliu (Nigeria); Karema Corine (Rwanda); Ahoranayezu Bosco (Rwanda); Jose Alvaro Leal Duarte (Sao Tome and Principe); Mame Birame Diouf (Senegal); Musa Sillah-Kanu (Sierra Leone); National Malaria Control Programme (South Africa); Zandie Dlamini for Simon Kunene (Swaziland); National Malaria Control Programme (Togo); Ebony Quinto (Uganda); Abdula Ali (Zanzibar, United Republic of Tanzania); Abdul-wahiyd Al-mafazy (Zanzibar, United Republic of Tanzania); Ritha Njau (United Republic of Tanzania); Rosemary Lusinde (United Republic of Tanzania); Fred Masaninga (Zambia); J. Mberikunashe (Zimbabwe). *WHO Eastern Mediterranean Region:* National Malaria Control Programme (Afghanistan); Zamani (Djibouti); Leila Faraji (Islamic Republic of Iran); Amed Akram Ahmed (Iraq); National Malaria Control Programme (Pakistan); Mohammad Al Zahrani (Saudi Arabia); Jamal Amran (Somalia); National Malaria Control Programme (Sudan); National Malaria Control Programme (Yemen). *WHO European Region:* Artavazd Vanyan (Armenia); Viktor Gasimov (Azerbaijan); Merab Iosava (Georgia); Usenbaev Nurbolot (Kyrgyzstan); Karimov Sayfuddin (Tajikistan); Seher Topluoglu (Turkey); Parida Umarova (Uzbekistan). *WHO Region of the Americas:* Ministry of Health (Argentina); Juan Carlos Arraya T. (Bolivia); Paola Marchesini (Brazil); Ministry of Health (Colombia); José Luis Garcés Fernández (Costa Rica); Ministry of Health (Dominican Republic); José Dávila Vasquez (Ecuador); Ministry of Health (El Salvador); Ministry of Health (Guatemala); Ministry of Health (Guyana); Ministry of Health (Haiti); Ministry of Health (Honduras); Ministry of Health (Mexico); Ministry of Health (Nicaragua); Ministry of Health (Panama); Ministry of Health (Suriname). MOH (Venezuela (Bolivarian Republic of)). *WHO Region of South-East Asia:* Md. Abdur Raquib (Bangladesh); Dechen Pemo (Bhutan); MOH (Democratic People's Republic of Korea); Johanes Don Bosco (Timor-Leste); GS Sonal (India); MOH (Indonesia); MOH (Myanmar); MOH (Nepal); MOH (Sri Lanka); Supawadee Konchom (Thailand). *WHO Region of Western Pacific:* Duong Socheat (Cambodia); MOH (China); Deyer Gopinath (Lao People's Democratic Republic); Azmi bin Abdul Rahim (Malaysia); Leo Makita, Zaixing Zhang, Kwabena Larbi (Papua New Guinea); Mario S. Baquilod (Philippines); Division of communicable disease control (Republic of Korea); Luke Honiola (Solomon Islands); MOH, Lasse Vestergaard (Vanuatu) and Nguyen Quang Thieu (Viet Nam).

The following WHO staff in regional and subregional offices assisted with the collection and validation of data, and reviewed epidemiological estimates and country profiles: Etienne Magloire Minkoulou (AFRO), Khoti Gausi (AFRO/eastern and southern inter-country support team), Samson Katikiti (AFRO/eastern and southern inter-country support team), Nathan Bakyaita (AFRO), Amadou Bailo Diallo (AFRO/central inter-country support team), Abderrahmane Kharchi (AFRO/western inter-country support team), Jean-Olivier Guintran (AFRO/western inter-country support team), Georges Alfred Ki-zerbo (AFRO), Soce Fall (AFRO), Ghasem Zamani (EMRO), Hoda Atta (EMRO), Karen Takse-Vester (EURO), Mikhail Ejov (EURO), Keith Carter (AMRO), Rainier Escalada (AMRO), Robert Montoya (AMRO), Prabhjot Singh (AMRO), Eva-Maria Christophel, Violeta Gonzales (WPRO), Oluwakemi Tesfazghi (WPRO), Krongthong Thimasarn (SEARO), and R. Rastogi (SEARO).

For Chapter 3 on interventions to control malaria, Manoj Menon (United States Centers for Disease Control and Prevention) and Louis Rosencrans, Tulane School of Public Health (USA), constructed the table of survey data and provided text on insecticide-treated nets (ITNs) and treatment. Abraham Flaxman, Nancy Fullman, Stephen Lim, and colleagues at the Institute of Health Metrics and Evaluation, University of Washington (USA), developed the model for ITN indicators, in collaboration with WHO and the United States Centers for Disease Control and Prevention and permitted use of the results from the model in this Report. Julie Rajaratnam and colleagues (Institute of Health Metrics and Evaluation) calculated mortality values for Zambia. John Milliner (US Agency for International Development) collected data on long-lasting insecticidal nets from manufacturers for RBM's Alliance for Malaria Prevention.

Additional information on the adoption and implementation of WHO policies and strategies for malaria control was provided by Amy Barrette, Stefan Hoyer, Jo Lines, Kamini Mendis, Sivakumaran Murugasampillay, Peter Olumese, Aafje Rietveld, Pascal Ringwald, Sergio Spinaci and Marian Warsame of the WHO Global Malaria Programme. Aafje Rietveld and Kamini Mendis developed the material on malaria elimination, further reviewed by Hoda Atta. Andrea Bosman and Silvia Schwarte contributed to Chapter 3 on deployment of ACTs.

We also thank Edward Addai, Awa Coll-Seck, Yosuke Kita, Marcel Lama, Daniel Low-Beer, and Rick Steketee who reviewed early drafts of several sections of the Report. The following persons at the United States Centers for Disease Control and Prevention reviewed the policy and other sections: Kwame Asamoa, Beatrice Divine, Scott J. Filler, Michael Lynch, Manoj Menon, Laurence Slutsker and Steven S. Yoon. The following persons contributed to the chapter on financing: Rajeev Ahuja (World Bank India Office), Laura Harley Andes, Matthew Sattah (President's Malaria Initiative), Awa Coll-Seck (RBM), Mitsuru Toda (Harvard University School of Public Health), Eline Korenromp and Ibrahima Coulibaly (Global Fund), Matt Schneider, Katie Leach-Kemon, Steve Lim (University of Washington, USA), Rick Steketee (Malaria Control and Evaluation Partnership in Africa), Karin Stenberg (WHO) and Ambachew Yohannes (UNITAID).

We thank Simone Colairo Valerio and Joan Griffith for administrative support. Elisabeth Heseltine edited the report.

Maru Aregawi, Richard Cibulskis and Ryan Williams designed the data-collection form and compiled and reviewed data provided by national malaria control programmes. Ryan Williams designed and managed the global malaria database, automated the production of country profiles and prepared maps and annexes. Policies and strategies for malaria control and epidemiological and financial data were analysed by Maru Aregawi, Richard Cibulskis and Mac Otten. Christopher Dye reviewed several chapters.

The principal source of financial support for the production of this WHO Report was the Government of Japan, without which it would have been impossible to produce the report.

The *World malaria report 2009* was produced by the Global Malaria Programme. Maru Aregawi, Richard Cibulskis, Ryan Williams and Mac Otten of the Surveillance, Monitoring and Evaluation Unit provided overall coordination.

Abbreviations

ACT   Artemisinin-based combination therapy
AIDS   Acquired immunodeficiency syndrome
API   Annual parasite incidence
DDT   Dichloro-diphenyl-trichloroethane
DHS   Demographic household survey
GBD   Global burden of diseases
GMP   Global Malaria Programme
HIV   Human immunodeficiency virus
IAEG   Inter-Agency and Expert Group on MDG Indicators
IRS   Indoor residual spraying
IPT   Intermittent preventive treatment
ITN   Insecticide-treated nets
LLIN   Long-lasting insecticidal nets
MDG   Millennium Development Goal
MERG   Monitoring and Evaluation Reference Group (for malaria)
MICS   Multiple indicator cluster survey
MIS   Malaria indicator survey
NMCP   National malaria control programme
RBM   Roll Back Malaria
RDT   Rapid diagnostic test
SPR   Slide positivity rate
SUFI   Scaling Up for Impact

Abbreviations of antimalarial medicines

AQ   Amodiaquine
AL   Artemether-lumefantrine
AM   Artemether
ART   Artemisinin
AS   Artesunate
CL   Clindamycine
CQ   Chloroquine
D   Doxycycline
DHA   Dihydroartemisinin
MQ   Mefloquine
NQ   Naphroquine
PG   Proguanil
PPQ   Piperaquine
PQ   Primaquine
PYR   Pyronaridine
QN   Quinine
SP   Sulfadoxine-pyrimethamine
T   Tetracycline
(d)   Days on treatment course

Abbreviations of WHO regions / offices

AFR   WHO African Region
AFRO   WHO Regional Office for Africa
AMR   WHO Region of the Americas
AMRO   WHO Regional Office for the Americas
PAHO   Pan-American Health Organization
EMR   WHO Eastern Mediterranean Region
EMRO   WHO Regional Office for the Eastern Mediterranean
EUR   WHO European Region
EURO   WHO Regional Office for Europe
SEAR   WHO South-East Asia Region
SEARO WHO Regional Office for South-East Asia
WPR   WHO Western Pacific Region
WPRO   WHO Regional Office for the Western Pacific

Summary

The *2009 World Malaria Report* summarizes information received from 108 malaria endemic countries and other sources and updates the analysis presented in the *2008 Report*. It highlights progress made in meeting the World Health Assembly (WHA) targets for malaria to be achieved by 2010 and 2015, and new goals on malaria elimination contained in the Global Malaria Action Plan (2008):

- International funding commitments for malaria control have increased from around US$ 0.3 billion in 2003 to US$ 1.7 billion in 2009 due largely to the emergence of the Global Fund and greater commitments by the US President's Malaria Initiative, the World Bank and other agencies. This increase in funding is resulting in dramatic scale-up of malaria control interventions in many settings and measurable reductions in malaria burden.

- An increased percentage of African households (31%) are estimated to own at least one insecticide-treated net (ITN) in 2008 compared to 2006 (17%), and more children under 5 years of age used an ITN in 2008 (24%) compared to previous years, but the percentage of children using a net is still below the WHA target of 80%. These weighted averages are affected by low ITN ownership in several large African countries for which resources for scale-up are only now being made available. Household ITN ownership reached more than 50% in 13 high burden African countries.

- Use of artemisinin-based combination therapies (ACTs) has increased compared to 2006 but remains very low in most African countries; in 11 of 13 countries surveyed during 2007–2008, fewer than 15% of children under 5 years of age with fever had received an ACT, well below the WHA target of 80%.

- More than one-third of the 108 malarious countries (9 African countries and 29 outside of Africa) documented reductions in malaria cases of > 50% in 2008 compared to 2000. The number of cases fell least in countries with the highest incidence rates.

- Ten countries are implementing nationwide elimination programmes of which six entered the elimination phase in 2009. Eight countries are in the pre-elimination stage and a further nine countries have interrupted transmission and are in the phase of preventing reintroduction of malaria.

In countries that have achieved high coverage of their populations with bed nets and treatment programmes, recorded cases and deaths due to malaria have fallen by 50% suggesting that Millennium Development Goals (MDG) targets can be achieved if there is adequate coverage of key interventions. While these results were observed in some island settings (Sao Tome and Principe and Zanzibar, United Republic of Tanzania), they were also seen in countries on the African mainland, including Eritrea, Rwanda, and Zambia.

There is evidence from Sao Tome and Principe, Zanzibar and Zambia that large decreases in malaria cases and deaths have been mirrored by steep declines in all-cause deaths among children less than 5 years of age, suggesting that intensive efforts at malaria control could help many African countries to reach, by 2015, a two-thirds reduction in child mortality as set forth in the MDGs.

Parasite resistance to antimalarial medicines and mosquito resistance to insecticides are major threats to achieving global malaria control. Well conducted surveillance of drug efficacy in endemic countries with support from WHO has shown early evidence of resistance to artemisinins, and WHO is leading a major resistance containment effort. Continued use of artemisinin monotherapy is a major factor in parasite resistance; yet, despite WHO's call for a halt to their use, marketing of artemisinin monotherapies continues in many countries.

International disbursements to malaria-endemic countries (US$ 0.65 billion in 2007, the latest year for which data are available), still fall short of the US$ 5 billion required annually to ensure high coverage and maximal impact world wide. Approximately 80% of external funds were targeted to the WHO African Region. The South-East Asia Region received the least money per person at risk for malaria and saw the lowest increase in external financing between 2000 and 2007. High levels of external assistance are associated with increased procurement of commodities and decreases in malaria incidence.

However, external funds for malaria control are disproportionately concentrated on smaller countries with lower disease burdens. More attention needs to be given to ensuring success in large countries that account for most malaria cases and deaths, and protecting the gains that have been made. This will require not only adequate financial resources but also the strengthening of health systems capable of delivering vector control interventions, providing diagnostics for the parasitologic confirmation of malaria alongside treatment with ACTs, and the development of routine surveillance systems for malaria as well as for parasite resistance to antimalarial medicines and mosquito resistance to insecticides.

Key points

● Background and context

With the target year 2010 in sight, malaria-endemic countries and the global community are attempting to achieve high coverage with effective interventions to attain both coverage and impact targets.

1. On World Malaria Day 2008, the United Nations Secretary General called for efforts to ensure universal coverage with malaria prevention and treatment programmes by the end of 2010.

2. The goal established by the Member States at the World Health Assembly and the Roll Back Malaria (RBM) Partnership is to reduce the numbers of malaria cases and deaths recorded in 2000 by 50% or more by the end of 2010 and by 75% or more by 2015.

3. In September 2008, RBM launched the Global Malaria Action Plan that defines the steps required to accelerate achievement of the Partnership's 2010 and 2015 targets for malaria control and elimination.

● Policies and strategies for malaria control

To reach the 2010 and 2015 targets, countries must reach all persons at risk for malaria with an insecticide-treated net (ITN) or indoor residual spraying (IRS) and provide laboratory-based diagnosis for all suspected cases of malaria and effective treatment of all confirmed cases.

Treatment

4. Prompt parasitological confirmation by microscopy or with a rapid diagnostic test (RDT) is recommended for all patients with suspected malaria, before treatment is started. Confirmed cases of uncomplicated *Plasmodium falciparum* malaria should be treated with an artemisinin-based combination therapy (ACT) and *P. vivax* malaria with chloroquine where it is effective, or an appropriate ACT in areas where *P. vivax* is resistant to chloroquine. Treatment of *P. vivax* should be combined with 14 days of primaquine to prevent relapse.

5. Treatment solely on the basis of clinical suspicion should be considered only when a parasitological diagnosis is not accessible. In 2008, 20 of 45 malaria-endemic countries in the WHO African Region and 51 of 64 countries outside the African Region reported having a policy of parasitological testing of suspected malaria cases in persons of all ages, and 78 countries reported a policy of treatment with ACT for *P. falciparum* malaria.

6. WHO recommends that oral artemisinin-based monotherapies be withdrawn from the market and replaced with ACTs. Thirty-seven countries still allow use of oral artemisinin-based monotherapies; most are located in the African Region, followed by the Region of the Americas and the South-East Asia Region.

7. Parasite resistance has rendered previous antimalarial medicines ineffective in most parts of the world, threatening malaria control. The highly effective artemisinin derivatives and their partner drugs are vulnerable to the same risk. Resistance of *P. falciparum* to artemisinins has been observed at the Cambodia-Thailand border.

Prevention

8. In 2008, 23 countries in the African Region and 35 outside that Region had adopted the WHO recommendation to provide bednets for all age groups at risk for malaria, not just women and children; this represents an increase of 13 countries since 2007.

9. IRS with WHO-approved chemicals (including DDT) remains one of the main interventions for reducing and interrupting malaria transmission by vector control in all epidemiological settings. In 2008, 44 countries, including 19 in the African Region, reported implementing IRS.

10. Intermittent preventive treatment (IPTp) is recommended for pregnant women in areas of high transmission. Thirty-three countries in the African Region, 3 in the Eastern Mediterranean Region and 1 in Western Pacific Region had adopted an IPTp policy by 2009.

● Progress in preventing malaria

Coverage with ITNs is increasing rapidly in some countries of Africa, household ITN ownership having risen to 31% in high-burden countries by the end of 2008.

11. Nearly 140 million long-lasting insecticidal nets (LLINs) were delivered to high-burden countries in the African Region in 2006–2008.

12. A model-based estimate showed that 31% of African households owned at least one ITN, and 24% of children under 5 years of age had used an ITN in 2008. Household ITN ownership reached ≥ 50% in 13 (37%) of 35 high-burden countries in the African Region by 2008. Surveys show that seven countries (Equatorial Guinea, Ethiopia [population living at < 2000 m], Gabon, Mali,

Sao Tome and Principe, Senegal and Zambia) had reached a household ITN ownership rate of ≥ 60% by 2007 or 2008.

13. The percentage of children < 5 years who had used an ITN the previous night, given household ownership of at least one ITN, was 51% (median; range, 14–68%) in six countries for which data were available in 2006–2007. As all six surveys were demographic and health surveys, which are usually conducted in the dry season; use in the wet season might be higher.

14. In two of four countries in the African Region in which repeated national surveys were carried out, household ITN ownership decreased by 13% and 37% within 24–36 months of mass distribution, suggesting that strong programmes for routine distribution of ITNs are needed. Routine monitoring of the durability of LLINs and of the longevity of the insecticide are needed in order to calculate the requirements for ITN maintenance.

● Progress in the diagnosis and treatment of malaria

ACT procurement is improving, and the percentage of children with fever who are treated with an ACT is rising. Nevertheless, countries received only about 50% of the ACTs needed to treat malaria cases at health facilities in the public sector in 2008.

15. In 18 high-burden WHO African Region countries for which data were available, 22% of the reported suspected malaria cases were confirmed with a parasite-based test in 2008.

16. Access to treatment, especially ACTs, was generally poor in African countries. Less than 15% of children under 5 years of age received an ACT when they had fever in 11 of 13 African countries for which survey data were available in 2007–2008.

17. Nine household surveys in 2007–2008 showed that 20% of pregnant women received a second dose of ITP.

● Impact of malaria control

Dramatic reductions in the numbers of childhood deaths from malaria and from all causes have been reported in some settings where high coverage has been reached with effective interventions.

18. Reductions of more than 50% in the numbers of reported malaria cases and deaths were observed in four high burden African countries (Eritrea, Rwanda, Sao Tome and Principe and Zambia) and one area (Zanzibar, United Republic of Tanzania). Reductions of > 50% were also observed in five low transmission African countries (Botswana, Cape Verde, Namibia, South Africa and Swaziland). In Sao Tome and Principe and Zanzibar (United Republic of Tanzania) reductions in the number of malaria cases and deaths were found within 2–3 years of widespread use of IRS, LLINs and ACTs. In Rwanda, a reduction was found with only LLINs and ACTs.

19. The numbers of inpatient deaths from all causes decreased by 53% in Sao Tome and Principe and 57% on the islands of Zanzibar (United Republic of Tanzania) after aggressive malaria control. In Zambia, child mortality rates from all causes fell by 35%, as measured both by the number of deaths recorded in health facilities and by < 5 mortality rates derived from the Demographic and Health Survey of 2007. These trends, if confirmed in non-island countries, suggest that intensive malaria control could help many African countries to reach, by 2015, a two-thirds reduction in child mortality, as set forth in the Millennium Development Goals.

20. In other WHO regions, the number of reported cases of confirmed malaria decreased by more than 50% in 29 of the 56 malaria-endemic countries between 2000 and 2008. The number of cases fell least in countries with the highest incidence rates, indicating that greater attention should be given to countries that account for most malaria cases and deaths outside Africa.

● Eliminating malaria

In September 2008, the RBM Partnership set a target of eliminating malaria in eight to ten countries by 2015 and afterwards in all countries that were in the pre-elimination phase in 2008.

21. Eight countries are in the pre-elimination stage of malaria control in 2009; 10 countries are implementing elimination programmes nationwide (six having entered the elimination phase in 2009), and a further nine countries (Armenia, Bahamas, Egypt, Jamaica, Morocco, Oman, Russian Federation, Syrian Arab Republic and Turkmenistan) have interrupted transmission and are in the phase of preventing re-introduction of malaria.

● Financing malaria control

The funds committed to malaria control from international sources have increased substantially, from approximately US$ 0.3 billion in 2003 to US$ 1.7 billion in 2009. The levels of domestic financing for malaria appear to have been maintained over this period.

22. Funds disbursed for malaria control increased from US$ 592 million in 2006 to US$ 652 million in 2007. Commitments for malaria control exceeded US$ 1 billion in 2008 and US$ 1.7 billion in 2009, suggesting that the funds continue to increase.

23. Of 108 malaria-endemic countries, 76 received external assistance for malaria control between 2000 and 2007. The highest per capita expenditure was seen in countries with smaller populations at risk.

24. Countries that received more than US$ 7 in external assistance per person at risk for malaria between 2000 and 2007 were more likely to report a reduction in the number of malaria cases than countries with a lower level of assistance.

Chapter 1.
Introduction

The renewed effort to control malaria worldwide and move towards elimination in some countries is founded on the latest generation of effective tools and methods for prevention and treatment. Increasing use of long-lasting insecticide nets (LLINs), artemisinin-based combination therapies (ACTs) and indoor residual spraying (IRS) of insecticide provides an unprecedented opportunity to control and, in selected countries, eliminate malaria.

To accelerate progress in malaria control, the 2005 World Health Assembly advanced the Roll Back Malaria (RBM) targets defined in 2000 by African Heads of State and set a coverage target of 80% or more for four key interventions: insecticide-treated nets (ITNs) for people at risk, appropriate antimalarial drugs for patients with probable or confirmed malaria, IRS for households at risk, and intermittent preventive treatment in pregnancy (in high-transmission areas) *(1)*. The Health Assembly specified that, as a result of these interventions, the numbers of malaria cases and deaths per capita should be reduced by 50% or more between 2000 and 2010, and by 75% or more between 2000 and 2015. These goals were affirmed in the Global Malaria Action Plan *(2)*.

Following a resolution of the Health Assembly to establish a World Malaria Day *(3)* as a yearly advocacy forum, international organizations, nongovernmental organizations, multilateral organizations and donors, private sector partners and research institutions commemorated the first World Malaria Day in 2008. The commemorations culminated in a call by the United Nations Secretary General for universal coverage with malaria control interventions.

Last year's *Report*, on the basis of data for 2006, showed that the increased political commitment from national governments and partners earlier in the decade had led to more financing and effective commodities to malaria-endemic countries. This was good news, as there were an estimated 880 000 deaths from malaria and about 250 million cases in 2006. The *2008 Report* also highlighted several success stories outside Africa, although the overall decrease in the number of confirmed cases was slow. In high-burden countries in Africa, relatively few successes were recorded. While progress in malaria control has been remarkable, a number of potential threats demand increased attention, including: resistance to insecticides and antimalarial medicines and lack of alternatives; insufficient funding to attain universal coverage; weak global and international purchasing and supply chains, which result in stock-outs of key commodities at national and health facility levels; and lack of monitoring and management information systems of effects in high-burden African countries.

Readers of this *Report* will want to know, in comparison to last year: have finances continued to grow, to enable scale up throughout Africa and globally? Have the commodities distributed by national governments ended up in households, benefitting children, women and other adults? Is the financing and the coverage by interventions having an effect?

This *Report* provides data for two additional years, 2007 and 2008. It describes the status of malaria control both outside as well as inside Africa. In addition, it describes the full chain, from financing and policies to number of commodities distributed, intervention coverage in households and, finally, impact. This third edition of the *World Malaria Report* covers progress in malaria control in five areas.

- **Chapter 2** addresses national policies and strategies on malaria control, established to reduce the burden of disease. It covers the adoption by countries of recommendations for malaria control, treatment and prevention promoted by WHO, with adjustments for their particular epidemiological settings.

- Progress in implementing treatment and control measures is compared to international targets for malaria control in **Chapter 3.** This chapter is based on data on the number of commodities distributed by ministries of health and those delivered by manufacturers and on survey data. The data were analysed to determine whether the commodities purchased, delivered and distributed ended up in households and at health facilities. The most recent surveys, 2006–2008, were analysed to see how successful national malaria programmes have been in reaching their intended targets, including universal coverage.

- **Chapter 4** summarizes the global burden of malaria, and reviews recent trends in the reported number of malaria cases and deaths. It also assesses the evidence for malaria control activities having an impact on malaria disease burden in each WHO Region.

- The status of elimination of malaria is described in **Chapter 5**, which presents progress in those countries that are preparing to enter the elimination phase (pre-elimination), those in the elimination phase and those that have eliminated malaria but are not yet certified by WHO (phase of prevention of reintroduction).

- **Chapter 6** summarizes trends in international and domestic financing for malaria and their relation to estimated resource requirements; how funds disbursed from external agencies have been allocated to different geographical regions, countries and programmes; and the relation between external financing, programme implementation and disease trends.

Profiles of 31 countries are then presented. Two or three countries with the highest malaria burdens were chosen from five of the six WHO Regions. The other profiles are those of the 20 countries with the highest burden in the African Region.

Following the profiles, annexes give data by country for malaria-related indicators.

References

1. Resolution WHA58.2. Malaria control. In: *Fifty-eighth World Health Assembly, Geneva, 16–25 May 2005. Volume 1. Resolutions and decisions, and list of participants.* Geneva, World Health Organization, 2005 (WHA58/2005/REC/1), 4–7. http://www.who.int/gb/ebwha/pdf_files/WHA58/WHA58_2-en.pdf.

2. *The global malaria action plan.* Geneva, World Health Organization, Roll Back Malaria, 2008. http://www.rollbackmalaria.org/gmap.

3. Resolution WHA60.18. Malaria, including proposal for establishment of World Malaria Day. In: *Sixtienth World Health Assembly, Geneva, 14–23 May 2007. Volume 1. Resolutions and decisions.* Geneva, World Health Organization, 2007 (WHA60/2007/REC/1).

Chapter 2.
Policies, strategies and targets for malaria control

This chapter summarizes the policies, strategies and targets for malaria control recommended by WHO. It includes three sections: 1) diagnosis and treatment of malaria; 2) malaria prevention by mosquito control; and 3) goals, indicators and targets.

2.1 Diagnosis and treatment of malaria, including preventive treatment

The two main objectives of an antimalarial treatment policy are:

1. to reduce morbidity and mortality by *i)* ensuring rapid, complete cure of the infection and thus preventing the progression of uncomplicated malaria to severe, potentially fatal disease, *ii)* malaria-related anaemia and, during pregnancy, *iii)* the negative impact of malaria on the fetus; and

2. to curtail the transmission of malaria by reducing the parasite reservoir of infection and infectivity.

Current WHO recommendations for diagnosis and treatment are shown in **Box 2.1**. Since publication of the *World Malaria Report 2008*, WHO has made several modifications to its malaria policy recommendations *(1)*:

i) Prompt parasitological confirmation by microscopy or alternatively by rapid diagnostic tests (RDTs) is recommended for all patients with suspected malaria before treatment is started. Treatment solely on the basis of clinical suspicion should be considered only when a parasitological diagnosis is not accessible.

ii) A fifth ACT, dihydroartemisinin-piperaquine, has been added to the treatment options.

iii) A single dose of primaquine is recommended in addition to ACT as an anti-gametocyte medicine in treatment of *P. falciparum* malaria, particularly as a component of a pre-elimination or an elimination programme, provided the risks for haemolysis in glucose-6-phosphate dehydrogenase (G6PD)-deficient patients have been considered.

Furthermore, in light of evidence of resistance to artemisinins, WHO urges more strongly the continued routine monitoring of therapeutic efficacy of antimalarial medicines and halting the use all monotherapies for the treatment of uncomplicated malaria *(2)*.

BOX 2.1

WHO recommendations for diagnosis and treatment of malaria

- Prompt parasitologic confirmation by microscopy or alternatively by rapid diagnostic tests (RDTs) is recommended in all patients suspected of malaria before treatment is started. Treatment solely on the basis of clinical suspicion should only be considered when a parasitological diagnosis is not accessible.

- Uncomplicated *Plasmodium falciparum* malaria should be treated with an artemisinin-based combination therapy (ACT); vivax malaria should be treated with chloroquine where it is effective, or an appropriate ACT, in areas where *P. vivax* resistance to chorloquine has been documented. Both chloroquine and ACTs should be combined with primaquine for 14 days in the treatment of *P. vivax* malaria, for the prevention of relapses, subject to considering the risk of haemolysis in patients with G6PD-deficiency.

- Five ACTs are currently recommended for use: artemether-lumefantrine, artesunate-amodiaquine, artesunate-mefloquine, artesunate-sulfadoxine pyrimethamine, and dihydroartemisinin-piperaquine. The choice of the ACT should be based on the efficacy of the combination in the country or area of intended use.

- Artemisinin derivatives should not be used as monotherapies for the treatment of uncomplicated malaria as this will promote resistance to this critically important class of antimalarials.

- A single dose of primaquine to be added as an anti-gametocyte medicine to ACT treatment of *P. falciparum* malaria, particularly as a component of pre-elimination or elimination programme, is recommended provided the risk of haemolysis in G6PD-deficient patients is considered.

- Severe malaria should be treated with a parenteral artemisinin derivative or quinine to be followed by a complete course of an effective ACT as soon as the patient can take oral medications. When intravenous or intramuscular treatment is not feasible, e.g. in peripheral health posts, patients should receive pre-referral treatment with an artemisinin suppository and be transferred to a health facility capable of providing definitive treatment with parenteral antimalarial medicines.

- In settings with limited health facility access, diagnosis and treatment should be provided at community level through a programme of community case management (home-based management) of malaria.

2.2 Malaria prevention through mosquito control

2.2.1 Aims

Malaria vector control is intended to protect individuals against infective mosquito bites and, at the community level, to reduce the intensity of local malaria transmission. The two most powerful and most broadly applied interventions are insecticide-treated nets (ITN) and indoor residual spraying (IRS). In some specific settings and circumstances (if the breeding sites are few, fixed, and easy to identify) these core interventions may be complemented by other methods such as larval control or environmental management. WHO recommendations for vector control are the following:

1. Because high coverage rates are needed to realize the full potential of either ITNs or IRS, WHO GMP recommends "universal coverage" of all people at risk in areas targeted for malaria prevention. In the case of ITNs, this means that all people at risk in areas targeted for malaria prevention should be covered with ITNs (3, 4).

2. ITNs should be either free of charge or highly subsidized. Cost should not be a barrier to making them available to all people at risk, especially young children and pregnant women (3).

3. Universal coverage with long-lasting insecticidal nets (LLINs) can be achieved and maintained by combining distribution through occasional campaigns with continuous distribution to pregnant women and infants at routine antenatal and immunization contacts (3).

4. Only LLINs recommended by the WHO Pesticide Evaluation Scheme (WHOPES) should be procured by national malaria programmes and partners for malaria control. These nets are designed to maintain their biological efficacy against vector mosquitoes for at least three years in the field under recommended conditions of use, obviating the need for regular insecticide treatment (5, 6).

5. IRS consists of the application of insecticides to the inner surfaces of dwellings, where endophilic anopheline mosquitoes often rest after taking a blood meal (4). IRS is applicable in many epidemiological settings, as long as operational and resource feasibility is considered in policy decisions. Twelve insecticides belonging to four chemical classes are currently recommended by WHO for IRS. An insecticide for IRS in a given area is selected on the basis of data on resistance, the residual efficacy of the insecticide, cost, safety and the type of surface to be sprayed. Special attention must be given to preserving susceptibility to pyrethroids, because they are the only class of insecticide currently used on ITNs.

6. Scientific evidence indicates that IRS is effective in controlling malaria transmission and thus reduces the related burden of morbidity and mortality as long as most houses and animal shelters (e.g. > 80%) in targeted communities are treated. IRS is effective only if the operation is performed correctly, which depends on the existence at national, provincial and district levels of adequate infrastructure and programme capacity for implementation, monitoring and evaluation (4).

7. DDT has comparatively long residual efficacy (≥ 6 months) against malaria vectors and plays an important role in the management of vector resistance. Countries can use DDT for IRS for as long as necessary and in the quantities needed, provided that the guide-lines and recommendations of WHO and the Stockholm Convention are met and until locally appropriate, cost-effective alternatives are available for a sustainable transition from DDT (7).

8. Resistance to insecticides, especially pyrethroids, is an urgent and growing threat to the sustainability of current methods of vector control. Monitoring and managing resistance to the insecticides used in both ITNs and IRS are vital (3, 4).

9. In most settings where IRS has been or is being deployed, ITNs or LLINs are already in use. Neither LLINs nor IRS alone will be sufficient to achieve and maintain interruption of transmission in holoendemic areas of Africa or in hyperendemic areas in other regions (3). Some observational evidence indicates that the combination of IRS and LLIN is more effective than either intervention alone, especially if the combination helps to increase overall coverage with vector control (8). More formal trials are being planned. In using the combination of IRS and ITNs, it is preferable to use a non-pyrethroid insecticide for IRS.

2.2.2 Resistance to antimalarial drugs

Antimalarial drug resistance is a major public health problem, which hinders the control of malaria. The rapid spread of resistance to these drugs over the past few decades has led to intensification of the monitoring of their efficacy, to ensure proper management of clinical cases and early detection of changing patterns of resistance in order to revise national malaria treatment policies. Surveillance of therapeutic efficacy over time is an essential component of malaria control. The results of tests for therapeutic efficacy (in vivo tests) provide the most important information for determining whether first- and second-line drugs are still effective and also provide evidence for ministries of health to update their national malaria treatment policies.

WHO's role in the global management of drug resistance has been twofold. Its normative and standard-setting role results in a harmonized approach to this global concern. In order to interpret and compare results within and between regions, and to follow trends over time, tests must be conducted with similar standardized procedures, and WHO has standarded the available methods. Since 1996, WHO has updated the protocol for assessing antimalarial drug efficacy on the basis of expert consensus and feedback from the field (9). WHO has also prepared a field manual on in vitro assays for the sensitivity of malaria parasites to antimalarial drugs (10) and a guideline on genotyping malaria parasites to distinguish between reinfection and recrudescence during therapeutic efficacy tests. Genotyping is now becoming mandatory with the longer follow-up of patients (11). Apart from its normative role, WHO GMP is also providing technical assistance to countries in both the surveillance of drug resistance and guidance on treatment policies. Routine surveillance systems put in place by countries and coordinated by WHO have shown that the failure rate of currently used ACTs is increasing on both sides of the Thai-Cambodian border, due mainly to local emergence of resistance to artemisinin derivatives. WHO is investigating this problem and implementing strategies to contain and prevent the dissemination of resistance further.

In response to the challenge posed by the emergence of resistance to antimalarial drugs, WHO has established a global database of information and the results of antimalarial drug efficacy tests at country level. The database is used by governments to review and update their treatment policies. The continuously updated database can also be made available to other stakeholders. The data will be analysed for a report on global monitoring in 2009, focusing on the efficacy of ACTs, which will describe WHO's work in monitoring resistance to antimalarial drugs, setting up the database, standardizing therapeutic efficacy tests, promoting more rational use of the available tests for evaluating resistance and showing how the results of these tests are used for updating national malaria treatment policies.

The indicators in Table 2.1 apply to countries with high, moderate and low transmission that are in the control phase but not to those in the pre-elimination or elimination phases. Indicators have not yet been developed for the phases of pre-elimination, elimination and prevention of reintroduction.

2.3   Goals, indicators and targets

The vision of the RBM Partnership is "a world free from the burden of malaria" *(12)*. As of 2007, the United Nations (through the MDGs), the World Health Assembly and the RBM Partnership had consistent goals for intervention coverage and impact for 2010 and 2015 *(13–15)*. Coverage is meant to reach ≥ 80% by 2010 with four key interventions: ITNs for people at risk, appropriate antimalarial medicines for patients with probable or confirmed malaria, IRS for targeted households at risk and intermittent preventive treatment in pregnancy (in moderate-to-high transmission settings). The global impact targets are a reduction in the number of malaria cases and deaths per capita by 50% or more between 2000 and 2010, and by 75% or more between 2000 and 2015.

The RBM partnership added three additional targets as part of the Global Malaria Action Plan in September 2008 *(16)*. The first is to reduce the global number of malaria deaths to near-zero preventable deaths by 2015. This target is more aggressive than the previous target of a 75% reduction in the number of malaria deaths by 2015, although there is no global consensus on how to measure preventable deaths. The second is that malaria should be eliminated in 8–10 countries by 2015 and afterwards in all countries that are in the pre-elimination phase today (2008). The third goal is, "in the long term, eradicate malaria worldwide by reducing the global incidence to zero through progressive elimination in countries".

The Inter-agency and Expert Group on MDG Indicators has established specific indicators for malaria *(13)*:

6.6   Incidence and death rates associated with malaria.

6.7   Proportion of children under 5 years sleeping under insecticide-treated bed nets.

6.8   Proportion of children under 5 years with fever who are treated with appropriate antimalarial medicines.

Table 2.1 draws together the work of RBM since 1998, the Abuja Declaration in 2000 *(14)*, the resolution of the Health Assembly in 2005 *(15)*, and various subsequent revisions of the MDGs for malaria and the RBM Global Action Plan for Malaria. It shows practical indicators recommended by WHO for use by national malaria programmes to measure coverage with malaria control interventions and epidemiological impact. Core national operational logistics and reporting indicators are also listed. The only substantial change from last year's indicator list is the addition of a new IRS indicator: percentage of at-risk population targeted by IRS. This indicator has no target but is intended to monitor the contribution of IRS to overall malaria control.

Table 2.1 Malaria indicators, targets and sources of data (17–19)

IMPACT MEASURE	INDICATOR	NUMERATOR	DENOMINATOR	DATA TYPE/SOURCE	TARGET
Malaria cases					
	1.1 Confirmed malaria cases (microscopy or RDT, per 1000 persons per year) [a]	Confirmed malaria cases per year (< 5 years or total)	Population (< 5 years or total)	Routine surveillance	Reduction in cases per capita: ≥ 50% by 2010, and ≥ 75% by 2015 in comparison with 2000
	1.2 Inpatient malaria cases (per 1000 persons per year) [b]	No. of inpatient malaria cases per year (< 5 years or total)	Population (< 5 years or total)	Routine surveillance	Reduction in cases per capita: ≥ 50% by 2010, and ≥ 75% by 2015 in comparison with 2000
Malaria transmission					
	1.3 Malaria test positivity rate (both microscopy and RDT) [a]	No. of laboratory-confirmed malaria cases	No. of suspected malaria cases with parasite-based laboratory examination	Routine surveillance	No target set, indicates level of control [c]
Malaria deaths					
	1.4 Inpatient malaria deaths (per 1000 persons per year)	No. of inpatient malaria deaths per year (< 5 years or total)	Population (< 5 years or total)	Routine surveillance	Reduction in deaths per capita: 50% by 2010 and ≥ 75% by 2015 in comparison with 2000 [d]
	1.5 Malaria-specific deaths (per 1000 persons per year)	No. of malaria deaths per year (< 5 years or total)	Population (< 5 years or total)	Verbal autopsy (surveys), complete or sample vital registration systems	
	For high-transmission countries 1.6 Deaths of children < 5 years old from all causes (per 1000 children < 5 years old per year)	No. of deaths in children < 5 years old from all causes	Population (< 5 years)	Household surveys, complete or sample vital registration systems	No target set

CONTROL STRATEGY	INDICATOR	NUMERATOR	DENOMINATOR	DATA TYPE/SOURCE	TARGET
Prompt access to effective treatment					
	2.1 Appropriate antimalarial treatment of children < 5 years within 24 hours of onset of fever [e–g] (MDG indicator 6.8)	No. of children < 5 years receiving appropriate antimalarial treatment (according to national policy) within 24 hours of onset of fever	No. of children < 5 years with fever in the past 2 weeks in surveyed households [e]	Household surveys	≥ 80%
Mosquito control with ITNs					
	2.2 ITN use by all persons or children < 5 years or pregnant women (MDG indicator 6.7) [h]	No. of persons (all ages) or children < 5 years or pregnant women who reported sleeping under an ITN during previous night	No. of persons (all ages) or children < 5 years old or pregnant women in surveyed households	Household surveys	≥ 80%
	2.3. "Administrative" ITN coverage [i]	No. of persons with ITN from numbers of ITN distributed [i]	No. of persons at risk for malaria	Routine NMCP data	≥ 80%
Mosquito control by IRS					
	2.4. Percentage of population at risk that is targeted for indoor-residual spraying (IRS)	No. of persons that are targeted for IRS	No. of persons at risk for malaria	Routine NMCP data	No target set. Indicates contribution of IRS to overall malaria control
	2.5. Households sprayed with insecticide among those targeted	No. of households sprayed at least once in one year according to national guidelines	No. of households targeted according to national guidelines	Routine NMCP data	100%
Prevention of malaria in pregnancy					
	For high-transmission countries 2.6. Pregnant women who received two doses of intermittent preventive therapy	No. of pregnant women who received two doses of intermittent preventive therapy	No. of pregnant women who made at least one ANC visit in one year	Routine antenatal clinic data	≥ 80%

C. OPERATIONAL INDICATORS USED AT HEALTH FACILITY, DISTRICT AND NATIONAL LEVELS, MEASURED USING ROUTINE HEALTH INFORMATION SYSTEMS

MONITORING	INDICATOR	NUMERATOR	DENOMINATOR	DATA TYPE/SOURCE	TARGET
Diagnosis					
	3.1. Percentage of outpatient suspected malaria cases that undergo laboratory diagnosis [j]	No. of outpatient suspected malaria cases that undergo laboratory diagnosis (by age group)	No. of outpatient suspected malaria cases that should be examined (by age group)	Routine surveillance data	≥ 90%
Appropriate treatment at health facilities					
	3.2. Percentage of outpatient cases that received appropriate antimalarial treatment according to national policy	No. of malaria cases receiving appropriate antimalarial treatment at health facility	No. of outpatient malaria cases expected to be treated at health-facility level with appropriate antimalarial medicine	Routine logistic data	100%
Routine distribution of mosquito nets					
	3.3. ITN distribution to vulnerable sub-groups	No. of ITNs distributed to vulnerable groups [k]	No. of persons in vulnerable groups targeted for receiving ITNs	Routine logistic data	≥ 80%
Antimalarial drug supplies					
	3.4. Health facilities without stock-outs of first-line antimalarial medicines, mosquito nets and diagnostics, by month	No. of health facilities without stock-outs of any first-line antimalarial medicines, ITNs and RDTs, by month [l]	No. of health facilities	Routine logistic data	100%
Reports for programme management					
	3.5. Completeness of monthly health facility reports on logistics or surveillance [m]	No. of health facility reports received each month, on logistics or surveillance	No. of health facility reports expected each month	Routine surveillance and logistic data	> 90%

From references *17–19*

RDT: rapid diagnostic test; MDG: Millennium Development Goal; ITN: insecticide-treated net; IRS: indoor residual spraying

[a.] Use only if > 90% of suspected cases have examination for parasites (microscopy or RDT).

[b.] Marker for severe malaria.

[c.] Malaria test positivity rate < 5% during the malaria season marks the readiness for transition from control stage to pre-elimination stage.

[d.] A new RBM target was introduced in the 2008 Global Malaria Action Plan: "near zero preventable malaria deaths" by 2015. This target is more ambitious than the target of 75% reduction in malaria deaths by 2015. There is no global consensus on how to measure preventable malaria deaths.

[e.] As malaria incidence is reduced, a smaller percentage of fevers will be due to malaria. With improved diagnosis, treatment can be targeted at confirmed cases. This indicator is currently under review.

[f.] In areas where *P. vivax* is dominant and in areas of low transmission, this indicator may be less useful.

[g.] The intention is to treat all persons with an appropriate antimalarial medicine; however, children are at greatest risk, especially in areas of high transmission.

[h.] Indicator should be calculated separately for all persons, children and pregnant women.

[i.] "Administrative" or operational ITN coverage is measured from the number of LLINs or ITNs distributed by ministries of health and partners. LLINs are the preferred type of ITN; they are assumed to protect for 3 years and conventional ITN for 1 year. One LLIN is assumed to protect two persons. This indicator mainly measures distribution and not hanging or use.

[j.] Laboratory diagnosis includes microscopy and RDT; this is also an indicator of the quality of surveillance.

[k.] e.g. pregnant women attending antenatal clinics, children attending in the context of the expanded programme on immunization.

[l.] This indicator has three subindicators: one each for antimalarial medicines, ITNs and RDTs.

[m.] This indicator can have one to three subindicators, depending on the data collection forms and reporting channels. For example, the inpatient data channel may be separate from the outpatient data channel, or logistics and disease surveillance data channels may be separate.

References

1. *Guidelines for the treatment of malaria.* Geneva, World Health Organization, in press (WHO/HTM/MAL/2009).

2. *Global malaria control and elimination: report of a meeting on containment of artemisinin tolerance.* Geneva, World Health Organization, 2008.

3. *Insecticide-treated mosquito nets: a WHO position statement.* Geneva, World Health Organization, Global Malaria Programme, 2007. http://apps.who.int/malaria/docs/itn/ITNspospaperfinal.pdf.

4. *Indoor residual spraying–Use of indoor residual spraying for scaling up global malaria control and elimination.* Geneva, World Health Organization, 2006.

5. *WHO recommended insecticide products for treatment of mosquito nets for malaria vector control.* WHO Pesticides Evaluation Scheme (WHOPES). Geneva, World Health Organization, 2009. http://www.who.int/whopes/Insecticides_ITN_Malaria_ok3.pdf.

6. *Report of the twelfth WHOPES working group meeting. Geneva, World Health Organization, 2009* (WHO/HTM/NTD/WHOWHOPES PES/20/ 2009.09.11). http://whqlibdoc.who.int/hq/2009/WHO_HTM_NTD _WHOPES_2009_1_eng.pdf.

7. *The use of DDT in malaria vector control.* WHO position statement. Geneva, World Health Organization, 2007.

8. Kleinschmidt I et al. Combining indoor residual spraying and insecticide-treated net interventions *American Journal of Tropical Medicine andHygiene,* 2009, 81:519–524.

9. Methods for surveillance of antimalarial drug efficacy. Geneva, World Health Organization, 2009. http://www.who.int/malaria/resistance.

10. Basco LK. *Field application of in vitro assays for the sensitivity of human malaria parasites to antimalarial drugs.* Geneva, World Health Organization, 2007. http://www.who.int/malaria/resistance.

11. *Methods and techniques for clinical trials on antimalarial drug efficacy: genotyping to identify parasite populations : Informal consultation organized by the Medicines for Malaria Venture and cosponsored by the World Health Organization, 29–31 May 2007, Amsterdam, The Netherlands.* Geneva, World Health Organization, 2008. http://www.who.int/malaria/resistance.

12. *RBM vision.* Geneva, World Health Organization, 2008. http://rbm.who.int/rbmvision.html.

13. *Official list of MDG indicators.* New York, United Nations, Interagency and Expert Group on MDG Indicators and United Nations Statistics Division, 2009. http://mdgs.un.org/unsd/mdg/Host.aspx?Content=Indicators/OfficialList.htm.

14. *The Abuja Declaration and the plan of action. An extract from the African Summit on Roll Back Malaria, Abuja, 25 April 2000.* Geneva, World Health Organization, 2000 (WHO/CDS/RBM/ 2000.1). http://www.rbm.who.int/docs/abuja_declaration.pdf.

15. Resolution WHA58.2. Malaria control. In: *Fifty-eighth World Health Assembly, Geneva, 16–25 May 2005. Volume 1. Resolutions and decisions, and list of participants.* Geneva, World Health Organization, 2005 (WHA58/2005/REC/1), 4–7. http://www.who.int/gb/ebwha/pdf_files/WHA58/WHA58_2-en.pdf.

16. *Global strategic plan 2005–2015.* Geneva, World Health Organization, Roll Back Malaria, 2008. http://rbm.who.int/gmap/index.html.

17. *Framework for monitoring progress and evaluating outcomes and impact.* Geneva, World Health Organization, Roll Back Malaria, 2000.

18. *Guidelines for core population-based indicators.* Geneva, World Health Organization, Roll Back Malaria Partnership, 2009. http://rbm.who.int/toolbox/tool_GuidelinesForCorePopulationBased-Indicators.html.

19. *World malaria report 2008.* Geneva, World Health Organization, 2008 (WHO/HTM/GMP/2008.1).

Chapter 3.
Interventions to control malaria

This chapter addresses the implementation of policies and coverage with interventions. The first part contains a description of how national programmes have adopted and implemented policies and strategies as compared with those recommended by WHO. Second, information is provided on global ACT supplies, the artemisinin market situation and oral artemisinin-based monotherapy medicines. The third section describes intervention coverage in high-burden countries in the WHO African Region. The fourth section gives the numbers of ITNs, ACTs and RDTs distributed, by WHO Region.

3.1 Adoption of policies and strategies for malaria control

Adoption of policies and strategies is reported to WHO by countries (see Annex 4.A). National adoption and implementation of policies by WHO Region is shown in **Table 3.1.** In 2008, 23 countries in the WHO African Region and 35 outside of the African Region had adopted the WHO policy recommendation to provide bed nets to all age groups at risk of malaria, an increase of 13 countries since 2007. In 2008, 44 countries, including 19 in Africa, reported implementing IRS. DDT use for IRS was reported by 12 countries: eight countries in the African Region, three in the South-East Asia Region and one in the Western Pacific Region. In 2008, 20 of 45 malaria endemic countries in the WHO Africa Region and 51 of 64 endemic countries in other regions reported having adopted a policy of providing parasitological diagnosis to all age groups. Twelve African countries are using RDTs at community level. Details of country policies are given in Annex 4.A. Thirty-three countries in the African Region, three in the Eastern Mediterranean Region and one in Western Pacific Region had adopted the policy by 2009.

3.2 Information on global ACT supplies and the artemisinin market situation

The sources of information on global adoption of the WHO policy on ACTs and their deployment, on artemether-lumefantrine supplies, on overall ACT sales, on the artemisinin market situation and on oral artemisinin-based monotherapy medicines are given below.

Information on adoption of the WHO policy on ACTs and their deployment:

- country adoption of ACTs: the WHO/GMP Antimalarial Drug Policies Database (http://www.who.int/malaria/treatmentpolicies.html) and

- country deployment of ACTs to general health services: compiled by the GMP Supply Chain Management Unit on the basis of reports from WHO regional and country offices.

Information on ACT sales for public sector use by manufacturers eligible for procurement by WHO in 2008 was obtained from various companies.

- Artemether-lumefantrine: Ajanta, Cipla, Novartis

- Artesunate + amodiaquine fixed-dose combination: Sanofi Aventis

- Artesunate + amodiaquine co-blisters: Cipla, Guilin, Ipca, Sanofi Aventis, Strides Arcolab

- Artesunate + mefloquine: data on number of treatment courses not available

- Artesunate + sulfadoxine-pyrimethamine: Cipla, Guilin

Information on the artemisinin market situation:

- Price fluctuations of artemisinin raw material: from the International Conference on Artemisinin Production and Marketing Needs: Meeting Global Demand, Bangkok, 25–26 June 2007, Medicines for Malaria Venture, WHO (http://www.mmv.org/article.php3?id_article=374) and the Artemisinin Forum 2008: Joint Meeting on Ensuring Sustainable Artemisinin Production: Meeting Global Demand, 24–26 November 2008 (http://www.mmv.org/article.php3?id_article=562).

Information on oral artemisinin-based monotherapy medicines:

- The position of pharmaceutical companies in relation to WHO recommendations on oral artemisinin-based monotherapy medicines: the WHO/GMP database at www.who.int/malaria/pages/performance/marketingmonotherapies.html.

- Countries and marketing authorization of oral artemisinin-based monotherapy medicines: the WHO/GMP database at www.who.int/malaria/pages/performance/monotherapycountries.html.

Table 3.1 Adoption and implementation of WHO-recommended policies and strategies for malaria control, by WHO Region, 2008

INTERVENTION	AFR	AMR	EMR	EUR	SEAR	WPR	TOTAL
Number of endemic countries [a]	43	23	13	9	10	10	108
Number of *P. falciparum* endemic countries	42	11	9	1	9	9	81
Insecticide-treated net (ITN)							
Targeting population – All	14	12	7	3	8	8	52
Distribution – Free	33	5	10	4	9	7	68
Indoor residual spraying (IRS)							
IRS is the primary vector control intervention	15	11	4	8	5	2	45
DDT is used for IRS (public health only)	8	0	0	0	3	1	12
Diagnosis and treatment							
ACT for treatment of *P. falciparum*	42	8	8	1	9	9	77
ACT is free of charge for children < 5 years in the public sector	23	4	10	1	8	6	52
Oral artemisinin-based monotherapies banned	17	5	10	1	8	3	44
Parasitological confirmation for all age groups	20	21	7	8	9	6	71
Diagnosis of malaria of inpatients based on parasitological confirmation	23	9	8	7	6	9	62
Pre-referral treatment at health facility level with quinine or artemether intramuscularly or artesunate suppositories	19	1	9	0	5	5	39
RDTs used at community level [b]	12	5	3	0	4	5	29
Oversight regulation of case management in the private sectors	14	2	6	3	4	4	33
Intermittent preventive therapy (IPT)							
Intermittent preventive therapy to prevent malaria during pregnancy	33	0	3	0	0	1	37

ACT: artemisinin-based therapy; RDT: rapid diagnostic test

[a] Includes countries in prevention of re-introduction phase

[b] Recommended by WHO in high transmission areas where there is poor access to health services

3.2.1 ACT policy adoption and deployment

By 2009, 77 of 81 *P. falciparum* malaria-endemic countries and territories had adopted ACTs for use in their national drug policy. As of 2008, French Guiana, Guatemala and Haiti were the only countries yet to adopt the policy of using ACT for treatment of *P. falciparum* malaria. Sixty countries are deploying these medicines in the general health services, with varying levels of coverage (**Fig. 3.1**).

3.2.2 Artemether-lumefantrine supplies

WHO is monitoring the global supply of and demand for the artemether-lumefantrine fixed-dose combination as part of the requirements of the Memorandum of Understanding signed with the manufacturer, Novartis, in 2001, to make Coartem® available at cost price for distribution in the public sector of malaria-endemic developing countries. The total supplies of this combination increased substantially, from 11.2 million treatment courses in 2005 to 62 million in 2006 and 66.3 million in 2007, with procurement of more than 78 million treatment courses in 2008. In the period 2006–2008, most artemether-lumefantrine was procured for young children weighing < 15 kg, and the smallest proportion was supplied for patients with a body weight of 25–34 kg (**Fig. 3.2**). Most countries that procure artemether-lumefantrine are located in the African Region (**Fig.3.3**).

Besides UNICEF, other agencies (Crown Agents, IDA Solutions, John Snow, Inc., Medical Export Group, Médecins Sans Frontières, Missionpharma, UNDP, UNOPS) have established direct procurement agreements with Novartis to supply Coartem® at the same prices negotiated by WHO. While overall artemether-lumefantrine supplies have increased since 2007, procurement of this medicine through WHO has proportionally decreased, while procurement through other agencies has proportionally increased (**Fig. 3.4**). Between December 2008 and May 2009, two additional preparations of artemether-lumefantrine, manufactured by Ajanta and Cipla, were prequalified by WHO.

3.2.3 Overall ACT sales

Public-sector sales of artemether-lumefantrine, artesunate + amodiaquine, and artesunate + sulfadoxine-pyrimethamine, manufactured by seven companies eligible for WHO procurement, are shown in **Figure 3.5**. During the period 2006–2008, procurement of fixed-dose combination ACTs progressively increased, and sales of co-blistered ACTs (**Fig. 3.6**), which represent a relatively small proportion of overall ACT sales to the public sector, showed a decreasing trend. Artemether-lumefantrine is the ACT that represents the largest volume of sales to the public sector, followed by artesunate + amodiaquine.

Figure 3.1 Adoption of policy and deployment of artemisinin-based therapy (ACT) by year, global data, 2001–2008

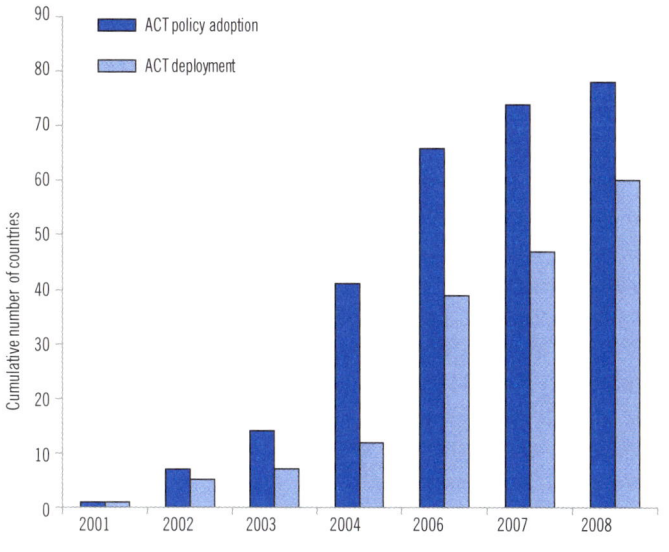

Figure 3.2 Procurement of artemether-lumefantrine for public sector use by weight-based dose package, global data, 2005–2008

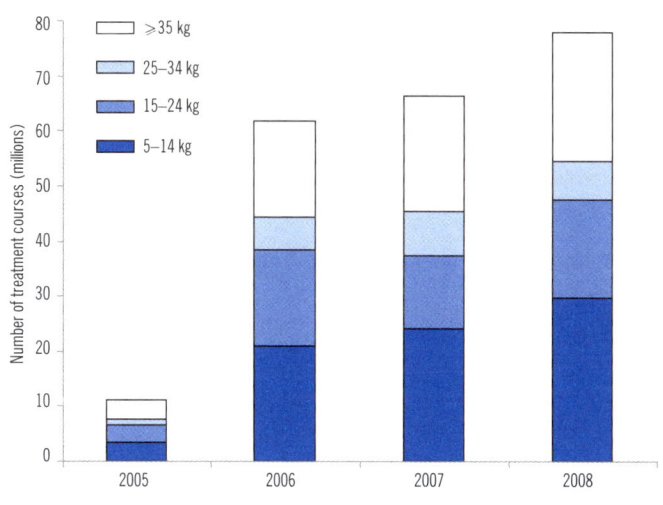

Figure 3.3 Public sector procurement of artemether-lumefantrine by year, by WHO Region, 2006–2008

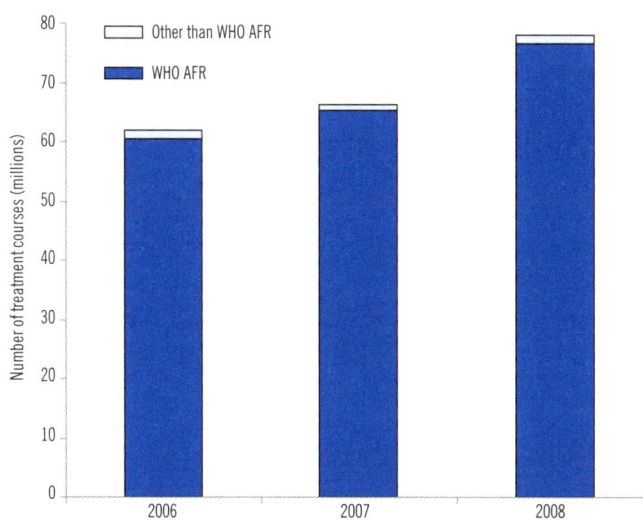

Figure 3.4 Number of artemether-lumefantrine treatment courses procured for public-sector use by procurement agency by year, global data, 2005–2008

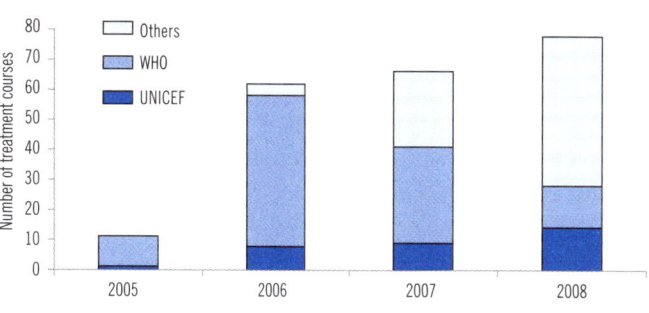

Figure 3.5 WHO-recommended artemisinin-based therapy courses procured for public sector use by year, global data

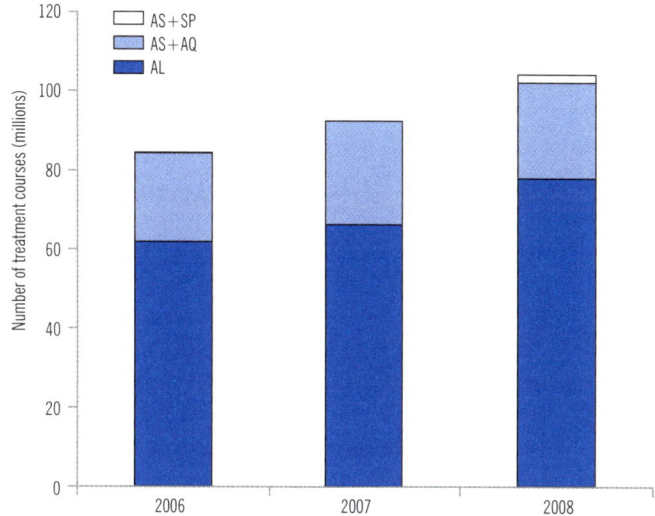

AL, artemether-lumefantrine; AS+AQ, artesunate + amodiaquine; AS+MQ, artesunate + mefloquine; AS+SP, artesunate + sulfadoxine/pyrimethamine

Figure 3.6 Co-blister packs and fixed-dose combination (FDC) artemisinin-based combination therapy procured for public-sector use by year; global data, 2006–2008

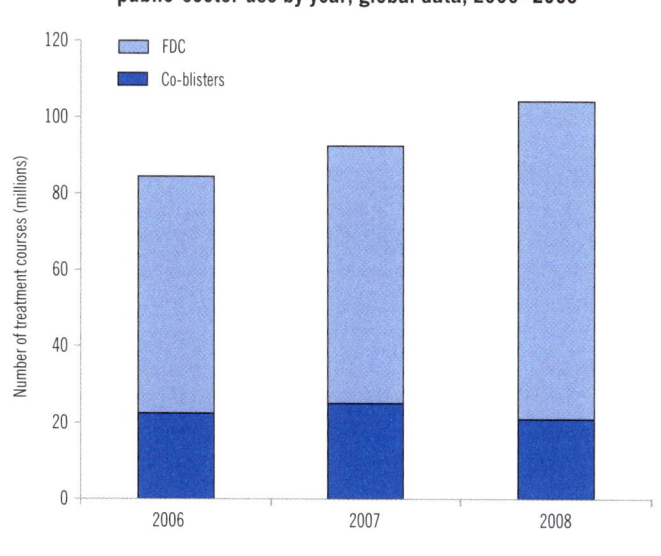

3.2.4 Artemisinin market situation

The major investments and the expansion in agricultural production of *Artemisia annua* and extraction of artemisinin in 2006–2007 were not matched by a similar increase in demand for artemisinin by ACT manufactures and suppliers of artemisinin-based active pharmaceutical ingredients. The resulting production surplus of artemisinin has led to a reduction in the prices of artemisinin raw material, even to below production costs, reaching as low as US$ 200 per kg by the end of 2007 and 2008. The subsequent withdrawal of many artemisinin producers and extractors from the market in 2008 is likely to create a shortage of artemisinin-based active pharmaceutical ingredients in 2010, when demand for ACTs will increase because of greater mobilization of funds from international agencies, including the Affordable Medicine Facility for malaria. To counteract these market dynamics, a new UNITAID-funded Initiative, based on credit-line facilities for artemisinin extractors, has been introduced. Production of artemisinin-based antimalarial medicines will remain dependent on agricultural production, as production of artemisinin with biotechnology from yeast culture will not become available until at least 2012.

3.2.5 Oral artemisinin-based monotherapy medicines

The presence of oral artemisinin-based monotherapies on the market continues to represent a threat to the therapeutic life of these medicines, by encouraging the development of resistance. To contain this risk and to ensure high cure rates of *P. falciparum* malaria, WHO recommends the withdrawal of oral artemisinin-based monotherapies from the market and use of ACTs instead. After publication of the *WHO Guidelines for the treatment* of malaria in January 2006, pharmaceutical companies were asked to stop producing and marketing the oral monotherapies. Major procurement and funding agencies as well as international suppliers cooperated with WHO by agreeing not to fund or procure these drugs. The recommendations were endorsed by all WHO Member States and are included in resolution WHA60.18 adopted by the 60th World Health Assembly in May 2007.

Since 2006, WHO GMP has convened several meetings in various countries to inform national drug regulatory authorities and representatives of the private sector about the WHO recommendations. As a result, a number of countries have taken regulatory measures to phase out the production and marketing of oral artemisinin-based monotherapies, including Benin, China, India, Pakistan and Viet Nam. The Indian experience is presented in **Box 3.1.**

To monitor implementation of the WHO recommendation to remove oral artemisinin-based monotherapies progressively from the market, WHO GMP is using a web-based system to compile data on both manufacturers' compliance and the regulatory steps taken by malaria-endemic countries. Twenty-two of 68 pharmaceutical companies identified by WHO by December 2008 had declared their intention to comply with the recommendation to stop production and marketing of the drugs, and another 12 have actually ceased production and marketing. While 24 malaria-endemic countries have either never registered or have taken regulatory measures to withdraw marketing authorizations for these medicines, and another 11 countries have declared their intention to comply with the WHO recommendation, 41 countries still allowed marketing of these products as of the end of 2008 (**Fig. 3.7**). Most of the countries that still allow the production and marketing of monotherapies are located in the African Region, followed by the regions of the Americas and South-East Asia.

Web-based WHO monitoring system for the implementation of WHA60.18

Information on manufacturing companies is available from:

http://apps.who.int/malaria/pages/performance/marketingmonotherapies.html.

Information on countries complying with the resolution is available from:

http://apps.who.int/malaria/pages/performance/monotherapycountries.html

World Health Assembly Resolution WHA60.18

In May 2007, the 60th World Health Assembly resolved to take strong action against oral artemisinin-based monotherapies and approved resolution WHA60.18, which:

• urges Member States to cease progressively the provision in both the public and private sectors of oral artemisinin-based monotherapies, to promote the use of artemisinin-combination therapies, and to implement policies that prohibit the production, marketing, distribution and the use of counterfeit antimalarial medicines;

• requests international organizations and financing bodies to adjust their policies so as progressively to cease to fund the provision and distribution of oral artemisinin monotherapies, and to join in campaigns to prohibit the production, marketing, distribution and use of counterfeit antimalarial medicines.

The full text of the resolution can be found at the following link: http://apps.who.int/gb/ebwha/pdf_files/WHA60/A60_R18-en.pdf.

BOX 3.1

Country example: India

Indian pharmaceutical companies export large quantities of artemisinin-based antimalarial medicines to African countries, and up to 70 companies marketing these medicines have been identified. In April 2006 and October 2008, two meetings were convened with Indian manufacturers to inform them about the risks for artemisinin resistance and about the WHO recommendations to phase out oral artemisinin-based monotherapies from the market. At the meeting in October 2008, which was chaired by the Drug Controller General of India, feasible mechanisms and timelines for the progressive withdrawal of oral artemisinin-based monotherapies from the Indian market were identified. In December 2008, the Drug Controller General of India requested the State Licensing Authorities to withdraw the production licenses and marketing authorization of these products over a 6-month period, affecting both their domestic and export markets.

Challenges to implementation of resolution WHA60.18 remain. As the private-sector pharmaceutical markets in many malaria-endemic countries are unregulated, pharmaceutical companies tend to ignore the WHO guidelines. Moreover, when responsible companies comply with the recommendation by withdrawing their oral artemisinin-based monotherapies from the market, they leave "niche markets", which are exploited by opportunistic companies manufacturing substandard products. More collaboration and involvement of national drug regulatory authorities is required to implement the resolution and to ensure complete elimination of oral artemisinin-based monotherapy medicines from all countries.

Compliance in some countries and positive responses from several manufacturers show that it is possible to phase out artemisinin-based monotherapies. The following timetable, based on the initial experience of countries that have succeeded, can be used as a guide.

ACTION	TASK	TIMELINE
STEP 1	Agreement on time frame of phasing out oral artemisinin-based monotherapies and introduction/implementation of artemisinin-based combination therapies	immediate
STEP 2	No more new marketing approvals for oral artemisinin-based monotherapies	immediate
STEP 3	No grand import licence for artemisinin or its derivatives to companies that are exclusively marketing oral artemisinin-based monotherapies	3–4 months
STEP 4	Large scale deployment of artemisinin-based combination therapies in the public sector	Time X
STEP 5	Promotion of widespread availability and affordability of ACTs in the private sector and communication campaigns to move prescribers and consumers away from monotherapies	Time Z
STEP 6	Withdrawal of manufacturing licences for oral artemisinin-based monotherapies as finished pharmaceutical products (FPP)	6 months after Time X
STEP 7	No export license for oral artemisinin-based monotherapies as FPP	6 months after Time X
STEP 8	Complete elimination of oral artemisinin-based monotherapies as FPP from the market	10–12 months after Time X

Figure 3.7   Countries' regulatory position on oral artemisinin-based monotherapy medicine by year and WHO Region, as of December 2008

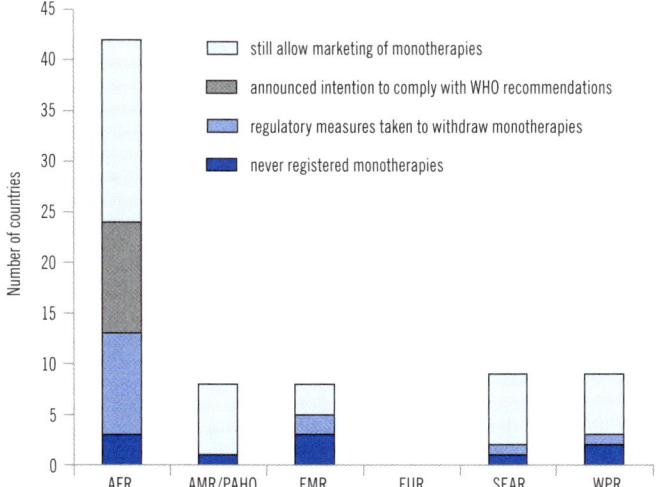

3.3   Intervention coverage in high-burden countries in the WHO African Region

This section describes coverage with interventions in 35 high-burden countries that comprised 87% of the population of African Region in 2008 and 99% of the population at risk. We have excluded low-burden countries: Botswana, Cape Verde, Namibia, South Africa, Swaziland and Zimbabwe.

3.3.1 Definitions

Three sources were used to estimate intervention coverage: logistics data reported by national programmes, the number of commodities delivered by manufacturers, and national surveys. Estimates for six interventions (ITNs, ACTs, IRS, parasite-based testing, RDTs and IPT for pregnant women) were derived from logistics or administrative data reported by ministries of health; these estimates are referred to as "operational" or "administrative" indicators and are summarized in **Box 3.2**.

The numerator for operational percentage coverage with ITNs is the number of persons covered by the ITNs distributed, assuming that one ITN covers two persons (1). As LLINs are assumed to last 3 years, the numerator includes the number of nets distributed over 3 years. The denominator is the population at risk, i.e. persons in a country who are at risk for malaria, as reported to WHO by national programmes. The percentage of the national population at risk was 100% for most countries in the African Region, except for e.g. Ethiopia and Kenya, where part of the country is considered by national experts as being at no risk (mostly areas at higher elevation). Persons living in areas of unstable transmission of malaria, where malaria is absent during most of the year but can occur as outbreaks, are still considered "at risk".

BOX 3.2

Six practical indicators obtained from routine data

1. **ITNs** – Operational ITN coverage: number of LLINs distributed in previous 3 years multiplied by 2 (assuming one long-lasting insecticidal net covers two persons) divided by population at risk for malaria.

2. **ACTs** – Percentage of reported malaria cases with access to ACTs: number of ACT treatment courses distributed divided by the number of reported malaria cases.

3. **IRS** – Percentage of population at risk protected by IRS: number of persons protected by IRS divided by population at risk.

4. **Parasite-based testing for malaria** – Percentage of suspected malaria cases tested by microscopy or RDT.

5. **RDTs** – Percentage of reported suspected malaria cases with access to RDTs: number of RDTs distributed divided by reported suspected malaria cases.

6. **IPT for pregnant women** – Percentage of women attending antenatal care at least once who received second dose of IPT: number of women receiving second dose of IPT divided by number who attended antenatal care at least once.

The numerators for ACT and RDT coverage are the numbers of ACT treatment courses and RDTs distributed at national level. The denominator for the ACT indicator was the number of reported malaria cases, and that for the RDT indicator was the number of reported suspected malaria cases.[1] Most ACTs and RDTs reported as distributed by ministries of health go to public-sector facilities. The denominator for IPT of pregnant women is the number of women making at least one antenatal care visit. The numerator is the number of pregnant women receiving a second dose.

3.3.2 Long-lasting insecticidal nets

Logistics. The numbers of LLINs distributed in countries reported from national programmes (public sector) and from manufacturers' data on the numbers of nets delivered to high-burden countries are compared in **Table 3.2** and **Figure 3.8**. Except in Nigeria, manufacturers reported delivering 25% more nets than the number of nets reported to have been distributed by national programmes in 2008. The difference could be due to the lag between delivery and distribution, inadequate record-keeping or other, unknown factors. In countries with large private sectors, ministry of health data might not include distribution by the private sector. For example, in Nigeria, manufacturers reported delivering 15 million LLINs, and the national programme reported distributing nearly 7 million. Some of the difference might be accounted for by delivery of nets to private-sector enterprises. The number of nets needed to cover all persons at risk in high-burden countries in 2008 was approximately 336 million (one half of the 671 million persons at risk, assuming that one net covers two persons). The cumulative number of LLINs delivered in 2006–2008 by manufacturers was 141 million, which represents 42% of the 336 million needed in 2008 (assuming a lifespan of 3 years). Data from ministries of health indicate that an estimated 35% of the nets needed were distributed.

Surveys. **Table 3.3** shows data on ITNs from the national surveys that were publicly available for 2006–2008 as of October 2009. Indicators from 2007–2008 surveys were available from reports to WHO and from preliminary reports of demographic and health surveys and malaria indicator surveys. Data were available (Table 3.3) for at least one indicator from 13 countries (49% of the at-risk population in the African Region) in 2008, from 9 countries (26% of the at-risk population) in 2007 and from 15 countries (27% of the at-risk population) in 2006. Table 3.3 shows both the weighted average and median for each year. The weighted average depended heavily on whether survey data were available for Nigeria (for 2008), the Democratic Republic of the Congo (for 2007) or neither of those countries (for 2006), as the ITN indicators for both countries are low, and their inclusion decreases the weighted average. The weighted average of household ITN ownership was 30%, and that of ITN use by children < 5 years was 24% in 2008. Seven countries (Equatorial Guinea, Ethiopia [population living at < 2000 m], Gabon, Mali, Sao Tome and Principe, Senegal and Zambia) had reached ≥ 60% household ITN ownership by 2007 or 2008, as also seen in Zanzibar, United Republic of Tanzania (**Fig. 3.9**).

The relation between ITN use by children < 5 years old and ITN household ownership from 35 surveys conducted in 2006–2007 from which data on both ITN use and household ITN ownership were available is shown in **Figure 3.10**. The figure also shows the relation between ITN use by persons of all ages and ITN household ownership in seven countries for which survey datasets were available to calculate use by persons of all ages (three in 2007 and four in 2006).

The percentage of children < 5 years old who had used an ITN the previous night, given household ownership of at least one ITN, was 51% (median; range, 14–68%) in six countries for which survey data were available in 2006–2007. As all six surveys were demographic and health surveys, which are usually conducted in the dry season, use in the wet season might be higher.

Figure 3.8 Reported numbers of long-lasting insecticidal nets (LLIN) delivered by manufacturers (manufacturers' data) and number distributed by ministries of health (MOH data), 2004–2008, 35 high-burden WHO African Region countries

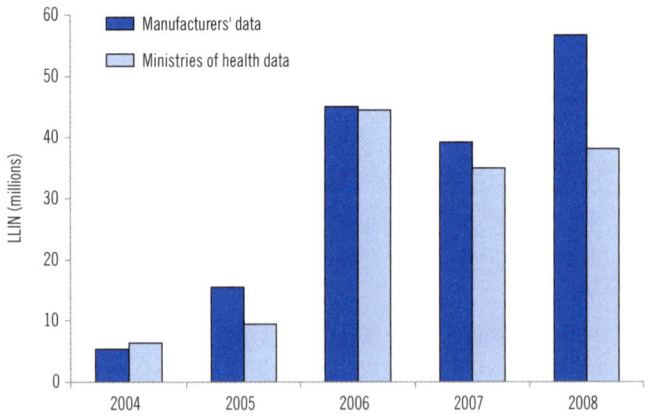

Figure 3.9 Household insecticide-treated net (ITN) ownership as measured by national surveys, 2007–2008, high-burden WHO African Region countries

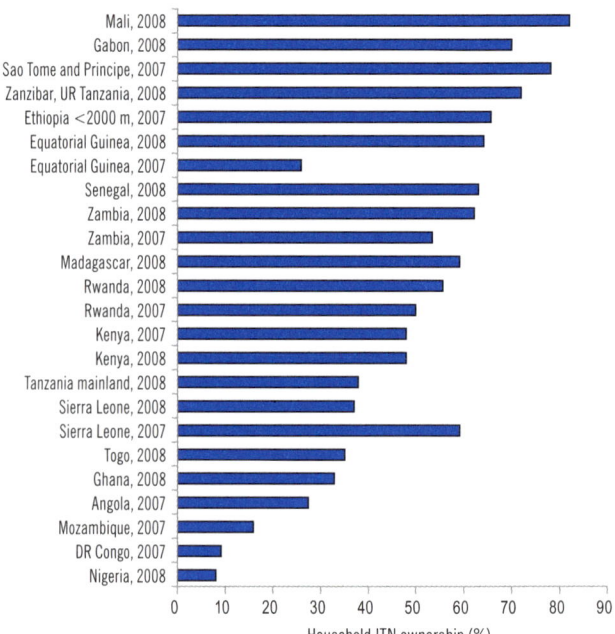

---

1. In most countries in the African Region in which there is little parasite-based testing of suspected malaria cases, the number of reported malaria cases and the number of reported suspected malaria cases are the same or similar. As the fraction of suspected cases tested for parasites increases, countries often start reporting confirmed cases alone or confirmed plus probable (untested) malaria cases as the official total of malaria cases.

Table 3.2 Number of long-lasting insecticidal nets (LLIN) reported to have been distributed by ministries of health, as reported to WHO, and numbers reported to have been delivered to countries by manufacturers, 2006–2008, high-burden African countries. These data, with survey data, were used to estimate ITN indicators (household ITN ownership and use) in a model

SUB-REGION / COUNTRY	Population at risk, 2008	Number of LLIN reported delivered by manufacturers					Number of LLIN reported to have been distributed, ministry of health data reported to WHO				
		2006	2007	2008	Cumulative 2006–2008	Operational ITN coverage, 2008* (%)	2006	2007	2008	Cumulative 2006-2008	Operational ITN coverage, 2008* (%)
Central											
Burundi	6 907 854	1 037 300	584 135	1 514 765	3 136 200	91	586 588	1 203 763	895 355	2 685 706	78
Central African Rep.	18 920 235	147 500	365 000	891 536	1 404 036	15	121 828	498 050	846 966	1 466 844	16
Cameroon	4 424 294	38 605	146 225	1 187 372	1 372 202	62	16 800	0	802 105	818 905	37
Chad	10 958 573	129 400	244 500	98 348	472 248	9	267 000	83 000	126 000	476 000	9
Congo	3 847 188	121 800	100 000	226 519	448 319	23	Data not av.				
DR Congo	64 703 615	1 750 841	3 317 755	8 506 216	13 574 812	42	2 981 026	2 385 684	5 788 513	11 155 223	34
Equatorial Guinea	519 697	28 330	166 000	105 150	299 480	115		152 992	65 913	218 905	84
Gabon	1 350 153	290 236	125 360	12 700	428 296	63	216 523	352 994	10 640	580 157	86
Rwanda	10 008 624	2 061 537	748 116	43 346	2 852 999	57	1 957 720	1 162 275	17 926	3 137 921	63
Sao Tome Principe	157 848	84 548	28 114	24 000	136 662	173	Data not av.				
South-East											
Angola	17 499 407	1 753 142	1 977 589	1 361 111	5 091 842	58	826 656	1 495 165	1 471 200	3 793 021	43
Eritrea	5 005 680	197 811	223 191	455 442	876 444	35	80 673	159 360	134 399	374 432	15
Ethiopia	57 948 997	12 294 218	4 639 411	1 935 148	18 868 777	65	8 606 640	4 475 301	3 316 696	16 398 637	57
Kenya	29 244 399	8 700 429	1 555 150	3 235 173	13 490 752	92	6 378 465	1 591 492	2 437 621	10 407 578	71
Madagascar	20 215 202	1 328 808	2 938 410	1 243 231	5 510 449	55	1 614 187	3 359 244	907 739	5 881 170	58
Malawi	14 288 374	273 466	997 465	378 494	1 649 425	23	120 000	255 266	858 026	1 233 292	17
Mozambique	21 812 550	567 000	1 386 233	2 484 777	4 438 010	41	313 102	1 586 534	2 086 367	3 986 003	37
UR Tanzania	41 463 923	39 200	193 000	1 021 387	1 253 587	6	549 244	322 516	927 461	1 799 221	9
Uganda	31 902 611	2 438 134	1 603 181	1 870 846	5 912 161	37	1 999 449	1 622 001	2 273 413	5 894 863	37
Zambia	12 154 060	806 564	3 226 109	671 119	4 703 792	77	1 162 578	2 458 183	1 188 443	4 809 204	79
West											
Benin	9 309 367	183 250	2 002 310	578 542	2 764 102	59	49 773	1 716 942	283 058	2 049 773	44
Burkina Faso	15 213 315	198 390	907 858	1 011 491	2 117 739	28	121 100	13 000	724 547	858 647	11
Côte d'Ivoire	19 624 238	350 200	394 200	1 591 308	2 335 708	24	336 000	0	0	336 000	3
Gambia	1 754 067	29 060	193 100	324 048	546 208	62	32 466	77 163	290 393	400 022	46
Ghana	23 946 817	3 268 898	2 015 509	2 663 727	7 948 134	66	2 268 336	1 934 460	257 717	4 460 513	37
Guinea	9 572 042	515 540	131 000	115 288	761 828	16	120 500	312 500	246 000	679 000	14
Guinea Bissau	1 745 835	147 083	12 000	129 773	288 856	33	182 906	91 700	2 064	276 670	32
Liberia	3 942 215	470 083	771 086	632 022	1 873 191	95	92 308	342 639	714 500	1 149 447	58
Mali	12 716 080	1 206 778	3 428 525	1 210 722	5 846 025	92	90 900	2 982 346	682 461	3 755 707	59
Mauritania	2 233 066	40 300	40 000	30 153	110 453	10	49 616	0	0	49 616	4
Niger	14 730 794	225 100	207 100	2 467 390	2 899 590	39	2 665 000	710 000	700 000	4 075 000	55
Nigeria	151 478 123	2 147 404	2 724 304	15 310 222	20 181 930	27	8 853 589	3 225 594	6 700 000	18 779 183	25
Senegal	12 687 625	462 000	1 487 810	1 103 037	3 052 847	48	400 000	0	1 572 261	1 972 261	31
Sierra Leone	12 687 625	1 546 220	193 230	638 126	2 377 576	37	1 301 164	319 199	541 265	2 161 628	34
Togo	6 762 422	154 700	123 000	1 618 370	1 896 070	56	65 235	43 946	1 261 706	1 370 887	41
Total annual	**671 736 915**	**45 033 875**	**39 195 976**	**56 690 899**	**140 920 750**	**42**	**44 427 372**	**34 933 309**	**38 130 755**	**117 491 436**	**35**
Total annual without Nigeria		**42 886 471**	**36 471 672**	**41 380 677**			**35 573 783**	**31 707 715**	**31 430 755**		
Total cumulative without Nigeria					**120 738 820**					**98 712 253**	

*based on 1 ITN per 2 persons

Manufacturers' data from John Milliner, USAID, as part of RBM Alliance for Malaria Prevention. National ministry of health data from that reported to WHO as part of the *World Malaria Report 2009*.
Operational coverage with ITNs was calculated from administrative data on number of LLIN delivered or distributed over 3 years times 2 (assuming one LLIN covers two persons) divided by the population at risk.

Table 3.3 Information on ITN ownership and use, parasitaemia and haemoglobin levels from national surveys, 2006–2008, high-burden African Region countries

COUNTRY	Population (million)	Month/year of survey	Type of survey	Aggregate data available	Dataset available for detailed analysis	ITN household ownership	ITN use, all ages	ITN use, < 5 years	ITN use, equity ratio	ITN use, lowest wealth quintile	ITN use, rural	Para-sitaemia %	Haemoglobin g/dl % <7	% <8
2008														
1 Angola	17	05/08–05/09	MICS	No	No	No data av.								
2 Equatorial Guinea	0.5		National	Yes	No	64		ND						
3 Ghana	24	09/08–11/08	DHS	Yes	No	33		28						
4 Gabon	1.4		National	Yes	No	70		55						
5 Kenya	38	11/08–02/09	DHS	Yes	No	48		39	1.4	35	48			
6 Madagascar	20		National	Yes	No	59		60						
7 Mali	13	04/08	National	Yes	No	82		79						
8 Mozambique	22	04/08	MICS	No	No	No data av.								
9 Nigeria	151	06/08–10/08	DHS	Yes	No	8		6			5			
10 Rwanda	10	12/07–04/08	DHS	Yes	No	56		56	2.1	47	55	2.6 (RDT)	8.3	
11 Sao Tome and Principe	0.16		DHS	No	No	No data av.								
12 Senegal	13	10/08–12/08	MIS	Yes	No	63		31						
13 Sierra Leone	6	04/08–06/08	DHS	Yes	No	37		26						
14 Togo	7	12/07–02/08	MOH-CDC	Yes	No	55		35						
15 Zambia	12	04/08–05/08	MIS	Yes	No	62		41	1.0	39	42	10.2		4.3
16 UR Tanzania, Mainland	41	10/07–03/08	AIS/MIS	Yes	Yes	38		25	3.1	22	32		2.7	7.5
Zanzibar, UR Tanzania			AIS/MIS	Yes	No	72		59	1.1	67	72		1.0	4.7
Number of countries with data						13		12	4	4	5	2	2	2
Median						56		37						
Weighted average						30		24						
Population, countries with surveys or data	376					337		336						
2007														
1 Kenya	38	06/07–07/07	MIS	Yes	No	48		39	1.5	29	39	7.6(BS) / 3.3 (RDT)		4.4
2 Mauritania	3	05/07–09/07	MICS	No	No	No data av.								
3 Nigeria	148	03/07–04/07	MICS	No	No	No data av.								
4 Rwanda	10	06/07–07/07	MIS	Yes	No	50		56						
5 DR Congo	63	01/07–08/07	DHS	Yes	Yes	9	4	6	5.2	2	4		3.4	9.0
6 Liberia	4	12/06–04/07	DHS	No	No	No data av.							ND	ND
7 Zambia	12	04/07–10/07	DHS	Yes	Yes	53	22	28	1.7	19	27		ND	ND
8 Sao Tome and Principe	0.2		National	Yes	No	78		54						
9 Mozambique	21	06/07–07/07	MIS	Yes	Yes	16		7	0.9	7	6	38.5 (BS)/ 51.5 (RDT)		11.9
10 Angola	17	11/06–04/07	MIS	Yes	Yes	28	12	17	0.8	17	19	19.5(RDT)	0.7	3.0
11 Sierra Leone	6	10/07–11/07	MIS	Yes	No	59		56						
12 Ethiopia	83	10/07–12/07	MIS	Yes	No	53		33	1.0	35	33	0.7		5.5
< 2000 m						66		42				0.9		6.6
> 2000 m						28		14				0.1		3.1
13 Equatorial Guinea	0.5		Other	Yes	No	26		42						
Number of countries with data						9	3	9	5	6				
Median						49		36						
Weighted average						36		25						
Population, countries with surveys or data	404					249		249						

* highest/ lowest wealth quintile

Table 3.3 *Continued*

COUNTRY	Population (million)	Month/year of survey	Type of survey	Aggre-gate data avail-able	Dataset avail-able for detailed analysis	ITNs						Para-sitaemia	Haemagloblin g/dl	
						ITN household ownership	ITN use, all ages	ITN use, < 5 years	ITN use, < 5 equity ratio	ITN use, lowest wealth quintile	ITN use, rural	%	% < 7	% < 8
2006														
1 Burkina Faso	14	03/06–05/06	MICS	Yes	Yes	23		10	5.7	5	6			
2 Central African Rep.	4	06/06–11/06	MICS	Yes	No	25		15						
3 Sao Tome and Principe	0.16		MICS	No	No	No data av.								
4 Zambia	12	04/06–05/06	MIS	Yes	No	44		23	1.6	19	21	22.1		13.8
5 Benin	9	08/06–11/06	DHS	Yes	Yes	25	14	32	1.8	22	30		6.7	13.8
6 Cameroon	18	05/06–06/06	MICS	Yes	Yes	4		3	3.8	1	2			
7 Côte d'Ivoire	19	08/06–10/06	MICS	Yes	Yes	10		3	4.6	1	2			
8 Ghana	23	08/06–11/06	MICS	Yes	Yes	10		18	1.0	21	21			
9 Guinea-Bissau	2	05/06–06/06	MICS	Yes	Yes	44		40	0.7	41	44			
10 Mali	12	05/06–12/06	DHS	Yes	Yes	50	21	27	1.2	26	26		8.7	19.3
11 Malawi	14	07/06–11/06	MICS	Yes	Yes	38		25	2.7	16	23			
12 Niger	14	01/06–05/06	DHS	Yes	Yes	43	4	7	2.6	5	6		6.1	15.3
13 Senegal	12	11/06–12/06	MIS	Yes	Yes	36	12	16	0.6	20	17		ND	ND
14 Togo	6	05/06–06/06	MICS	Yes	Yes	40		38	0.9	41	40			
15 Uganda	30	04/06–10/06	DHS	Yes	Yes	16	7	9	1.4	10	8		5.8	12.0
16 Gambia	1.7	12/05–03/06	MICS	Yes	Yes	46		28	1.2	21	28			
Number of countries with data						15	5	15	14	14	14			
Median						31	12	23	1.5	19	21			
Weighted average						26		17						
Population, countries with surveys or with data	192					173		190						

MICS: multiple indicator cluster service; DHS: demographic health survey; MOH: ministry of health; CDC: Centers for Disease Control and Prevention (USA); MIS: malaria indicator survey; AIS: AIDS indicator survey; RDT: rapid diagnostic test; BS: blood spot; N/A: not applicable; ND: no data

Surveys that were not DHS, MIS, or MICS, but were reported to cover the national at-risk population were included.

Estimating household ITN ownership and ITN use by chidren < 5 years old, by country and year, from both survey and administrative data. Flaxman and colleagues at the Institute for Health Metrics and Evaluation at the University of Washington (USA), in collaboration with WHO and the United States Centers for Disease Control and Prevention, have constructed a model to combine data from surveys, manufacturers and ministries of health to obtain annual estimates of ITN ownership and use *(2)*. The method for the model is shown in **Box 3.3**. The weighted average estimate of household ITN ownership was 31%, and ITN use by children < 5 years old was 24% in all 35 high-burden countries in 2008 (**Table 3.4** and **Fig. 3.11**). These estimates were partially driven by very low household ITN ownership in the Democratic Republic of the Congo and Nigeria, two populous countries. Table 3.4 shows household ITN ownership by country in 2004–2008. As of 2008, 13 (37%) countries had reached ≥ 50% household ITN ownership, and 10 (29%) had reached ≥ 60%. Because this model can provide an estimate of ITN coverage for each country each year, it provides information that complements the data gathered directly in surveys.

Coverage and effectiveness of LLINs over time after mass distribution. Four countries have conducted surveys ≥ 12 months after the month of mass ITN distribution to children and pregnant women. In Sierra Leone, household ITN ownership declined 37%

within 2–3 years after mass campaign. In Togo, ownership declined 13% and ITN use in children <5 years old declined 20% within three years of the campaign (**Table 3.5**), although differences in survey methods could have accounted for some of the difference. The Ministry of Health in Togo in collaboration with the United States Centers for Disease Control and Prevention retrieved LLINs 36 months after their distribution during the mass campaign and found that between 30% and 40% of the nets collected did not pass the WHO bioassay for killing mosquitoes or had at least one hole that was ≥ 10 cm in diameter *(3)*. Multi-country studies for the WHO Pesticide Evaluation Scheme have identified surprisingly large country-to-country variations in mean net life *(4)*. Decreased ownership, use and net durability (physical and insecticide) might be reducing the effectiveness of ITNs in field situations. These data suggest that routine ITN systems after mass distribution may not have been adequate to sustain the high, equitable coverage that was achieved during the mass campaign. Waning ITN ownership and use, as well as limitations of net durability (physical and insecticide) might reduce the public health impact of this important malaria control tool.

In contrast, household ITN ownership coverage was maintained for 15 months in Rwanda (50% in the 2007 malaria indicator survey and 56% ,15 months after the campaign) and for 30 months in Kenya (51% immediately after campaign and 48%, 30 months later) (Table 3.5).

BOX 3.3

Summary of model for estimating coverage with ITNs

Background

Most of the information on the distribution and coverage of ITNs consists of annual data on the numbers of long-lasting insecticidal nets delivered to countries by manufacturers; annual data on the distribution of both long-lasting insecticidal and non-long-lasting insecticidal nets by national malaria control programmes to health facilities and operational partners; and periodic data on household net ownership and use by children under the age of 5. While data from manufacturers and national malaria control programmes provide important information on the supply and distribution of ITNs, the only direct measurement of whether ITNs are reaching and are being used by households is from surveys, which are, at best, conducted only every 3–5 years. It is therefore not possible to track properly the scale-up of control programmes to reduce the burden of malaria. The challenge is to impute, in an objective and replicable way, missing survey coverage from information from manufacturers and national malaria control programmes. The method should ideally resolve the issue that data from manufacturers, national malaria control programmes and households capture the stock and flow of nets at different points of the supply and distribution chain. For example, surveys measure the stock of nets in households at a specific time, whereas manufacturer data represent flows to a country over 1 year.

Model

A Bayesian inference-based compartmental model was developed to make annual estimates between 1999 and 2008 of ITN coverage, defined as the proportion of households owning at least one ITN, and ITN use by children under 5, defined as the proportion of children under the age of 5 years sleeping under an ITN during the wet season. Briefly, the model is based on the precise relations between net supply, distribution and ownership over time; for example, for a net to be owned by a household, it must have been distributed or purchased sometime in the past, and before that it must have been manufactured and sent to the organizations responsible for distribution or to the commercial sector for household purchase.

The compartmental model, with parameters describing the supply, distribution, ownership and discard of nets by households, is shown below. In this model the "supply" compartment reflects both public and commercial supply, and "distribution" includes public distribution as well as the purchase of nets by households from the commercial sector. The model includes a discrete 1-year step and allows flows into a compartment to be part of flows out of the compartment for the same year. This model ensures that estimates of supply, distribution, ownership and discard of nets are consistent over time. Compartmental model parameters are limited to long-lasting insecticidal nets, as manufacturer delivery data is available only for these nets and also because the stock of non-long-lasting nets is essentially equivalent to the flow of non-long-lasting ITNs in this model, given that they must be re-treated yearly. On the basis of previous studies the primary assumption is that a long-lasting insecticidal net is no longer active after four years and is not included in the household stock.

The compartmental model gives an estimate of the total number of long-lasting insecticidal nets in households in each country over time. We add to this a parameter that accounts for non-long-lasting ITNs in households to determine the total number of ITNs in households. We estimate the number ITNs per capita in each country by dividing by the estimated total population. A negative binomial distribution is used to estimate the distribution of ITNs per household; that is, the fraction of households with zero, one, two or three or more ITNs. The parameters of the model and the steps used to determine ITN ownership coverage are estimated by Bayesian inference; it provides a way of assessing uncertainty about the inputs and outputs of the model. As the model is further refined it is possible that default values for parameters – or the way they are handled – may change, which could influence the results.

ITN use by children under 5

An important factor that determines use of nets by children under 5 is the season in which surveys are conducted; people are more likely to sleep under ITNs when the risk for mosquito bites is higher. A regression model was used to estimate ITN use by children under 5 from ITN ownership coverage and the proportion of the total population represented by children under 5, while controlling for the season (wet or dry) in which the survey was conducted, from all available survey data (47 surveys). The regression parameters were then applied to the Bayesian inference-based compartmental model estimates of ITN ownership coverage to predict ITN use by children under 5 during the wet season.

Stocks

$S(t)$ = ITNs in national supply for distribution at time t
$H1(t)$ = 1 year old LLINs in households at time t
$H2(t)$ = 2 year old LLINs in households at time t
$H3(t)$ = 3 year old LLINs in households at time t
$H4(t)$ = 4 year old LLINs in households at time t

Flows

$m(t)$ = LLINs delivered to national supply by manufacturers during time period t
$d(t)$ = LLINs distributed by agencies to households during time period t
$l1(t)$ = number of 1 year old LLINs discarded by a household during time period t
$l2(t)$ = number of 2 year old LLINs discarded during time period t
$l3(t)$ = number of 3 year old LLINs discarded during time period t

Figure 3.10 Correlation between household insecticide-treated net (ITN) ownership and ITN use by children < 5 years old (35 surveys) and persons of all ages (7 surveys); 2006–2008, high-burden WHO African Region countries

a) *ITN use by children < 5 years old vs. household ITN ownership*

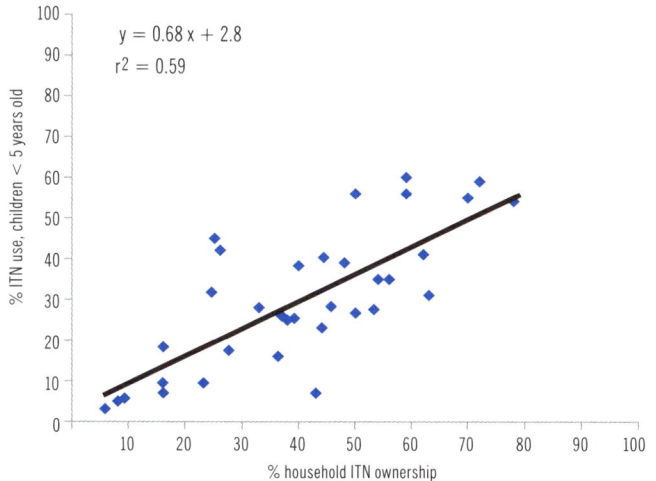

$y = 0.68 x + 2.8$
$r2 = 0.59$

b) *ITN use by persons of all ages vs. household ITN ownership*

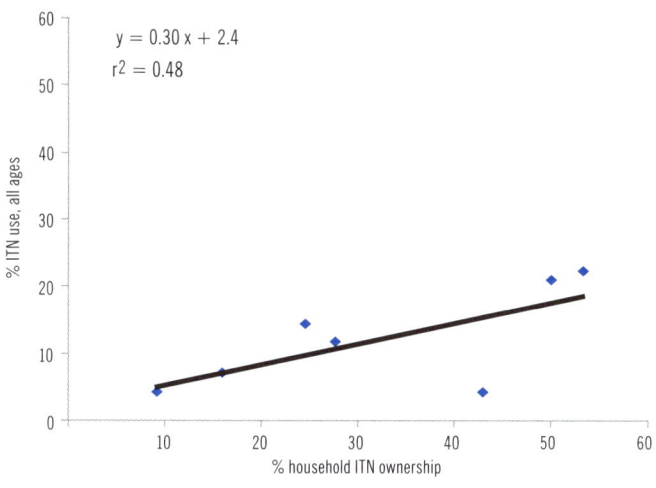

$y = 0.30 x + 2.4$
$r2 = 0.48$

Figure 3.11 Percentage household ownership of insecticide-treated nets (ITNs) estimated from model, 2000–2008, 35 high-burden WHO African Region countries

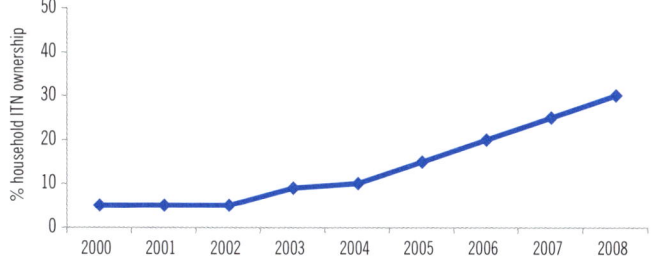

Table 3.4 Model-based estimates of percentage household insecticide-treated net (ITN) ownership, by year, high-burden African Region countries, 2004–2008; ordered by estimate of ownership in 2008

COUNTRY	MODEL ESTIMATES OF HOUSEHOLD ITN OWNERSHIP						
	2004	2005	2006	2007	2008	2008 lower limit	2008 upper limit
Sao Tome and Principe	21	18	39	76	91	76	99
Mali	4	10	38	69	80	76	86
Zambia	3	7	17	40	70	60	80
Madagascar	11	22	46	54	69	58	78
Ethiopia	3	7	16	39	66	57	75
Equatorial Guinea	2	3	17	42	65	58	75
Eritrea	3	5	8	27	64	57	72
Liberia	77	67	64	59	64	29	93
Rwanda	3	6	24	53	61	44	82
Guinea-Bissau	8	17	35	52	60	42	73
Kenya	20	36	48	48	57	29	80
Niger	11	16	30	48	55	41	70
Togo	12	30	57	59	54	41	73
Senegal	41	58	43	45	49	37	62
Sierra Leone	17	20	29	37	48	41	54
Gambia	19	35	38	30	37	22	53
Benin	8	15	30	35	36	19	57
UR Tanzania	16	20	26	39	36	25	47
Malawi	4	5	14	40	34	31	37
Ghana	31	28	37	37	33	19	49
Central African Rep.	5	6	15	24	31	25	37
Uganda	7	13	23	26	25	11	43
Angola	3	7	17	22	24	15	34
Mozambique	5	6	14	20	23	14	33
Burundi	7	7	10	15	21	15	28
Cameroon	6	9	13	17	20	10	31
Burkina Faso	6	12	22	22	18	9	26
DR Congo	9	12	20	20	16	10	25
Congo	3	5	8	12	15	10	22
Côte d'Ivoire	3	6	8	10	11	5	20
Gabon *							
Mauritania	1	3	5	8	9	6	13
Chad	4	4	5	6	9	4	13
Guinea	1	2	3	5	8	6	10
Nigeria	2	2	3	4	7	6	9
TOTAL	7	9	17	25	31	29	33

* Revision of Gabon data was made too late to be fully incorporated in this Report. Estimated household ITN ownership was 80% in 2008.

3.3.3 Indoor residual spraying

The number of persons protected by IRS more than doubled between 2006 and 2008, from 15 to 59 million (**Fig. 3.12**). This represented 9% of the at-risk population in the African Region in 2008. Seven countries protected > 10% of their at-risk populations with IRS in 2008: Botswana (38%), Equatorial Guinea (56%), Ethiopia (51%), Madagascar (32%), Mozambique (30%), Namibia (16%) and Zambia (47%).

3.3.4 Rapid diagnostic tests

In 2009, WHO recommended that persons of all ages with suspected malaria undergo diagnostic testing. In 2008, 22% of suspected malaria cases were tested in 18 of 35 countries reporting. **Figure 3.13** shows the percentage tested by year. Nine countries (Angola, Burundi, Equatorial Guinea, Gabon, Liberia, Madagascar, Niger, Rwanda, Senegal) reported testing > 50% of suspected malaria cases.

RDTs distributed. The number of RDTs delivered increased rapidly in 2007 and 2008, from near zero in 2005 (Fig. 3.13). The total number of RDTs distributed in 2008, however, corresponded to only 13% of all malaria cases reported in the 12 countries reporting, indicating a continuing gap in malaria diagnostic capacity.

3.3.5 Treatment

The number of ACTs distributed at country level increased significantly between 2004 and 2006, while the rate of increase in 2006–2008 was lower (**Fig. 3.14**). This is due at least partly to the low approval rate of grants for malaria activities in rounds 5 and 6 of the Global Fund, which influenced procurement of ACTs in 2006 and 2007. Data from manufacturers showed an 18% increase in ACT sales to the public sector in 2008 as compared with 2007.

Access to ACTs in the public sector can be estimated from operational or administrative data. If it is assumed that all ACTs reported by ministries of health were used for public sector facilities, enough ACTs were distributed to treat 48% of persons with malaria attending those facilities. **Figure 3.15** show the percentages of reported malaria cases with access to ACTs (ratio of ACTs distributed to reported malaria cases in 2008) by country. Fourteen of 35 countries reported distributing enough ACTs to treat at least 50% of reported malaria cases in the public sector; five countries reported distributing enough ACTs to treat all reported malaria cases in 2008 (**Table 3.6**).

Data from surveys in 2006–2008 on access to ACT are shown in **Table 3.7**. Preliminary reports from 10 countries were available in 2008, providing data primarily for two treatment indicators: percentage of children treated with any antimalarial medicine, and percentage of children treated with ACTs. The weighted average percentage of children with fever in the 2 weeks preceding the survey who received any antimalarial medicine was 32%. The percentage of children with fever who received an ACT was 16%, but data were available from only seven countries. Of 13 countries with survey-based data on ACT coverage in 2007 or 2008, the percentage of children with fever receiving ACT exceeded 15% in only two (Gabon, with 25%, and the United Republic of Tanzania, with 22%).

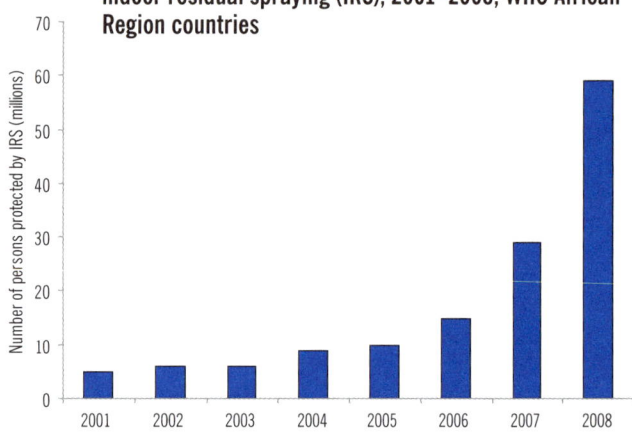

Figure 3.12 Numbers of persons protected with at least one round of indoor residual spraying (IRS), 2001–2008, WHO African Region countries

Figure 3.13 High-burden WHO African Region countries, 2004–2008

a) Number of rapid diagnostic tests (RDTs) distributed

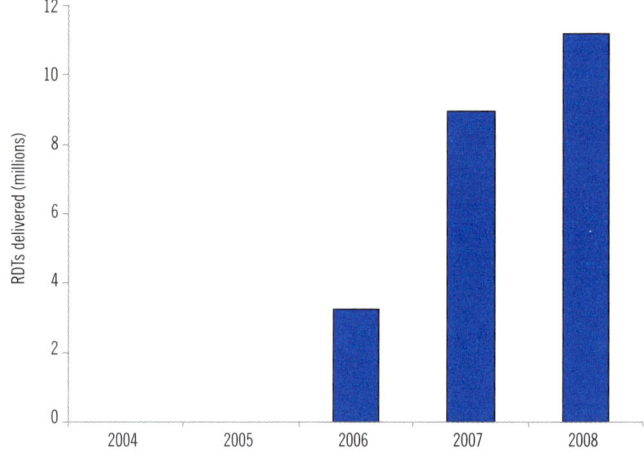

b) Percentage of reported malaria cases tested (microscopy or RDTs)

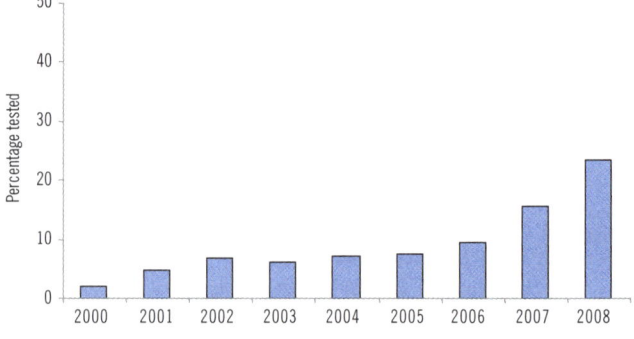

Figure 3.14 Numbers of ACT treatment courses distributed by countries, high-burden WHO African Region, 2003–2008

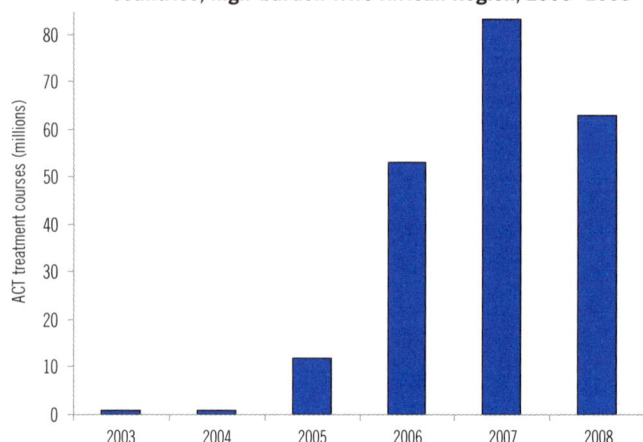

Table 3.5 Trends of household ownership and use of insecticide-treated nets (ITNs) by children < 5 years old in countries with at least two surveys after mass distribution of nets; Togo, Sierra Leone, Rwanda, and Kenya, 2004–2008

TYPE OF SURVEY	Dates of survey	Duration after campaign	(%) Household ownership any net	(%) Household ITN ownership, at least 1	(%) ITN use in children <5 years old
TOGO: mass distribution conducted in December 2004 to children 9–59 months and pregnant women					
CDC	Jan.–Feb. 2005	+ 1 month (dry)	66	63	44
CDC	Sept. 2005	First rainy season after campaign	64	60	53
MICS	May–Jun. 2006	+ 1.5 year (between dry/wet)	46	40	38
CDC	Dec. 2007–Feb. 2008	+ 3.0 year (between wet/dry)	55	55	35
% decline, last survey compared with first survey			17%	13%	20%
SIERRA LEONE: mass distribution conducted in November 2006 to children 9–59 months and pregnant women					
DataDyne	Jan. 2007	+ 1 month (dry)			51
CDC	Nov. 2007	+ 1 year	64	59	53
DHS	Apr.–Jun. 2008	+ 2.5 year (dry)	40	37	26
% decline, last survey compared with first survey			38%	37%	49%
RWANDA: mass distribution conducted in September 2006 to children 9–59 months and pregnant women					
MIS 2007	Jun.–Jul. 2007	+ 9 months	–	50	56
DHS 2008	Dec. 2007–Feb. 2008	+ 16–18 months	59	56	56
% decline, last survey compared with first survey				– 12%	0%
KENYA: mass distribution was conducted in two phases in July and September 2006 to children 9–59 months and pregnant women					
MOH-CDC 2006	Oct.–Nov. 2006	+ 1–2 months	54	51	52
MIS 2007	Jun.–Jul. 2007	+ 1 year	63	48	39
DHS 2008	Nov. 2008–Feb. 2009	+ 2 years	–	48	39
% decline, last survey compared with first survey				6%	25%

MOH = ministry of health; CDC = US Centers for Disease Control and Prevention; DHS= Demographic and Health Survey; MICS = Multiple Indicator Cluster Survey; MIS = Malaria Indicator Survey; DataDyne is a technical non-governmental organization.

Intermittent preventive treatment of pregnant women. For 10 of the 35 high-burden countries (Burkina Faso, Central African Republic, Equatorial Guinea, Gabon, Ghana, Niger, Nigeria, Senegal, Togo and Uganda), consistent data were available on both the second dose of IPT (numerator) and the number of women who had attended antenatal care at least once (denominator) for 2007 and 2008. Data on IPT for pregnant women from surveys in 2007–2008 were available for nine countries with a total population of 217 million. In 2007–2008, the percentage of women who received two doses of treatment during pregnancy ranged from 3% in Angola to 66% in Zambia; the weighted average was 20%.

3.3.6 Quality of administrative data on LLINs, ACTs, RDTs and diagnostic testing

The quality of the management information available was poor in many countries, especially for ACTs (see missing data in Table 3.7). For example, some countries rounded the estimated numbers of LLINs and ACTs distributed to the thousands, indicating incomplete data recording systems. Inadequate management information systems are likely to lead to inadequate monitoring of stock-outs of nets, ACTs and RDTs in health facilities. Poor management information

Figure 3.15 Estimated percentage of reported malaria cases with access to artemisinin-based combination therapy (ACT). Ratio of number of ACTs distributed to number of reported malaria cases, national data, 2008, high-burden WHO African Region countries

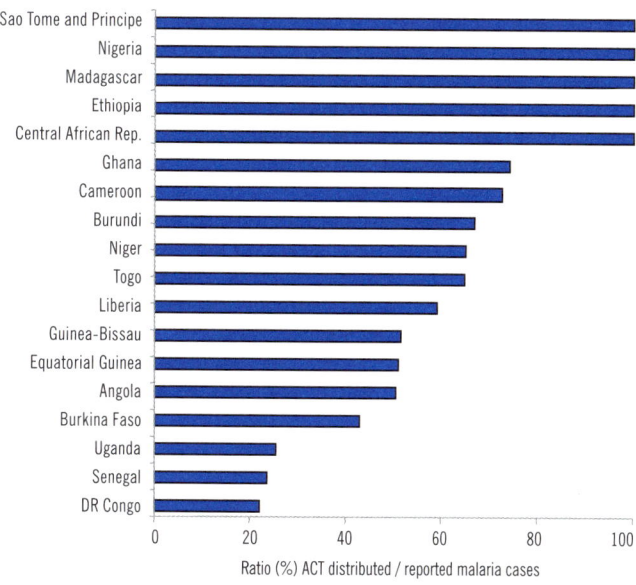

Countries without data are not shown

COUNTRY	POPULATION (million)	TREATMENT			IPT in pregnancy (births in past 2 years)	
		% with any antimalarial	% with any anti-malarial within 24 h	% with any ACT	2 (or more) doses of IPT during pregnancy	2 (or more) doses of IPT at least one of which was during an ANC visit
2008						
Angola	17	No data available				
Equatorial Guinea	0.5	16		3		
Gabon	0.0	48		25		
Ghana	24	24		12		
Kenya	38	24		ND		
Madagascar	20	No data available		ND		
Mali	13	No data available				
Mozambique	22	No data available				
Nigeria	151	33	15	ND		7
Rwanda	10	6	0	5		
Sao Tome and Principe	0.16	No data available				
Senegal	13	ND		ND		
Sierra Leone	6	30		ND		
Togo	7	37		11		
Zambia	12	43	29	13	66	60
UR Tanzania, Mainland	41	57	39	22	30	30
Zanzibar, UR Tanzania		38	37	10	55	52
Number of countries with data		**10**	**4**	**7**	**2**	**3**
Median		**32**		**12**		
Weighted average		**32**		**16**		
Population, countries with surveys or with data	375	310		95		
2007						
Kenya	38	24	15	8	13	
Mauritania	3	No data available				
Nigeria	148	No data available				
Rwanda	10				18	17
Democratic Rep. Congo	63	30	17	1	7	5
Liberia	4	59	26	9	12	
Zambia	12	38	21	11	66	63
Sao Tome and Principe	0.2	No data available	ND	ND		
Mozambique	21	23	18	ND	16	
Angola	17	29	13	3	3	3
Sierra Leone	6	No data available				
Ethiopia	83	10	4	4		
< 2000 m		12	5			
> 2000 m		2	1			
Equatorial Guinea	0.5	No data available				
Number of countries with data		**7**	**7**	**6**	**7**	**4**
Median		**29**	**17**	**6**		
Weighted average		**22**	**12**	**4**	**14**	
Population, countries with surveys or with data	404	237	237	216	164	
2006						
Burkina Faso	14	48	41	0	1	
Central African Rep.	4	No data available				
Sao Tome and Principe	0.2	No data available				
Zambia	12	53	32	10	59	57
Benin	9	54	42	0	3	
Cameroon	18	59	39	2	6	
Côte d'Ivoire	19	36	26	3	8	
Ghana	23	61	48	4	28	
Guinea-Bissau	2	46	27	2	7	
Mali	12	48	22	ND	11	4
Malawi	14	25	21	0	47	
Mauritania	1.3	21	10	1		
Senegal	12	20	9	6	51	49

Table 3.6 *Continued*

| COUNTRY | POPULATION (million) | TREATMENT | | | IPT in pregnancy (births in past 2 years) | |
		% with any antimalarial	% with any anti-malarial within 24 h	% with any ACT	2 (or more) doses of IPT during pregnancy	2 (or more) doses of IPT at least one of which was during an ANC visit
2006 *continued*						
Togo	6	48	38	1	18	
Uganda	30	61	29	3	18	16
Gambia	1.7	63	52	0	33	
Number of countries with data		**15**	**15**	**13**	**13**	**4**
Median		**48**	**29**	**2**	**18**	
Weighted average		**47**	**31**	**3**	**22**	
Population, countries with surveys or with data	**192**	**187**	**187**		**172**	

ND, no data; SP=sulfadoxine-pyramethamine; ANC=antenatal clinic; ACT=arteminsin-based combination therapy

Table 3.7 Outpatient malaria cases, number of suspected malaria cases tested, number ACT treatment courses received, number of RDT received, along with three key indicators comparing those data elements, 2006-2008, high-burden WHO African Region countries.

| SUB-REGION / COUNTRY | 2007 | | | 2008 | | |
	% Outpatient malaria cases tested	Ratio (%) RDT/ outpatient malaria cases	Ratio (%) ACT received/outpatient malaria cases	% Outpatient malaria cases tested	Ratio (%) RDT/ outpatient malaria cases	Ratio (%) ACT received/outpatient malaria cases
Central						
Burundi	47		75	50		67
Cameroon			184			73
Central African Republic			510			533
Chad	13			13		
Congo						
Democratic Rep. Congo	17	0	19	30	0	22
Equatorial Guinea				72	9	51
Gabon	68		234	70		
Rwanda	100	NA		100	NA	
South-East						
Angola	51	16	53	77	3	51
Eritrea	NA	NA		NA	NA	
Ethiopia	88	276		35	164	211
Kenya						
Madagascar	18	66	57	65	360	255
Malawi						
Mozambique						
Uganda	21		80	16	4	25
UR Tanzania	0	2				
Zambia		6			44	
West						
Benin						
Burkina Faso	3			2	3	43
Côte d'Ivoire						
Gambia						
Ghana				22		74
Guinea	2	5	3			
Guinea Bissau	17			29		52
Liberia	96		70	122		59
Mali			72			
Mauritania				1		
Niger	45	9	55	72	26	65
Nigeria		0	327		5	423
Sao Tome and Principe	NA	NA	176	NA	NA	181
Senegal	19			71	69	23
Sierra Leone				20		
Togo	52			22	65	65
Total	**14**	**9**	**39**	**22**	**13**	**48**

NA = not applicable. The RDT indicator does not work well when a high percentage of reported malaria cases are confirmed. The indicator for percentage of outpatient malaria cases tested does not work well if the number of suspected malaria cases is not reported. Sao Tome and Principe and Eritrea reported confirmed malaria cases only and not suspected malaria cases.

systems may contribute to inadequate stock-out monitoring, low ACT coverage, a low percentage of suspected malaria cases being tested and inadequate routine distribution of LLINs. National malaria control programmes should strengthen their management information systems and link them to supervision and quarterly performance assessments to improve programme effectiveness.

3.3.7 Summary of coverage with all interventions

Table 3.8 shows summary coverage indicators for all key interventions and diagnostics in high-burden countries. The number of commodities distributed and coverage with all interventions have been increasing. By 2007–2008, 37% of 35 high-burden countries had reached 50% household ITN ownership or more. In 2008, 24% of children < 5 years old had used an ITN the previous night. IRS is increasing but covers only 9% of the population at risk. IRS protects an important percentage (> 10%) of the population in seven countries.

Less progress has been made on treatment, diagnostics and IPT of pregnant women. The percentage of children with fever treated with an ACT was ≥ 15% in only two (Gabon and the United Republic of Tanzania) of 13 countries for which survey data were available for 2007–2008. Only 14 countries reported distributing enough ACT to treat at least 50% of reported malaria cases in the public sector, and only five countries reported distributing enough ACT to treat all reported malaria cases in 2008. Only 13% of the RDTs needed to test all reported malaria cases was distributed in 2008. Based on limited survey data, IPT coverage of pregnant women was 20%.

3.4 Intervention coverage in countries outside the WHO African Region

In regions other than the African Region, effective coverage with interventions is more difficult to measure, for several reasons. First, the target population for each intervention (treatment, IRS, ITNs) may be different within a country and is not standard for all countries. For example, interventions such as IRS and ITN are often targeted to hard-to-reach or mobile populations who are most at risk (e.g. migrants, workers in mining and forest areas). Secondly, surveys are less useful in areas with focalized malaria and are conducted less often.

Despite these limitations, operational coverage with interventions was estimated by using the population at high risk (> 1 malaria case per 1000 population) as the denominator and the numbers of ITNs and ACT doses distributed as the numerators. The reporting systems of many national malaria programmes do not, however, distinguish between procurement and delivery of ITNs, drugs and other commodities.

Administrative or operational coverage with ITNs was low in all regions, ranging from 1% to 5%. Analysis by country showed that ITN coverage was relatively high (> 20%) in Suriname (58%), Malaysia (54%), Sudan (55%), Vanuatu (41%), the Lao People's Democratic Republic (37%), Bangladesh (31%), Solomon Islands (25%), Bhutan (23%), Cambodia (23%), China (23%) and Tajikistan (19%) The IRS coverage of the high-risk population was more than 50% in Bhutan, Malaysia and Tajikistan, whereas that in India, Pakistan, the Philippines, Solomon Islands and Sudan was 20–40%. Regional trends in coverage with IRS are shown in **Figure 3.16**.

Table 3.8 Summary of intervention coverage, 2008, high-burden African countries

ITN COVERAGE		TREATMENT AND DIAGNOSTICS	
All ages		**Treatment**	
Operational ITN coverage with LLINs delivered by manufacturers	42	% fever cases in children < 5 years treated with any antimalarial, survey data	32
Operational ITN coverage with LLINs distributed, national programme data	35	% fever cases in children < 5 years treated with ACT, survey data	16*
		% ACT coverage in public sector (ACT distributed / reported malaria cases), administrative and disease surveillance data	48
Children < 5 years old		**Intermittent preventive treatment of pregnant women**	
Weighted average of ITN use by children < 5 years from surveys in 12 countries in 2008	24	% pregnant women receiving at least 2 doses during last pregnancy (previous 2 years), survey data	20**
Estimate of ITN use by children < 5 years old from model	24		
Household ownership		**Diagnostics**	
Weighted average of household ITN ownership from surveys in 13 countries in 2008	30	% reported malaria cases tested, disease surveillance data	22
Estimate of household ITN ownership from model (all countries)	31	% RDT delivered / reported malaria cases, administrative and disease surveillance data	13

* Data from only 7 countries representing 95 million persons.

** Data from only 9 countries in 2007-2008 representing 217 million persons.

Surveys showed that ITN ownership was low (< 20% of households) in Djibouti, Somalia and Sudan and also in Viet Nam (19%). In the Cambodia Malaria Survey 2007, 96% of households owned a net and 88% of children under 5 had slept under a net the previous night. However, most were untreated nets: only 36% of households owned an ITN and 28% of children slept under an ITN the previous night.

In most countries outside the African Region, access to first-line treatment was adequate to treat all reported confirmed malaria cases. All countries except some in the South-East Asia Region had distributed more than two treatment courses per confirmed case.

Table 3.9 shows the numbers of ITNs, ACT and RDTs distributed globally by national programmes in 2004–2008 by WHO region. The number of ITNs distributed in regions outside Africa increased steadily, from 5 million in 2005 to 22 million in 2008. The number of ACT treatment courses distributed increased to 10 million in 2008. The number of RDTs distributed has increased progressively, to 12 million in 2008.

Figure 3.16 Coverage with indoor residual spraying (IRS) of high-risk populations in WHO regions outside Africa, national programme data, 2001–2008

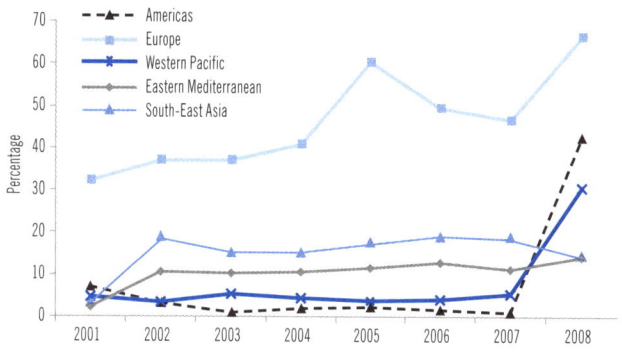

Table 3.9   Numbers of insecticide-treated nets (ITNs), artemisinin-based therapies (ACTs) and rapid diagnostic tests (RDT) reported by national programmes to have been distributed, by year, by WHO region

WHO REGION	2004	2005	2006	2007	2008
Number of ITNs					
Eastern Mediterranean	2 194 030	2 223 164	3 268 398	6 456 000	7 699 772
European	22 952	25 919	15 150	29 438	29 494
Americas	0	597 277	732 552	638 246	777 012
South-East Asia	1 939 995	3 578 065	7 127 021	7 803 354	10 587 135
Western Pacific	905 126	2 809 881	2 882 557	3 243 781	3 843 482
Outside African	5 062 103	9 234 306	14 025 678	18 170 819	22 936 895
African	14 720 440	25 869 098	52 451 596	40 098 395	45 316 731
Total	19 782 543	35 103 404	66 477 274	58 269 214	68 253 626
Number of ACT treatment courses					
Eastern Mediterranean	0	0	5 667 856	5 354 398	6 289 371
European	151	81	28	7	2
Americas	89 960	95 099	136 839	85 131	1 915 200
South-East Asia	4 528	78 900	604 241	959 118	1 308 199
Western Pacific	646 025	635 805	776 033	494 431	600 175
Outside African	740 664	809 885	7 184 997	6 893 085	10 112 947
African	1 213 541	12 245 271	53 666 521	83 196 974	62 637 244
Total	1 954 205	13 055 156	60 851 518	90 090 059	72 750 191
Number of RDTs					
Eastern Mediterranean			226 200	153 700	714 600
European	151	81	28	7	2
Americas					
South-East Asia		1 200 000	2 862 000	9 452 500	10 068 000
Western Pacific	32 150	318 000	368 425	683 300	1 556 168
Outside African	32 301	1 518 081	3 456 653	10 289 507	12 338 770
African	0	100 000	3 328 091	9 149 939	11 500 855
TOTAL	**32 301**	**1 618 081**	**6 784 744**	**19 439 446**	**23 839 625**

References

1. *Long-lasting insecticidal nets for malaria prevention: a manual for malaria programme managers.* Geneva, World Health Organization, Global Malaria Programme, 2007. http://www.who.int/malaria/whomalariapublications.htm#2007.

2. Flaxman A et al. (2009) Rapid scaling-up of insecticide-treated bed net coverage in Africa and its relationship with development assistance for health: a systematic synthesis of supply, distribution and household survey data. Submitted for publication, October 2009.

3. Ministry of Health, Togo, and Stephan Smith, United States Centers for Disease Control and Prevention, Malaria Branch. *Togo bednet durability—2008.* Presentation at annual meeting of the RBM Alliance for Malaria Prevention, January 2009.

4. *Report of the twelfth WHOPES working group meeting.* Geneva, World Health Organization, 2009 (WHO/HTM/NTD/WHOWHOPESPES/ 20/2009.09.11). http://whqlibdoc.who.int/hq/2009/WHO_HTM_NTD_WHOPES_2009_1_eng.pdf.

Chapter 4.
Impact of malaria control

This chapter summarizes the global burden of malaria and provides assessments of the evidence that malaria control activities have had an impact on malaria disease burden in each WHO Region.

4.1 Global estimates of malaria cases and deaths in 2008

The global numbers of malaria cases and deaths in 2008 were estimated by one of the two methods described in the *World Malaria Report 2008 (1)* (Annex 1). In brief, the numbers of malaria cases were estimated: *i)* by adjusting the number of malaria cases for completeness of reporting, the extent of health service use and the likelihood that cases are parasite-positive; when the data permit, this is generally the preferred method and was used for countries outside Africa and for selected African countries; or *ii)* from an empirical relation between measures of malaria transmission risk and case incidence; this procedure was used for countries in Africa where a convincing estimate could not be made from reports.

The numbers of malaria deaths were estimated: *i)* by multiplying the estimated number of *P. falciparum* malaria cases by a fixed case fatality rate for each country, for countries where malaria accounts for a relatively small proportion of all deaths and where reasonably robust estimates of case incidence could be made, primarily outside Africa; or *ii)* from an empirical relation between measures of malaria transmission risk and malaria-specific mortality rates, primarily for countries in Africa where estimates of case incidence could not be made from routine reports.

4.1.1 Cases

In 2008, there were an estimated 243 million cases of malaria (5th–95th centiles, 190–311 million) worldwide (**Table 4.1**). The vast majority of cases (85%) were in the African Region, followed by the South-East Asia (10%) and Eastern Mediterranean Regions (4%). The totals are similar to those reported in the *World Malaria Report 2008 (1)* (for the year 2006), except that the number of cases in the Region of the Americas is lower because of updated information from household surveys and other information on the number of cases detected by surveillance systems. The number of cases in the South-East Asia Region is higher, owing to updated household survey information for Bangladesh and Indonesia on where patients seek treatment for fever. The estimates also reflect progress in reducing the number of cases in several countries, but because most reductions have been seen in smaller countries, they do not yet have much influence on the regional and global totals. The estimates are accompanied by large uncertainty intervals, which overlap those of previous estimates.

4.1.2. Deaths

Malaria accounted for an estimated 863 000 deaths (5th–95th centiles, 708–1003 million) in 2008, of which 89% were in the African Region, followed by the Eastern Mediterranean (6%) and the South-East Asia Regions (5%). The estimated numbers of deaths are similar to those reported in the *World Malaria Report 2008 (1)* (for the year 2006), but the number of deaths in Africa is lower by 34 000, primarily because of a reduction in the total number of deaths from all causes among children under 5 years of age *(2)*. The number of malaria deaths is assumed to follow this trend, although evidence on trends in malaria-specific mortality is not available for most of the countries in which a reduction in under-5 mortality is documented.

Table 4.1 Estimated numbers of malaria cases (in millions) and deaths (in thousands) by WHO Region, 2008

WHO REGION	CASES				DEATHS			
	Point	Lower	Upper	P. falciparum (%)	Point	Lower	Upper	Under 5 (%)
AFR	208	155	276	98	767	621	902	88
AMR	1	1	1	32	1	1	2	30
EMR	9	7	11	75	52	32	73	77
EUR	0	0	0	4	0	0	0	3
SEAR	24	20	29	56	40	27	55	34
WPR	2	1	2	79	3	2	5	41
Total	**243**	**190**	**311**	**93**	**863**	**708**	**1003**	**85**

The number of deaths due to malaria is also higher in the Eastern Mediterranean Region, owing to increases in envelops for mortality from all causes in children under 5 in Somalia and Sudan *(2)*, although specific evidence of a rise in malaria mortality is lacking. The number of deaths in the South-East Asia region is higher owing to the increased estimate of the number of cases that was due to better information on where fever cases seek treatment; there is no specific evidence of an upward trend in the number of malaria deaths. The estimates are accompanied by large uncertainty intervals, which overlap those of previous estimates.

4.2   Assessing the impact of malaria interventions

4.2.1 Investigating trends in the incidence of malaria

The reported numbers of malaria cases and deaths are used as core indicators for tracking the progress of malaria control programmes. The main sources of information on these indicators are the disease surveillance systems operated by ministries of health. Data from such systems have two strengths. First, case reports are recorded continuously over time and can thus reflect changes in the implementation of interventions or climate conditions. Secondly, routine case and death reports are often available for all geographical units of a country. Changes in the numbers of cases and deaths reported by countries do not, however, necessarily reflect changes in the incidence of disease in the general population, because: *i)* not all health facilities report each month, and so variations in case numbers may reflect fluctuations in the number of health facilities reporting rather than a change in underlying disease incidence; *ii)* routine reporting systems often do not include patients attending private clinics or morbidity treated at home, so disease trends in health facilities may not reflect trends in the entire community; and *iii)* not all malaria cases reported are confirmed by slide examination or RDT, so that cases reported as malaria may be other febrile illnesses *(3)*. When reviewing data supplied by ministries of health in malaria-endemic countries, we attempted to minimize the influence of these sources of error and bias by pursuing the following strategy:

- Focusing on confirmed cases (by microscopy or RDT) to ensure that malaria and not other febrile illnesses are tracked. For high-burden countries in the WHO African Region, where little case confirmation is undertaken, the number of inpatient malaria cases is reviewed because the predictive value of an inpatient diagnosis is considered to be higher than outpatient diagnoses based only on clinical signs and symptoms; in such cases, the analysis may be heavily influenced by trends in severe malaria rather than trends in all cases.

- Monitoring the number of laboratory tests undertaken. It is useful to measure the annual blood examination rate, which is the number of laboratory tests undertaken per 100 people at risk per year, to ensure that potential differences in diagnostic effort or completeness of reporting are taken into account. The annual blood examination rate should ideally remain constant or be increased if attempting to discern decreases in malaria incidence.[1] When reviewing the number of malaria admissions and deaths, the health facility reporting rate should remain constant and should be high, i.e. > 80%.

- Monitoring trends in the malaria (slide or RDT) positivity rate. This rate should be less severely distorted by variations in the annual blood examination rate than trends in the number of confirmed cases. For high-burden African countries, when the number of malaria inpatients is being reviewed, it is also informative to examine the percentage of admissions or deaths due to malaria, as this proportion is less sensitive to variation in reporting rates than the number of malaria inpatients or deaths.

- Monitoring the number of cases detected in the surveillance system in relation to the total number of cases estimated to occur in a country.[2] Trends derived from countries with high case detection rates are more likely to reflect trends in the broader community. When examining trends in the number of deaths, it is informative to compare the total number of deaths occurring in health facilities with the total number of deaths estimated to occur in a country.

- Examining the consistency of trends. Unusual variation in the number of cases or deaths that cannot be explained by climate or other factors or inconsistency between trends in cases and in deaths can suggest deficiencies in reporting systems.

- Monitoring changes in the proportion of cases due to *P. falciparum* or the proportion of cases occurring in children < 5. While decreases in the incidence of *P. falciparum* malaria may precede decreases in *P. vivax* malaria, and there may be a gradual shift in the proportion of cases occurring in children < 5, unusual fluctuations in these proportions may point to changes in health facilities reporting or to errors in recording.

The aim of these procedures is to rule out data-related factors, such as incomplete reporting or changes in diagnostic practice, as explanations for a change in the incidence of disease and to ensure that trends in health facility data reflect changes in the wider community. The conclusion that trends inferred from health facility data reflect changes in the community has more weight if: *i)* the changes in disease incidence are large, *ii)* coverage with public health services is high and *iii)* interventions promoting change, such as use of ITNs, are delivered throughout the community and not restricted to health facilities.

---

1. Some authorities recommend that the annual blood examination rate should exceed 10% to ensure that all febrile cases are examined; however, the observed rate depends partly on how the population at risk is estimated, and trends may still be valid if the rate is < 10%. Some authorities have noted that 10% may not be sufficient to detect all febrile cases. It is noteworthy that the annual blood examination rate in the Solomon Islands, a highly endemic country, exceeds 60%, with a slide positivity rate of 25%, solely by passive case detection.

2. The *World Malaria Report 2008* described methods for estimating the total number of malaria cases in a country based on the number of reported cases and taking into account variations in health facility reporting rates, care-seeking behaviour for fever as recorded in household surveys and the extent to which suspected cases are examined in laboratory tests.

4.2.2 Assessing coverage with malaria interventions

Data on the number of ITNs distributed by malaria programmes and populations covered by IRS are supplied annually by ministries of health to WHO as part of reporting for the *World Malaria Report*. Such information may contain inaccuracies or gaps, particularly for earlier years. Hence, if data for earlier years are missing, it might be inferred incorrectly that preventive activities have recently been intensified. Nevertheless, for many countries, data from ministries of health are the only source of information on preventive activities and are consistent over the years. Data from nationally representative household surveys are available for selected countries, but these surveys are usually not undertaken frequently enough to allow assessment of trends in intervention coverage or to provide contemporary information. Information on access to treatment is less complete than data on ITNs and IRS, as few countries supply information on the number of courses of antimalarial medicines distributed in relation to the number of cases treated in the public sector. Information on preventive activities or treatment provided by the private sector is almost completely absent. It is therefore not always possible to obtain a complete picture of the extent of control activities in a country. Similarly, information on other factors that can affect malaria incidence is often not available, such as climate variations, deforestation or improved living conditions.

4.2.3 Establishing a link between malaria disease trends and control activities

In establishing a causal link between malaria disease trends and control activities, one should consider what the disease trends would have been without application of the control activities and then assess whether the decrease in malaria observed is greater than that expected without control activities. A robust view of what would have happened without control activities (i.e. counterfactual) cannot be established from the data currently available; however, it can be expected that, without a change in control activities, the malaria incidence might fluctuate in response to short-term climate variations but would otherwise show little change, as improved living conditions, environmental degradation or long-term climate change have only gradual effects (although there may be local exceptions). Thus, a plausible link with control efforts can be established if the disease incidence decreases at the same time as control activities increase, if the magnitude of the decrease in malaria incidence is consistent with the magnitude of the increase in control activities (a 50% decrease in the number of cases is unlikely to occur if malaria control activities cover only 10% of the population at risk) and if the decreases in malaria incidence cannot readily be explained by other factors.

Countries for which there is evidence from good-quality surveillance data of a large, sustained decrease (> 50% or 25%) in the number of cases since 2000 are presented below by WHO region. Information on the scale of malaria control interventions is also summarized, to identify countries with preventive programmes that cover > 50% of the population at high risk and countries that undertake extensive case detection and treatment. Countries in which there is evidence of both a sustained decrease in cases since 2000 and extensive control activities are highlighted as providing evidence of an impact of malaria control activities. Selected high-burden countries in the African Region are discussed individually. For other regions, the results of the analysis are shown in a standard set of graphs, as described in **Box 4.1**.[3]

BOX 4.1

Explanation of graphs

Population at risk: the population at high risk for malaria is that living in areas where the incidence is 1 or more per 1000 per year (defined at the second or lower administrative level). The population at low risk for malaria is that living in areas with fewer than 1 case of malaria per 1000 per year (see Methods in Annex 1).

Percentage of cases due to *P. falciparum*: percentage of confirmed cases in which *P. falciparum* or a mixed infection was detected

Annual blood examination rate: number of slide examinations undertaken each year in relation to the population at risk for malaria, expressed as a percentage.

Confirmed cases reported as a percentage of total estimated: total number of confirmed cases in relation to the estimated number of malaria cases in a country. The estimated number of cases is calculated by taking into account: *i)* the completeness of reporting from health facilities, *ii)* the extent to which people with fever use public health facilities for treatment and *iii)* the extent to which public health facilities undertake case confirmation (see technical notes). The line in the centre of the bar represents the point estimate of the percentage of estimated cases captured by the surveillance system. The width of the bars reflects uncertainty around the estimate of the number of cases.

Change in number of reported cases: the number of confirmed malaria cases is shown on the vertical axis, with each country indexed at 100 in 2000 (or a later year if data were not available for 2000); i.e. a value of 200 in 2005 indicates that the number of cases in 2005 was twice that reported in 2000 and represents a 100% increase. Countries with evidence of a decrease are generally those in which there has been a consistent decrease in the number of cases and consistency in reporting of malaria cases (e.g. stable annual blood examination rate). Countries for which there is little evidence of a decrease are those that do not show a decrease in the number of cases or where there have been irregular variations in surveillance data (e.g. annual blood examination rate falling, or unexplained variations in the percentage of cases due to *P. falciparum*).

IRS and ITNs delivered. The vertical scale shows the percentage of the population at risk for malaria potentially covered by preventive programmes with IRS and ITNs. It is assumed that each bed net delivered can cover two people, that conventional nets are retreated regularly and that each net is not replaced for 3 years. IRS is assumed to target a different population from that receiving bed nets. The percentage of the population potentially covered is therefore the maximum possible covered by the interventions delivered. The denominator is the population living at high risk for malaria, as the number of malaria cases in areas of low risk is small. The scale of preventive efforts in any year is calculated as: 100 x (number of ITNs delivered in past 3 years + number of people protected by IRS in current year)/population at high risk. Note that this indicator can exceed 100% if interventions are also applied to populations at low risk.

---

3. Countries in the prevention of re-introduction phase with only sporadic cases are excluded from the analysis.

4.3   African Region

4.3.1 *High burden countries*

This section updates the trends in morbidity and mortality from malaria presented in the *World Malaria Report 2008*. As the quality of the information received from most of the 35 high-burden countries in the WHO African Region was poor, trends could be analysed for only four of these countries, Eritrea, Rwanda, Sao Tome and Principe, Zambia and for the Zanzibar area of the United Republic of Tanzania. The four countries were among the ten with the highest rates of ITN ownership, as estimated in Chapter 3, the percentage of households owning at least one ITN exceeding 60% in 2008. A household survey undertaken in Zanzibar at the end of 2007 showed that 72% of households owned at least one ITN.

Eritrea. Eritrea had a population of 3.8 million in 2001 and reported a total of 126 000 malaria cases in that year. More than 1.1 million nets were distributed between 2001 and 2008 (an average of 139 000 per year), with LLIN distribution starting in 2005. In 2004, 73% of households in areas of high transmission owned an ITN and 59% of children 0–5 years slept under a net *(4)*. A malaria indicator survey in 2008 showed that 71% of households owned at least one ITN, and 39% of children < 5 years slept under an ITN (Eritrea Ministry of Health, unpublished data). Annual rounds of IRS protected approximately 238 000 people per year between 2001 and 2006. An average of 28 000 courses of ACT were distributed annually between 2006–2008, which was sufficient to treat all cases of *P. falciparum* malaria in outpatients.

The number of malaria outpatients fell by more than 90% between 2001 and 2008 (**Fig. 4.1**). The number of patients admitted to hospital for any reason increased by 44% between 2001 and 2008, but the number of malaria inpatients decreased by 68%. There were 86% fewer deaths from malaria among inpatients in 2008 than in 2001. A review of the evidence suggested that the observed decreases in the numbers of cases and deaths were due to malaria control interventions and not solely to environmental or other factors *(4)*.

Rwanda. Two sources of information on trends in the numbers of malaria cases and deaths were available from Rwanda: the results of a study by the Ministry of Health and WHO on the impact of malaria control in 2001–2008 on the basis of information from 19 health facilities in all 10 provinces and nationwide case records from surveillance activities in 2001–2007[4], as reported to WHO.

Approximately 765,000 ITNs (not LLINs) were distributed between 2001 and 2005 for a population of 8–9 million; 185,000 LLINs were added in 2005. During a nationwide campaign targeting children < 5 years in 2006, 1.96 million LLINs were distributed, and a further 1.16 million LLINs were distributed in 2007, increasing the percentage of the population potentially covered by nets to 70%. ACTs were distributed nationwide between September and October 2006, at the same time as the mass distribution of LLINs. A malaria indicator survey in 2007 showed that 50% of households owned an ITN and

56% of children < 5 slept under an ITN. A demographic and health survey conducted in 2007–2008 showed that 56% of households owned an ITN and 56% of children < 5 slept under a net.

The numbers of malaria cases and deaths appeared to decrease rapidly after the distribution of LLINs and ACT in 2006 (**Fig. 4.2**). In the 19 health facilities visited for the impact study in 2009, the annual number of confirmed malaria cases (all ages) in 2008 was 53% lower than the average for 2001–2005 (data not available by age group). The number of malaria inpatients was 52% lower, and the number of malaria deaths was 41% lower in 2008 than in 2001–2005 among children < 5 years old (target age group of the ITN campaign).

A similar trend is seen in an aggregation of surveillance data nationwide for 2001–2007. The annual number of confirmed malaria cases (all ages) in 2007 was 31% lower than in 2001–2005, the number of admissions for malaria was 43% lower, and the number of malaria deaths was 66% lower among children < 5 years old.[4] The slide positivity rate fell from an average of 52% between 2001 and 2005 to 22% in 2007. The annual blood examination rate increased from 8% in 2001 to 16% in 2007. Health facility reporting rates were high throughout the period, averaging 92%, the lowest value being obtained in 2006.

In summary, mass distribution of ITNs to children < 5 and to pregnant women, distribution of ACTs to public-sector facilities and increased rates of household ITN ownership and use by children exceeding 50% were associated with approximately 50% decreases in the numbers of confirmed outpatient cases, inpatient cases and deaths due to malaria over 24 months.

Sao Tome and Principe. The population of Sao Tome and Principe was 160 000 in 2008. IRS protected 140 000 people in 2005, 126 000 in 2006 and 117 000 in 2007. By 2007, nationwide ITN coverage was among the highest in Africa: 78% of households owned at least one ITN, and 54% of children < 5 years of age slept under an ITN. ACT was introduced for treatment of malaria in 2005, and the number of treatment courses distributed in 2005–2008 was enough to cover all reported cases.

The annual number of confirmed malaria cases in 2005–2008 was 84% lower than in 2000–2004, and the slide positivity rate fell from 47% between 2000 and 2004 to < 13% between 2005 and 2008 (**Fig. 4.3**). The number of admissions due to malaria was 87% lower in 2005–2008 than in 2000–2004, while the percentage of admissions for malaria fell from an average of 62% in 2000–2004 to 23% in 2005–2008. Similarly, the number of malaria inpatient deaths in 2005–2008 was 86% lower than in 2000–2004, and the percentage of deaths due to malaria in health facilities fell from 23% to 4%. The number of deaths from malaria among children < 5 fell by 89%, while the number of deaths from all causes among children < 5 decreased by 59%. By 2008, the numbers of inpatient malaria cases and deaths and outpatient malaria cases had decreased by > 90% in comparison with 2000–2004. All-cause inpatient deaths declined by 53%.

In Sao Tome and Principe, therefore, a strong association is seen between interventions and impact, albeit on a relatively small scale *(5)*.

---

4. As a new information system was introduced in 2008, it is difficult to compare data from the national health information system for 2008 with those for previous years.

Figure 4.1 Malaria inpatient cases and deaths by year, all ages, 2001–2008, Eritrea

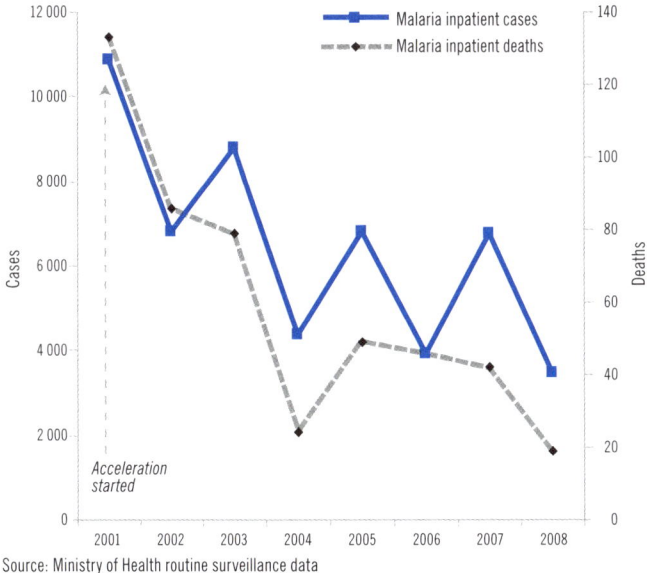

Source: Ministry of Health routine surveillance data

Figure 4.2 Malaria inpatient cases and deaths among children < 5 by year and outpatient all-cause and confirmed malaria cases in all ages, 19 health facilities, 2001–2008, Rwanda

a) *Malaria inpatient cases/deaths, children <5 years old*

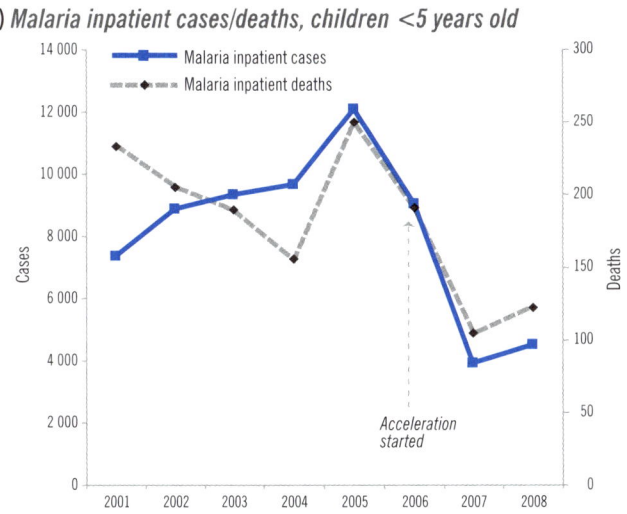

* Mass distribution of ITN to children < 5 years old and pregnant women and distribution of ACT to public health facilities

b) *Outpatients: all-cause cases and malaria test positivity rate, all ages*

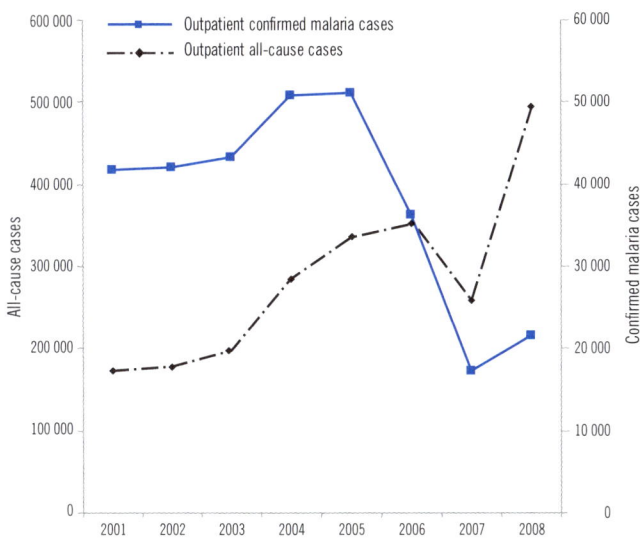

Figure 4.3 Malaria inpatient cases and deaths, all ages, by year, 2000–2008, Sao Tome and Principe

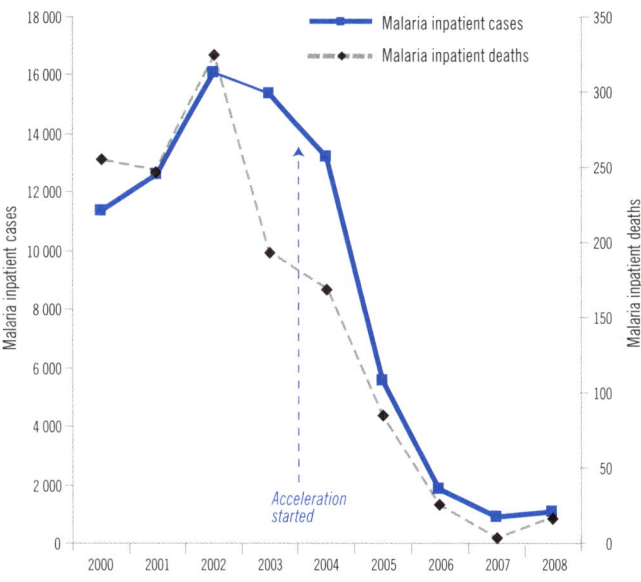

Source: Ministry of Health routine surveillance data

Figure 4.4 Malaria inpatient cases and deaths by year, all ages, first and second quarter each year, 2001–2008, Zambia

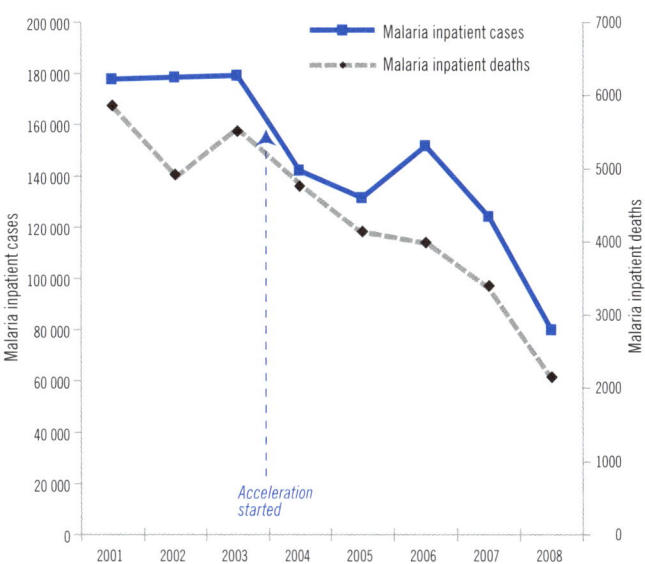

Source: Ministry of Health routine surveillance data

Zambia. Data on malaria trends in Zambia are more comprehensive than those for most countries, because: *i)* records from the health management information system were more or less complete between 2001 and the first half of 2008, and *ii)* two nationally representative household surveys that included testing for malaria parasites and anaemia were undertaken in 2006 and 2008.

Zambia had a population of 12.6 million in 2008. During 2002–2005, 1.26 million LLINs were distributed, enough to protect about 2.5 million people (assuming one net protects two people). An additional 4.8 million LLINs were distributed between 2006 and 2008 – enough to protect 9.6 million people, or 76% of the population. IRS covered an average of 0.9 million persons between 2003 and 2005, 2.4 million in 2006 (mostly in urban areas), 3.3 million in 2007 and 5.7 million in 2008. ACT was made available nationwide in 2004. The number of ACT treatment courses distributed increased from 1.2 million in 2004 to 3.1 million in 2008, coverage increasing from 29% of the malaria cases reported in public health facilities to 100%.

A nationally representative household survey in 2006 found that 44% of households owned an ITN, and 23% of children < 5 slept under an ITN. In 2008, these proportions had risen to 62% of households and 41% of children < 5. Approximately 47% of the population (mostly urban) were protected by IRS; 13% of children with fever in the previous 2 weeks had received ACTs, and 16% had received other antimalarial medicines.

A switch to a new health management information system during the third and fourth quarters of 2008 resulted in some incompleteness of reporting for those quarters. Therefore, data for the first two quarters of each year (the peak malaria season in most years) are presented. These surveillance data show that the numbers of malaria inpatients and deaths were 55% and 60% lower, respectively, in 2008 than the average for 2001–2002 for all ages (**Fig. 4.4**). The numbers of admissions and deaths from diseases other than malaria or anaemia decreased by 0% and 6%, respectively.

The scale of change observed in health facility data on inpatient cases is consistent with that from household surveys. The parasite prevalence among children < 5 decreased by 53% between 2006 and 2008 (from 21.8% to 10.2%), and the percentage of children with severe anaemia (< 8 g/dl haemoglobin) decreased by 68% (from 13.3% to 4.3%). The numbers of inpatient malaria cases and deaths among children < 5 decreased by 57% and 62%, respectively, while the number of admissions for anaemia decreased by 47%.

The magnitude of the decrease in numbers of inpatient deaths from all causes among children < 5 was similar to that of the decrease in mortality among children aged 1–59 months observed in the 2007 demographic and health survey (**Fig. 4.5**). A possible reason for the similarity between inpatient and population trends might be the geographically homogeneous ITN coverage: the 2008 malaria indicator survey showed that ITN coverage in Zambia was similar for the poorest (63%) and richest quintiles (65%) and in urban (59%) and rural areas (64%).

Zanzibar, United Republic of Tanzania. The islands of Zanzibar had a population of 1.2 million in 2008. ACT was made freely available in all public health facilities in September 2003. Approximately 245 000 LLINs were distributed in 2006, enough to cover 40% of the population, while a further 213 000 were distributed in 2007–2008. ITN household ownership was 72% and ITN use by children was 59%

Figure 4.5 Trends in 1–59-month child mortality rate
from a demographic and health survey (DHS) compared with inpatient all-cause and malaria deaths from routine health information system, 1999–2007, Zambia. Mortality rates in children 1–59 months in 2-year intervals from DHS data are shown in black squares (95% confidence interval shown as line)

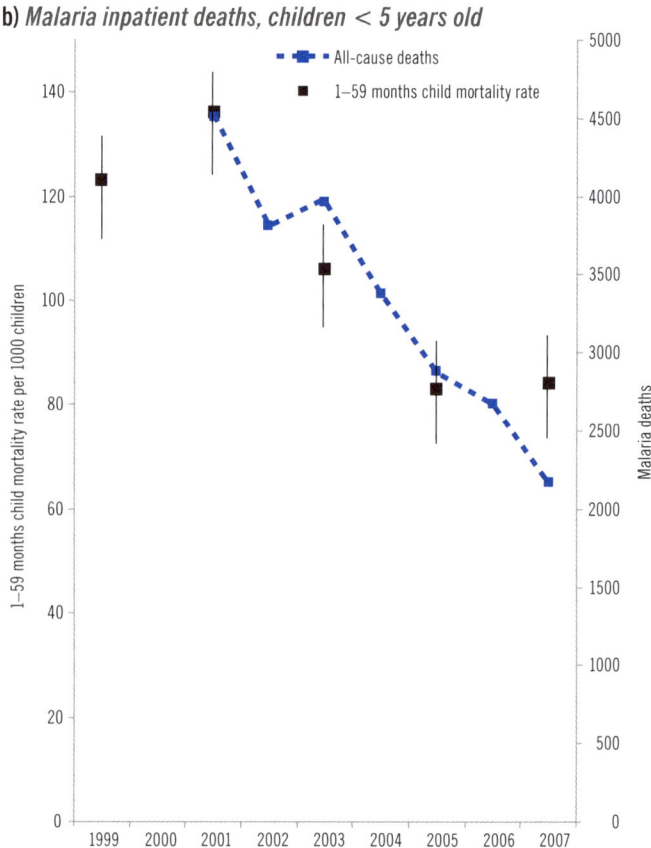

a) *All-cause inpatient deaths, children < 5 years old*

b) *Malaria inpatient deaths, children < 5 years old*

* Mortality rates from DHS data were calculated by Julie Rajaratnam, Linda N. Tran and Alison Levin-Rector at Institute for Health Metrics and Evaluation

Figure 4.6 Malaria inpatient cases and deaths, all ages, by year, 1999–2008, six of seven hospitals in Zanzibar, United Republic of Tanzania

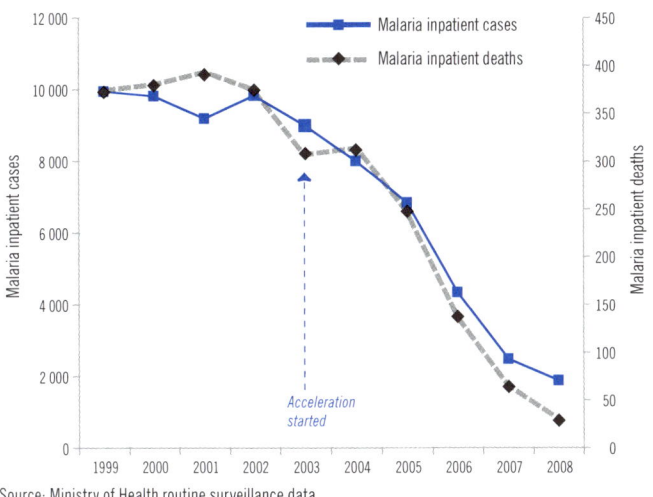

Source: Ministry of Health routine surveillance data

at the end of 2007. One round of IRS was carried out in 2006, followed by a further two rounds in 2007 and a single round in 2008. Each round covered nearly all households.

The numbers of inpatient cases and deaths from malaria decreased substantially between 2003 and 2008, and in 2006–2008, the numbers of malaria admissions and deaths were 70% lower than the numbers recorded in 2001 and 2002 (**Fig. 4.6**). By 2008, the numbers of inpatient malaria cases and deaths were lower by 80% and 92%, respectively. In contrast the number of admissions for conditions other than malaria was 20% higher.

Before acceleration of malaria control activities in 2005, 52% of cases and 53% of deaths among all inpatients were diagnosed as malaria. The number of inpatient deaths from all causes among children decreased by 57% and that of cases by 48% in 2008 as compared with 1999–2003, before acceleration. While the decrease in the number of admissions for malaria is dramatic and its timing is associated with high coverage with antimalarial interventions, it is uncertain how much of the decrease is due to improved diagnosis of cases, as fewer cases were diagnosed symptomatically and consequently fewer non-malarial fevers were classified as malaria. (A total of 650,000 RDTs were distributed by the Zanzibar malaria control programme between 2005 and 2006.) Other evidence for an impact of malaria interventions comes from a detailed investigation in one district, where, among children < 5, there were substantial reductions in *P. falciparum* prevalence, malaria-related admissions, blood transfusions, crude mortality and malaria-attributed mortality after introduction of ACTs in 2003 *(6)*.

4.3.2 Low-transmission countries in the African Region

In Botswana, Cape Verde, Namibia, South Africa, Swaziland and Zimbabwe, malaria is highly seasonal, and transmission is of much lower intensity than in the rest of sub-Saharan Africa. The vast majority of cases are due to *P. falciparum* (**Fig. 4.7b**). Five countries (Botswana, Cape Verde, Namibia, South Africa and Swaziland) demonstrated decreases > 50% in the numbers of confirmed cases and deaths due to malaria between 2000 and 2008 (**Fig. 4.7e**), although the decrease in cases appears to have levelled off, the numbers of cases remaining at 10–25% of those in 2000. The reasons are not yet clear, but the few cases remaining may be more difficult to prevent, detect and treat. Four of these countries (Botswana, Namibia, South Africa and Swaziland) also reported large decreases in the number of deaths due to malaria (**Table 4.2**) while Cape Verde reported only 2 deaths in 2008. In Zimbabwe, an increase in the number of confirmed malaria cases from 16 990 in 2004 to 92 900 in 2008 was associated with a sixfold increase in the number of slides examined; in contrast, the total of all reported malaria cases, which includes unconfirmed cases, decreased from 1.8 million in 2004 to 1 million in 2008. The increase in the number of slides examined is a positive development but makes it difficult to assess trends in the number of cases.

The scale of IRS has remained fairly constant over the past 8 years; South Africa and Swaziland protect 80% and 100% of their population at risk per year, while Botswana, Namibia and Zimbabwe protected 91%, 26% and 20% of those populations between 2000 and 2008, respectively. Namibia delivered 630 000 LLINs between 2006 and 2008, enough to cover 92% of the population at high risk (a ratio of one LLIN per two persons at risk); Swaziland reached about 47% of the population at risk by delivering about 85 000 LLINs during the same period; and the number of ITNs delivered in Botswana was negligible. South Africa adopted ACTs for first-line treatment of malaria in 2001, and their introduction, with improved mosquito control (including spraying with DDT), has been associated with a decrease in malaria cases. Botswana, Namibia and Swaziland adopted ACTs after 2005. Zimbabwe adopted a policy of treating *P. falciparum* cases with ACTs in 2008, but the programme has not yet reported deployment to public health facilities. The malaria programme in Cape Verde focuses on case detection and treatment.

In summary, five of the six low-transmission countries in the African Region (Botswana, Cape Verde, Namibia, South Africa and Swaziland) showed > 50% decreases in the numbers of malaria cases and deaths between 2000 and 2008. Each of these countries implemented widescale malaria programmes, but a drought affecting Namibia, South Africa, Swaziland and Zimbabwe between 2001 and 2003 might also have contributed to an initial decrease. It is not possible to determine whether the number of cases in Zimbabwe is increasing, stable or decreasing, but preventive activities appeared to cover > 50% of the population at high risk in 2008.

Table 4.2 Reported numbers of deaths due to malaria in southern African low-transmission countries

COUNTRY	2000	2001	2002	2003	2004	2005	2006	2007	2008
Botswana		29	23	18	19	11	40	6	12
Namibia		1728	1504	1106	1185	1325	571	181	171
Swaziland		62	46	30	25	17	27	14	5
South Africa	458	119	96	142	89	64	87		
Zimbabwe			1844	1044	1809	1916	802	285	

Figure 4.7   WHO African Region, low transmission countries

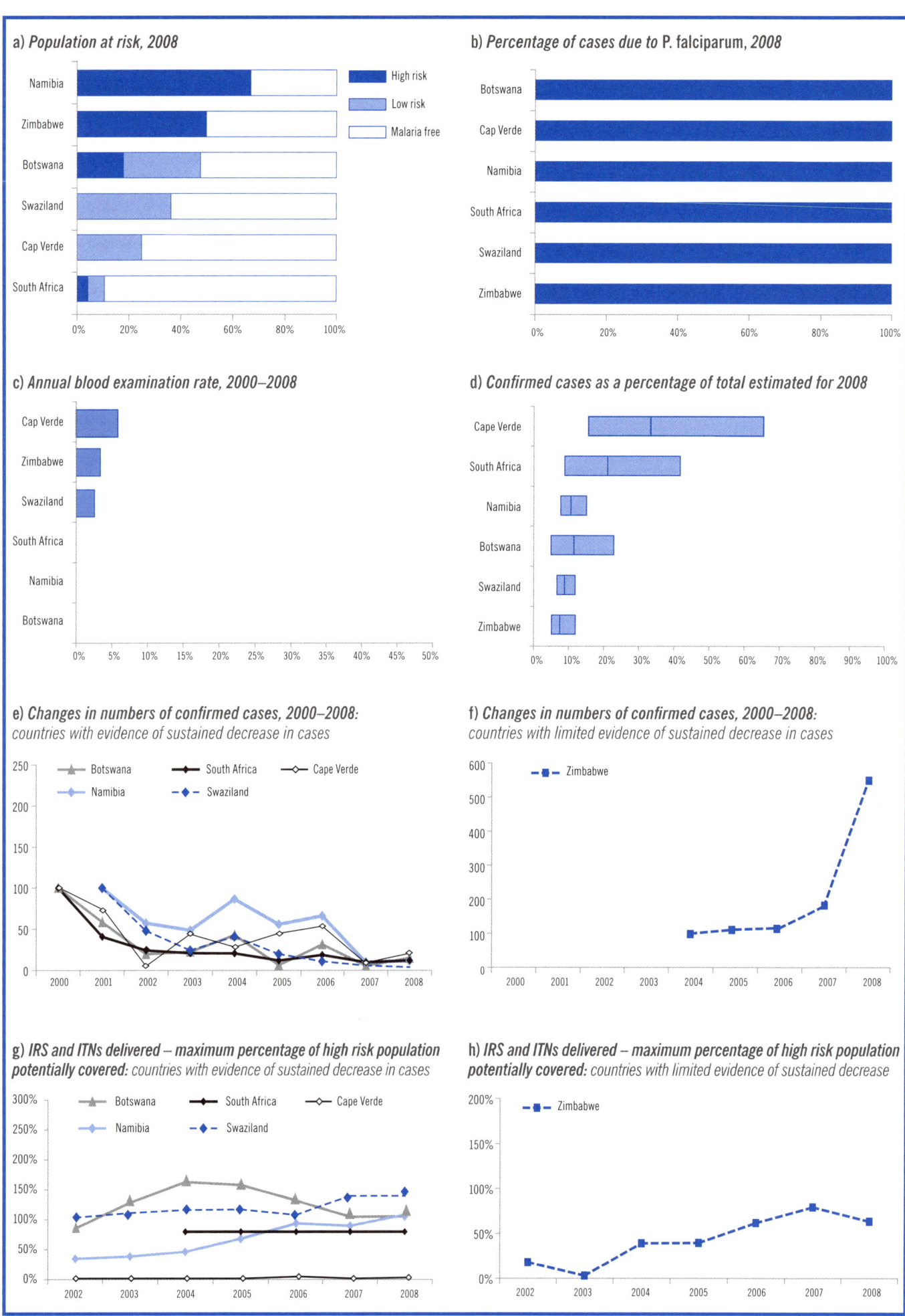

a) *Population at risk, 2008*

b) *Percentage of cases due to* P. falciparum, *2008*

c) *Annual blood examination rate, 2000–2008*

d) *Confirmed cases as a percentage of total estimated for 2008*

e) *Changes in numbers of confirmed cases, 2000–2008:* countries with evidence of sustained decrease in cases

f) *Changes in numbers of confirmed cases, 2000–2008:* countries with limited evidence of sustained decrease in cases

g) *IRS and ITNs delivered – maximum percentage of high risk population potentially covered:* countries with evidence of sustained decrease in cases

h) *IRS and ITNs delivered – maximum percentage of high risk population potentially covered:* countries with limited evidence of sustained decrease

Figure 4.8   WHO Region of the Americas by IRS in 2006

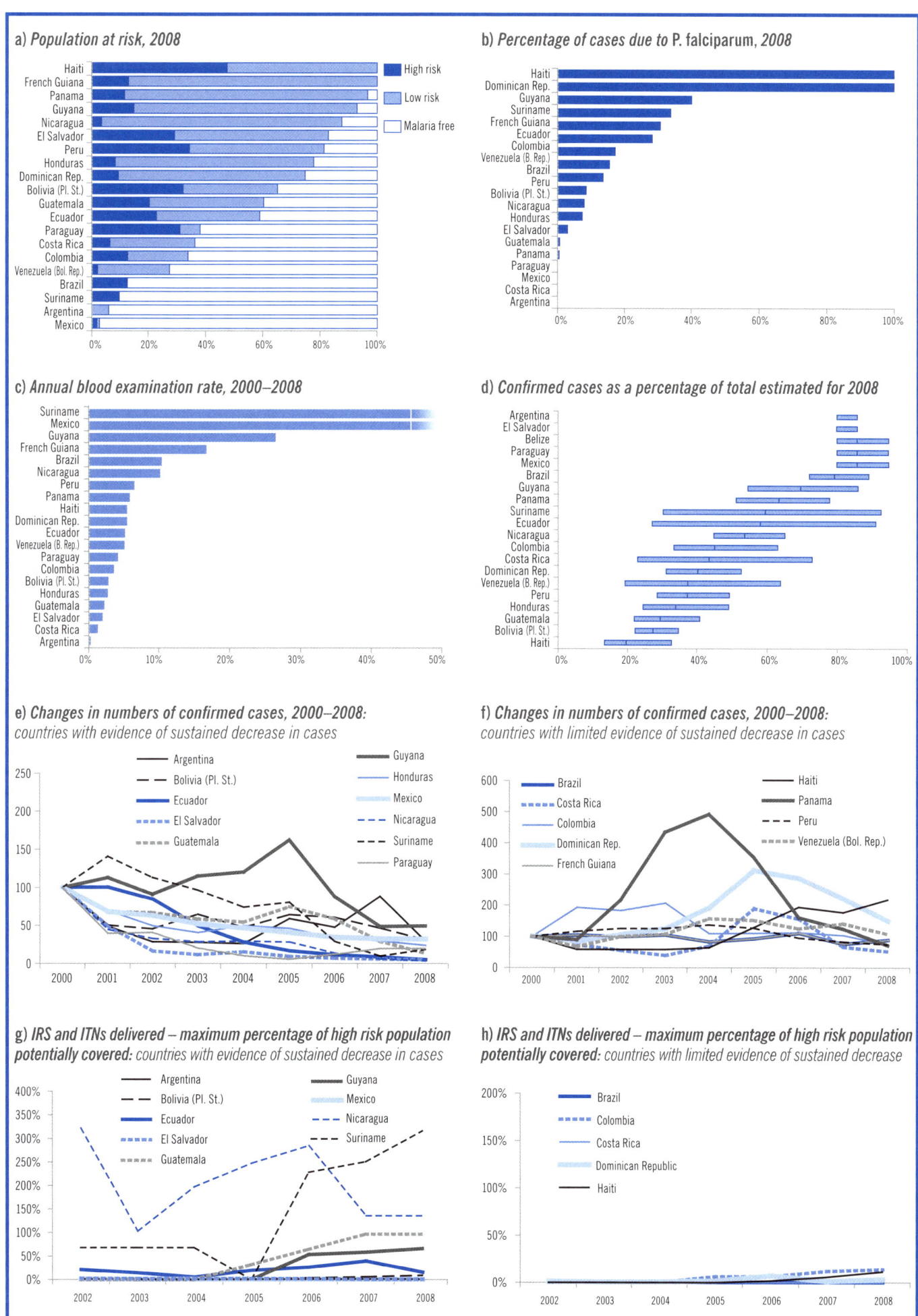

a) *Population at risk, 2008*

b) *Percentage of cases due to* P. falciparum, *2008*

c) *Annual blood examination rate, 2000–2008*

d) *Confirmed cases as a percentage of total estimated for 2008*

e) *Changes in numbers of confirmed cases, 2000–2008:* countries with evidence of sustained decrease in cases

f) *Changes in numbers of confirmed cases, 2000–2008:* countries with limited evidence of sustained decrease in cases

g) *IRS and ITNs delivered – maximum percentage of high risk population potentially covered:* countries with evidence of sustained decrease in cases

h) *IRS and ITNs delivered – maximum percentage of high risk population potentially covered:* countries with limited evidence of sustained decrease

Figure 4.9 WHO South-East Asia Region

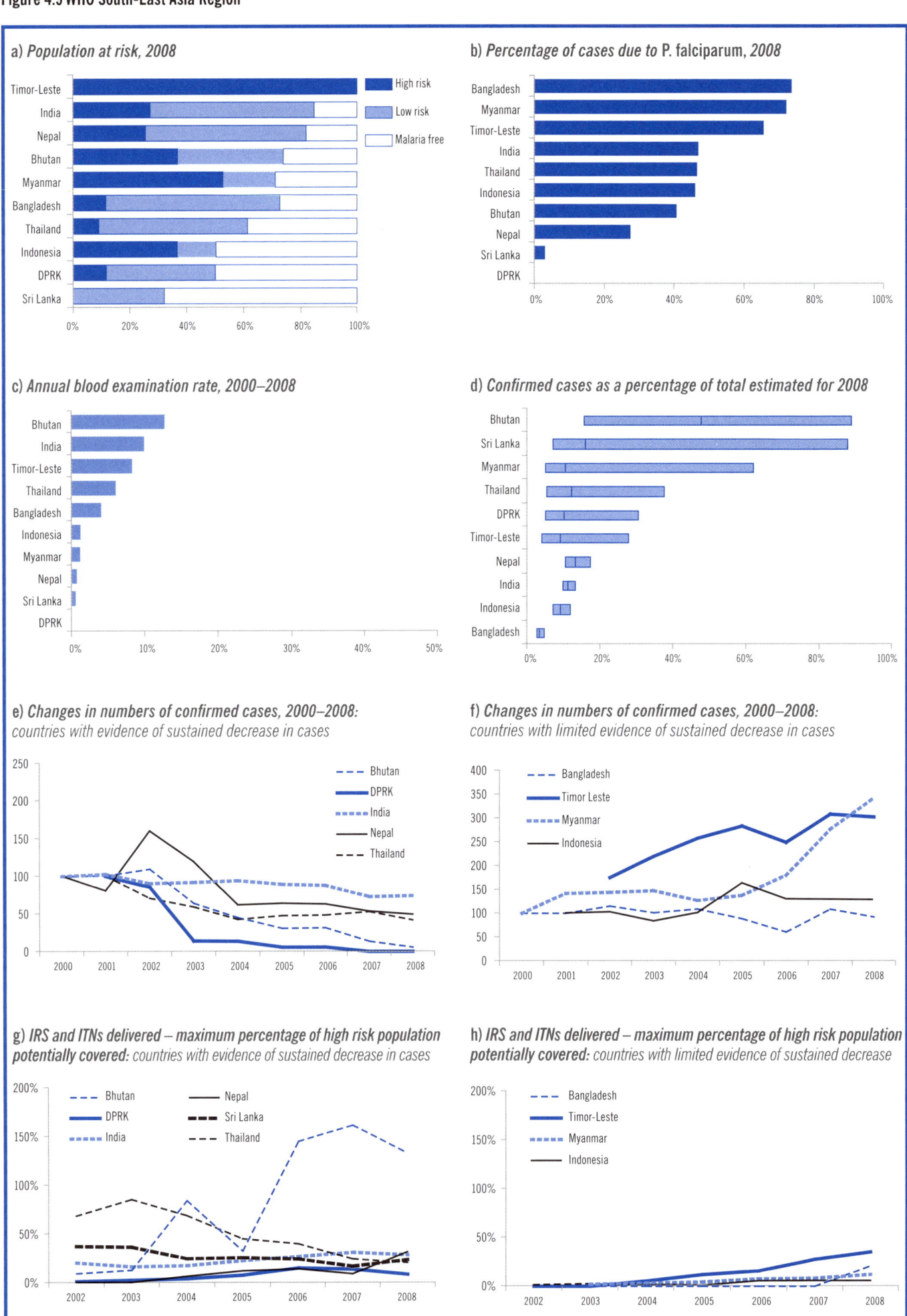

a) *Population at risk, 2008*

b) *Percentage of cases due to* P. falciparum, *2008*

c) *Annual blood examination rate, 2000–2008*

d) *Confirmed cases as a percentage of total estimated for 2008*

e) *Changes in numbers of confirmed cases, 2000–2008:* countries with evidence of sustained decrease in cases

f) *Changes in numbers of confirmed cases, 2000–2008:* countries with limited evidence of sustained decrease in cases

g) *IRS and ITNs delivered – maximum percentage of high risk population potentially covered:* countries with evidence of sustained decrease in cases

h) *IRS and ITNs delivered – maximum percentage of high risk population potentially covered:* countries with limited evidence of sustained decrease

Figure 4.10 WHO European Region

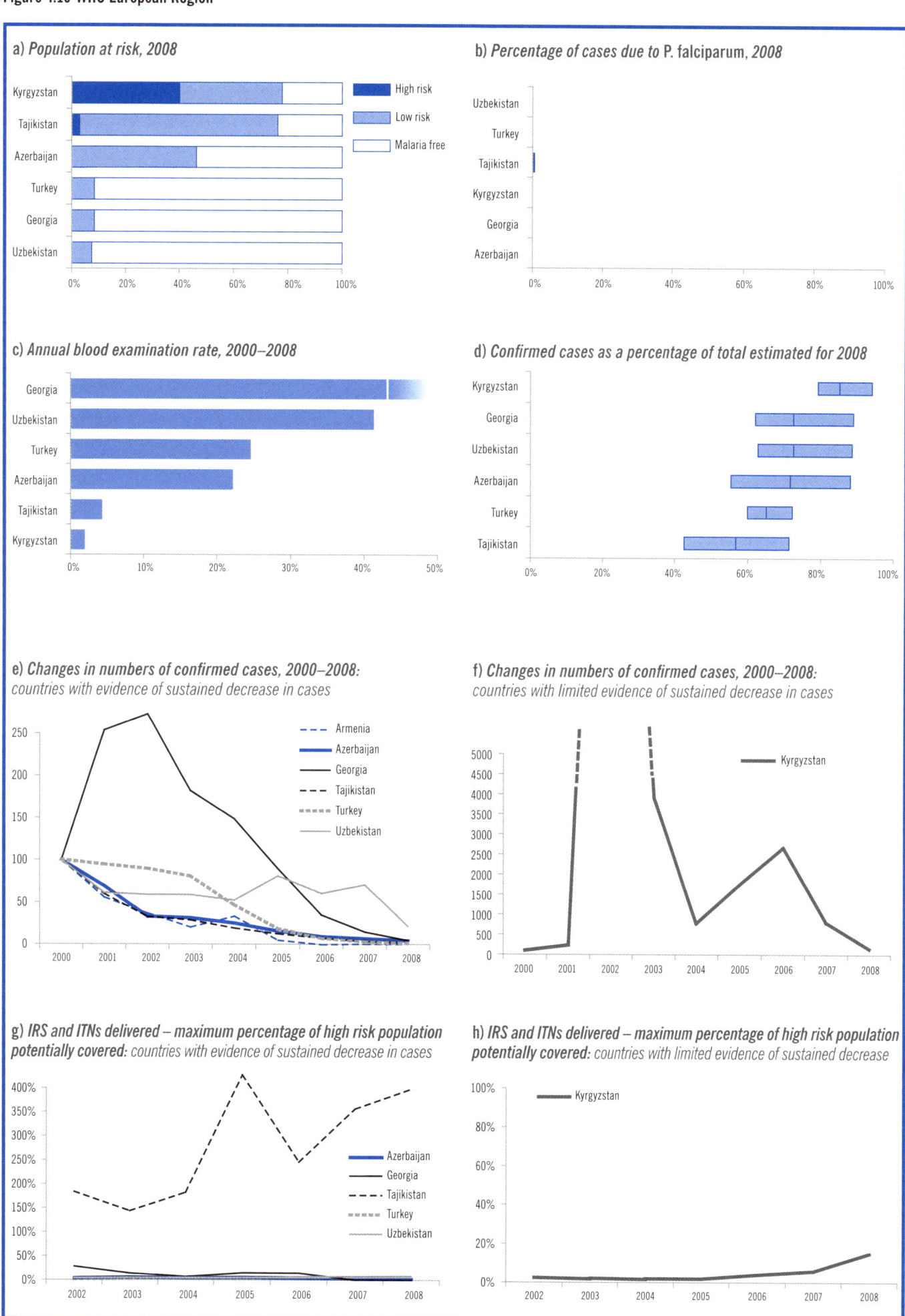

a) *Population at risk, 2008*

b) *Percentage of cases due to P. falciparum, 2008*

c) *Annual blood examination rate, 2000–2008*

d) *Confirmed cases as a percentage of total estimated for 2008*

e) *Changes in numbers of confirmed cases, 2000–2008:*
countries with evidence of sustained decrease in cases

f) *Changes in numbers of confirmed cases, 2000–2008:*
countries with limited evidence of sustained decrease in cases

g) *IRS and ITNs delivered – maximum percentage of high risk population*
potentially covered: countries with evidence of sustained decrease in cases

h) *IRS and ITNs delivered – maximum percentage of high risk population*
potentially covered: countries with limited evidence of sustained decrease

Figure 4.11 WHO Eastern Mediterranean Region

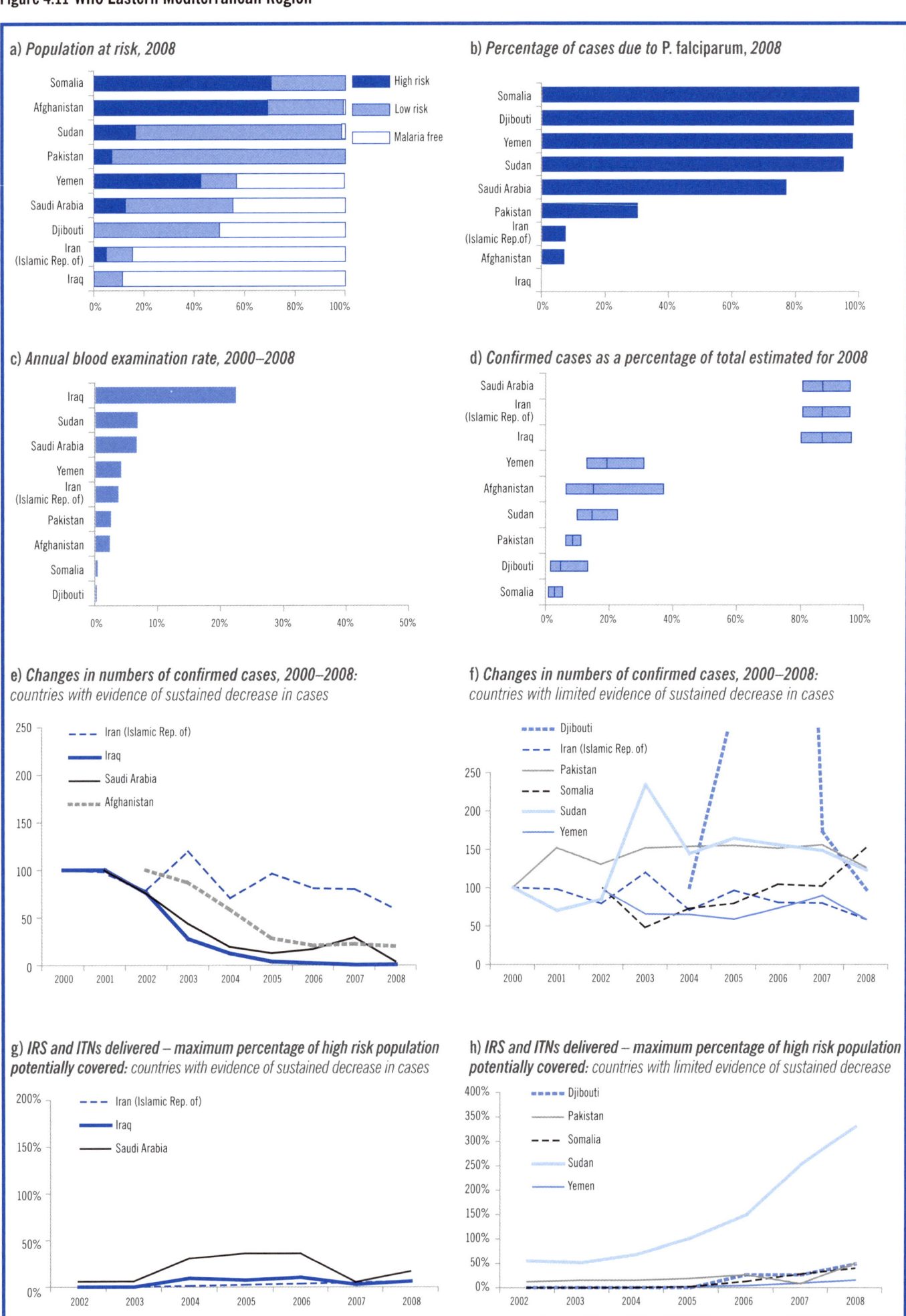

a) *Population at risk, 2008*

b) *Percentage of cases due to* P. falciparum, *2008*

c) *Annual blood examination rate, 2000–2008*

d) *Confirmed cases as a percentage of total estimated for 2008*

e) *Changes in numbers of confirmed cases, 2000–2008:*
countries with evidence of sustained decrease in cases

f) *Changes in numbers of confirmed cases, 2000–2008:*
countries with limited evidence of sustained decrease in cases

g) *IRS and ITNs delivered – maximum percentage of high risk population potentially covered:* countries with evidence of sustained decrease in cases

h) *IRS and ITNs delivered – maximum percentage of high risk population potentially covered:* countries with limited evidence of sustained decrease

Figure 4.12 WHO Western Pacific Region

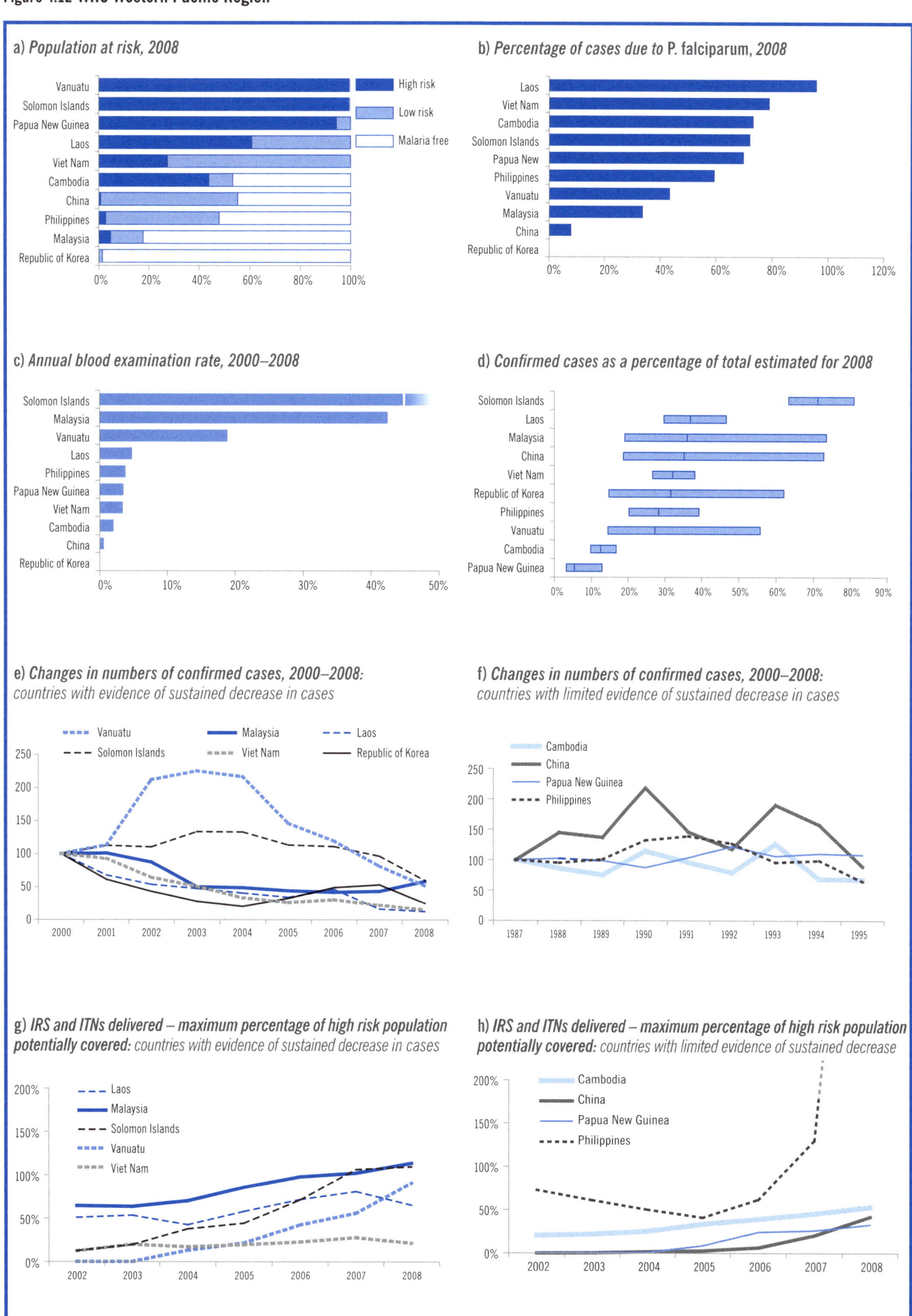

a) *Population at risk, 2008*

b) *Percentage of cases due to* P. falciparum, *2008*

c) *Annual blood examination rate, 2000–2008*

d) *Confirmed cases as a percentage of total estimated for 2008*

e) *Changes in numbers of confirmed cases, 2000–2008:* countries with evidence of sustained decrease in cases

f) *Changes in numbers of confirmed cases, 2000–2008:* countries with limited evidence of sustained decrease in cases

g) *IRS and ITNs delivered – maximum percentage of high risk population potentially covered:* countries with evidence of sustained decrease in cases

h) *IRS and ITNs delivered – maximum percentage of high risk population potentially covered:* countries with limited evidence of sustained decrease

4.4 Region of the Americas

Malaria transmission occurs in 21 countries of the Region, with almost 3 of every 10 persons at varying degrees of risk for malaria transmission. *P. vivax* accounted for 77% of all cases reported in 2008, but the percentage of cases due to *P. falciparum* was almost 100% in Haiti and the Dominican Republic (**Fig. 4.8b**). The number of cases reported in the Region decreased from 1.14 million in 2000 to 572 000 in 2008. Reductions of > 50% were reported in 12 countries (Argentina, Belize, Bolivia, Ecuador, El Salvador, Guatemala, Guyana, Honduras, Mexico, Nicaragua, Paraguay and Suriname) (**Fig. 4.8e**). Four of the countries (Argentina, El Salvador, Mexico and Paraguay) are in the elimination or pre-elimination phase, with active follow up of suspected cases. In five others (Belize, Guyana, Guatemala, Nicaragua and Suriname), control activities are implemented extensively among populations at risk for malaria; three of these countries (Guyana, Nicaragua and Suriname) also have high rates of annual blood examinations, which indicate good access to malaria treatment. Five countries (Brazil, Colombia, Costa Rica, Panama and Peru) reported fluctuations in the number of cases between 2000 and 2008, which may be associated with reductions in recent years. Brazil has greatly extended the availability of diagnosis and treatment through a network of more than 40 000 health workers, who reach individual households. The number of confirmed cases in French Guiana showed little change between 2000 and 2008. Three countries (Dominican Republic, Haiti and Bolivarian Republic of Venezuela) reported increased numbers of cases between 2000 and 2008, although the increase in Haiti is associated with an increased rate of annual blood examinations.

Thus, nine countries – Argentina, Belize, El Salvador, Guatemala, Guyana, Mexico, Nicaragua, Paraguay and Suriname – experienced a > 50% decrease in the number of cases, associated with intense malaria programme activity.

4.5 South-East Asia Region

Ten of the 11 countries of the region are malaria-endemic; there has been no indigenous transmission of malaria in the Maldives since 1984. Approximately 8 of 10 people in the region live at some risk for malaria, of whom 3 of 10 live at high risk (areas with a reported incidence of > 1 case per 1000 population per year). In 2008, 2.4 million laboratory-confirmed malaria cases and 2408 deaths were reported, whereas the estimates were about 24 million cases and 40 000 deaths, respectively. Four countries accounted for 97% of the estimated cases in the region in 2008 (Bangladesh, 10%; India, 55%; Indonesia, 15% and Myanmar, 17%). Most cases in the region are due to *P. falciparum*, although the proportion varies by country; transmission is due almost entirely to *P. falciparum* in Myanmar and Timor-Leste but due exclusively to *P. vivax* in the Democratic People's Republic of Korea (**Fig. 4.9b**). Reductions of more than 50% in the number of reported cases between 2000 and 2008 were seen in five countries (Bhutan, the Democratic People's Republic of Korea, Nepal, Sri Lanka and Thailand; **Fig. 4.9e**). Reductions of > 25% but < 50% were seen in one country (India). There was evidence of widescale implementation of antimalarial interventions in two countries that showed decreases in the number of cases (Bhutan and Thailand), although the decrease in Thailand levelled off in 2006 as the number of persons potentially reached by malaria prevention programmes decreased. Two countries in the pre-elimination stage actively follow up all suspected cases (Democratic People's Republic of Korea and Sri Lanka). The scale of preventive interventions appears to be small in India and Nepal, with less than 50% of the population at high risk covered. The remaining malaria-endemic countries reported no change or an increase in the number of cases (Bangladesh, Indonesia, Myanmar and Timor-Leste), and the scale of control activities appeared to be small in relation to the total population at risk.

In summary, four countries (Bhutan, the Democratic People's Republic of Korea, Sri Lanka and Thailand) experienced a decrease in the number of malaria cases, which was associated with malaria programme activity, although the decrease in Thailand appears to have levelled off between 2006 and 2008.

4.6 European Region

Locally acquired malaria cases were reported in 6 of the 53 Member States of the region in 2008: Azerbaijan, Georgia, Kyrgyzstan, Tajikistan, Turkey and Uzbekistan. Transmission of *P. falciparum* is confined to Tajikistan, with only two cases reported in 2008; in other countries, transmission is due exclusively to *P. vivax*, although imported cases of *P. falciparum* may occur. In all affected countries, malaria transmission is seasonal, occurring between June and October, and shows a marked focal distribution. The number of reported cases of malaria in the Region has been reduced substantially, from 32,474 in 2000 to 660 in 2008, only Kyrgyzstan failing to register a decrease of > 50% in the number of cases since 2000. In Kyrgyzstan, the number of cases rose from 12 in 2000 to 2744 in 2002, before falling to 18 in 2008 (**Fig. 4.10e,f**). Tajikistan and Turkey accounted for 80% of the reported cases in the Region in 2008.

Intensive control activities are implemented throughout the Region. IRS is the primary means of vector control in all countries and is applied with strict total coverage of all residual and new foci of malaria, with a view to interrupting transmission over the target area as soon as possible and preventing its re-establishment. The intensity of activity is not evident from **Figure 10g**, as the denominator used is the total population at risk rather than that living in active foci. ITNs are also used for protection, particularly in Tajikistan. The use of larvivorous *Gambusia* fish is promoted by almost all affected countries in rice-growing areas.

Blood slides are taken from clinically suspected malaria cases for active and passive case detection. All cases detected are treated, and information on their origins is obtained to facilitate epidemiological classification of malaria foci. Particular attention is given to situations in which there is a risk for spread of malaria between neighbouring countries and regions. In 2005, all nine malaria-affected countries in the region endorsed the Tashkent Declaration (7), the goal of which is to interrupt malaria transmission by 2015 and eliminate the disease within the region. Since 2008, national strategies on malaria have been revised to reflect the new elimination challenges.

In summary, all the malaria-endemic countries in the European Region have active malaria control programmes, and five of six countries reported sustained decreases of > 50% in the number of cases. Kyrgyzstan was the only country that did not show a sustained decrease in the number of cases since 2000, but only 18 cases were reported in 2008.

4.7   Eastern Mediterranean Region

The region contains six countries with areas of high malaria transmission (Afghanistan, Djibouti, Pakistan, Somalia, Sudan and Yemen), and three countries with low, geographically limited malaria transmission and effective malaria programmes (Islamic Republic of Iran, Iraq and Saudi Arabia). *P. falciparum* is the dominant species of parasite in Djibouti, Saudi Arabia, Sudan and Yemen, but the majority of cases in Afghanistan and Pakistan and almost all cases in the Islamic Republic of Iran and Iraq are due to *P. vivax* (**Fig. 4.11b**). The Eastern Mediterranean region reported 890 000 confirmed cases in 2008, from an estimated regional total of 8.6 million cases. Four countries accounted for 90% of the estimated cases: Afghanistan, 7%; Pakistan, 18%; Somalia, 10% and Sudan, 62%. Four countries reported downward trends in malaria frequency (Afghanistan, Islamic Republic of Iran, Iraq and Saudi Arabia), and in the last three there is evidence of intense control activities, these countries having been classified as in the elimination or pre-elimination stage (**Fig. 4.11e**). Other countries in the region have not registered consistent decreases in the number of cases (Djibouti, Pakistan, Somalia, Sudan and Yemen), although Sudan has extended the coverage of malaria preventive activities to more than 50% of the population at risk for malaria and any change in cases may be masked by changes in reporting practices.

In summary, three countries (Islamic Republic of Iran, Iraq and Saudi Arabia) showed evidence of a sustained decrease in the number of cases associated with widescale implementation of malaria control activities.

4.8   Western Pacific Region

The epidemiology of malaria in the Western Pacific Region is highly heterogeneous. Transmission is intense and widespread in the Pacific countries of Papua New Guinea, Solomon Islands and, to a lesser extent, Vanuatu; however, malaria is highly focal in the countries and areas of the Greater Mekong subregion, such as Cambodia, Yunnan (China), the Lao People's Democratic Republic and Viet Nam, occurring in remote forested areas and disproportionately affecting ethnic minorities and migrants. Malaria is also restricted to particular geographical locations in Malaysia, the Philippines and the Republic of Korea. Most countries have both *P. falciparum* and *P. vivax*, but transmission is entirely due to *P. vivax* in the Republic of Korea and central areas of China (**Fig. 4.12b**). Approximately 240 000 confirmed cases were reported from the Western Pacific Region in 2008, while 1.75 million cases were estimated for the region in 2008. Two countries accounted for 82% of the estimated cases in 2008 (Papua New Guinea, 68%; and Cambodia, 15%). Three countries reported decreases in the numbers of confirmed cases of > 50% between 2000 and 2008 (the Lao People's Democratic Republic,

the Republic of Korea and Viet Nam), and three countries reported decreases of 25–50% (Malaysia, Solomon Islands and Vanuatu) (**Fig. 4.12e**). In all six countries, there is evidence of widescale implementation of malaria control activities. No evidence for a sustained decrease in the number of cases was found in Cambodia, China, Papua New Guinea or the Philippines. Evidence of increased preventive or curative activities was seen in all these countries, particularly the Philippines, but this has either been too recent for effects to be apparent in the long term, or weaknesses in surveillance systems have meant that changes are not detected.

In summary, six countries in the Western Pacific Region showed evidence of a sustained decrease in the number of cases associated with widescale implementation of malaria control activities (Lao People's Democratic Republic, Malaysia, Republic of Korea, Solomon Islands, Vanuatu and Viet Nam).

4.9   Conclusions

4.9.1 WHO African Region

Reductions in the number of reported malaria cases and deaths of ≥ 50% have been observed in four high-burden countries of the WHO African Region (Eritrea, Rwanda, Sao Tome and Principe and Zambia) and one area (Zanzibar, United Republic of Tanzania). Reductions achieved in 2007 were maintained in 2008. Reductions of > 50% were also observed in five low transmission African countries (Botswana, Cape Verde, Namibia, South Africa and Swaziland). All the reductions were associated with intense malaria programme activity. The role of the climate and other factors in promoting change cannot be excluded; in particular, a drought in 2001–2003 may have contributed to an initial decrease in southern African countries. Nevertheless, decreases have been seen consistently for more than five years in seven countries or areas (Botswana, Eritrea, South Africa, Sao Tome and Principe, Swaziland, Zambia and Zanzibar, United Republic of Tanzania) and are unlikely to be due entirely to climate variation. In Rwanda, large decreases in the number of cases were observed soon after a rapid scale-up of malaria control activities, and these also are unlikely to be due to climate factors, although it would be valuable to test this hypothesis formally.

In Botswana, Cape Verde, Namibia, Sao Tome and Principe, South Africa and Swaziland, large initial decreases in the numbers of cases appear to have levelled off, the numbers of cases remaining at 10–25% of those seen in 2000. The reasons are not yet clear, but the few cases remaining may be more difficult to prevent, detect and treat, and it may be necessary to strengthen the programmes further.

When comparisons are possible, correspondence is seen between the trends in data from health facilities, household surveys and individual studies. The magnitude of the change seen in data from health facilities in the numbers of confirmed malaria cases, admissions for anaemia and overall numbers of childhood deaths is consistent with changes in parasite prevalence, prevalence of severe anaemia and mortality rates for children < 5 reported from household surveys. The magnitude of the decreases seen in the numbers of cases and deaths in health facilities is also consistent with the impact expected from controlled trials of the interventions. These observations suggest that surveillance data can be used to monitor the impact of interventions.

It is important, however, to ensure completeness of reporting and to choose indicators for monitoring trends that are highly specific for malaria (i.e. confirmed malaria cases or malaria admissions).

All 10 countries in the African Region that were reviewed had > 50% coverage with vector control activities. Some evidence of changes in the malaria burden in other countries with high coverage rates has been published, but the studies – in Equatorial Guinea (8), the Gambia (9) and Kenya (10) – were confined to limited geographical areas, and the generalizability of the results is uncertain. More studies are needed to measure the impact of high coverage in the countries identified in Chapter 3, particularly high-transmission areas in western and central Africa.

The main reason for the lack of additional evidence for a change in the malaria burden has been weak disease surveillance systems. Although many governments and partners have scaled-up malaria control interventions massively, their impact is not being measured consistently and continuously. The ability of malaria-endemic countries to monitor changes in the numbers of confirmed malaria cases, admissions for severe malaria and malaria-associated deaths must be strengthened. Inadequate monitoring can lead to poor adjustment of strategies, inefficient use of funds and inadequate "learning" for malaria programmes. Once malaria transmission has been reduced, national programmes must be able to detect malaria resurgence quickly and respond with appropriate resources. As experience suggests that malaria transmission decreases heterogeneously, robust surveillance systems are essential to identify residual transmission foci and target additional resources to those areas. Strengthening of surveillance systems will require investment in diagnostic services, reporting systems and capacity-building to manage systems and undertake appropriate data analysis and dissemination.

In countries where malaria control has been scaled-up, not only have the rates of malaria cases, hospitalizations and deaths dropped dramatically, but overall child mortality rates are also in steep decline. National disease surveillance data from Eritrea, Sao Tome and Principe, Rwanda, Zambia and Zanzibar, United Republic of Tanzania, showed a > 50% reduction in malaria cases and deaths in health facilities after the introduction of accelerated malaria control. In Sao Tome and Principe and Zanzibar, these gains were mirrored by a > 50% decrease in inpatient cases and deaths from all causes among children < 5 years of age. In Zambia, child mortality rates from all causes fell by 35%, as measured both by the number of deaths recorded in health facilities and by < 5 mortality rates derived from the Demographic and Health Survey of 2007. The magnitude of these decreases is similar to that found in a recent study on Bioko Island, Equatorial Guinea, in which population-based mortality among children < 5 had decreased by 66% in the fourth year after the start of intensive malaria control (8). If this finding is confirmed by additional studies, intensive malaria control can be considered an important intervention for helping African countries to reach the MDG target of reducing child mortality by 2015.

4.9.2 Other WHO Regions

A > 50% decrease in the reported number of cases of malaria was found between 2000 and 2008 in 29 of the 56 malaria-endemic countries outside Africa (**Table 4.3**), and downward trends of 25–50%

were seen in five other countries, most of which showed longer-term decreases of > 50%. The European Region has been the most successful, as almost all countries have reduced their case loads. Most small countries in the South-East Asia Region also reported substantial progress in reducing their malaria burden, while in other regions, large decreases in the number of malaria cases were observed in countries with strong political and financial support and well-developed health systems at central and peripheral levels.

Of the 34 countries that showed a decrease of > 25% in the number of cases, there was evidence of extensive control activities in 27 (in comparison with 4 of 22 for which there was limited evidence of a decrease). In 10 countries, the decrease in the number of cases was associated with an increase in preventive activities to > 50% of the population at high risk and strengthened case management (Guyana, Guatemala, Nicaragua and Suriname in the Region of the Americas; Bhutan and Thailand in the South-East Asia Region; and the Lao People's Democratic Republic, Malaysia, Solomon Islands and Vanuatu in the Western Pacific Region). In 15 countries, the decrease was associated mainly with intensive case detection and treatment, combined with rapid response to outbreaks (Argentina, El Salvador, Mexico and Paraguay in the Region of the Americas; Azerbaijan, Georgia, Tajikistan, Turkey and Uzbekistan in the European Region; the Islamic Republic of Iran, Iraq and Saudi Arabia in the Eastern Mediterranean Region; the Democratic People's Republic of Korea and Sri Lanka in the South-East Asia Region; and the Republic of Korea in the Western Pacific Region).

The magnitude and consistency of the changes observed in these countries are unlikely to be due to variations in case reporting, and, while factors such as climate variation, the environment or improved living conditions may have had some influence on the number of cases, they are unlikely to be entirely responsible for the change. It was not possible to link the scale and timing of interventions precisely with the changes in disease incidence in the analyses undertaken here; that would require disaggregation of the information on numbers of cases and control activities by month and subnationally. Until more detailed analyses can be undertaken, the association between implementation of control activities and changes in disease incidence is suggestive but not conclusive.

The size of the decrease observed in health facility data may not be seen in the wider community; however, with changes as large as those observed and with typically ≥ 40% of affected persons attending public health facilities, some impact can be expected in the wider community. The analytical approach used might result in an underestimate of the impact of control efforts in countries in which the effect is not noticeable at national level or in which the impact is more recent and cannot yet be distinguished from changes due to year-to-year climate variations or possible changes in reporting practices.

The countries that saw > 50% decreases in the numbers of cases comprised only 4% of the total estimated cases outside Africa in 2006 (850 000 cases out of 34 million estimated). The countries with the highest malaria burdens in each region (such as Bangladesh, Brazil, Cambodia, Colombia, Indonesia, Myanmar, Pakistan, Papua New Guinea and Sudan) were less successful in reducing the numbers of cases of malaria nationally. The scale of interventions in relation to populations at risk appears to be particularly small in the South-East Asia Region, presumably because of the additional challenges of implementing programmes on a larger scale, requiring not only considerable financial resources but also time to build systems for, e.g. the distribution of commodities (ITNs, insecticide, diagnostic tools, medicines and equipment), training staff, mobilizing communities, quality control and supervision. Nevertheless, some of these countries have reported successful control in some parts of their territory, due either to targeted efforts in some communities or to phasing implementation over a wide scale. Further work is needed to determine if current levels of investment and programme implementation are likely to yield more positive results in the near future. Current evidence suggests, however, that, while smaller countries are making considerable progress towards reaching the MDGs and other malaria targets, more attention should be given to ensuring success in the countries that account for most malaria cases and deaths.

Table. 4.3   Summary of progress in reducing the number of malaria cases between 2000 and 2008

Decrease in cases > 50%	Decrease in cases > 25%	Limited evidence of decrease
African Region		
Botswana		Angola
Cape Verde		Benin
Eritrea		Burkina Faso
Namibia		Burundi
Rwanda		Cameroon
Sao Tome and Principe		Central African Republic
South Africa		Chad
Swaziland		Comoros
Zambia		Congo
		Côte d'Ivoire
		DR Congo
		Equatorial Guinea *
		Ethiopia**
		Gabon
		Gambia *
		Ghana
		Guinea
		Guinea-Bissau
		Kenya *
		Liberia
		Madagascar***
		Malawi
		Mali
		Mauritania
		Mozambique
		Niger
		Nigeria
		Senegal
		Sierra Leone
		Togo
		Uganda
		UR Tanzania*
		Zimbabwe

Decrease in cases > 50%	Decrease in cases > 25%	Limited evidence of decrease
Region of the Americas		
Argentina		**Brazil**
Belize		Colombia
Bolivia (Plurinational State of)		Costa Rica
Ecuador		Dominican Republic
El Salvador		French Guiana
Guatemala		Haiti
Guyana		Panama
Honduras		Peru
Mexico		Venezuela (Bolivarian Rep. of)
Nicaragua		
Paraguay		
Suriname		
South-East Asia Region		
Bhutan	India	Bangladesh
DPRK		Indonesia
Nepal		Myanmar
Sri Lanka		Timor-Leste
Thailand		
European Region		
Armenia		**Kyrgyzstan**
Azerbaijan		
Georgia		
Tajikistan		
Turkey		
Uzbekistan		
Eastern Mediterranean Region		
Afghanistan	**Islamic Rep. of Iran**	Pakistan*
Iraq		Somalia
Saudi Arabia		**Sudan***
		Yemen*
Western Pacific Region		
Lao People's Dem. Rep.	**Malaysia**	Cambodia
Rep. of Korea	**Solomon Islands**	China
Viet Nam	**Vanuatu**	Papua New Guinea
		Phillipines*

The assessment of whether a country has evidence of decreases in cases or widespread coverage of programmes was made according to the data available to WHO at the time of publication of this Report. It is possible that additional evidence of decreases in cases or widespread coverage of programmes is available at country level.

Countries in bold show evidence of wide scale implementation of malaria control activities to more than 50% of the population at high risk.

* The country reports some progress sub-nationally where interventions have been intensified.

** A ministry of health/WHO study, 2001–2007 previously reported a 50% decrease in cases and deaths, but national data as reported to WHO in 2008 are inconsistent; further investigation is required.

*** Data submitted in 2008 were different from data published in the *World Malaria Report 2008*. Therefore observed decreases of more than 50% in cases and deaths need further investigation.

References

1. *World malaria report 2008*. Geneva, World Health Organization, 2008 (WHO/HTM/GMP/2008.1).

2. Provisional WHO estimates of child mortality to be published in *World health statistics 2008*.

3. Cibulskis RE et al. Estimating trends in the burden of malaria. *American Journal of Tropical Medicine and Hygiene,* 2007, 77 (suppl. 6):133–137.

4. Graves PM et al. Effectiveness of malaria control during changing climate conditions in Eritrea, 1998–2003. *Tropical Medicine and International Health,* 2008, 13:218–228.

5. Teklehaimanot HD et al. Malaria in São Tomé and Principe: on the brink of elimination after three years of effective antimalarial measures. *American Journal of Tropical Medicine and Hygiene,* 2009, 80:133–140.

6. Bhattarai A et al. Impact of artemisinin-based combination therapy and insecticide-treated nets on malaria burden in Zanzibar. *PLoS Medicine,* 2007, 6:e309.

7. *The Tashkent Declaration: the move from malaria control to elimination in the European Region*. Copenhagen, World Health Organization Regional Office for Europe, 2005. www.who.euro.int/document/e89355.pdf

8. Kleinschmidt I et al. Steep increase in child survival after four years of integrated malaria control in Bioko Island, Equatorial Guinea. *American Journal of Tropical Medicine and Hygiene,* 2008, 79 (Abstract 790):54.

9. Ceesay SJ et al. Changes in malaria indices between 1999 and 2007 in The Gambia: a retrospective analysis. Lancet, 2008, 372:1545–1554.

10. O'Meara WP et al. Effect of a fall in malaria transmission on morbidity and mortality in Kilifi, Kenya. *Lancet,* 2008, 372:1555–1562.

Chapter 5.
Elimination of malaria

This chapter describes the state of malaria elimination in the world, to illustrate progress towards the elimination targets. It provides a summary of the progress being made in countries that have embarked on eliminating malaria, including their progression through the different phases from pre-elimination to certification of elimination by WHO. The chapter also provides a brief background to the WHO strategies and guidelines, as well as a historical perspective of malaria elimination in these countries.

5.1   Background

From a country perspective, interruption of local mosquito-borne malaria transmission or elimination of malaria is the ultimate goal of malaria control. Malaria elimination has been achieved progressively in parts of the world since the recorded history of the disease. By the mid-19th century, malaria had been eliminated from several countries in temperate zones in which it had been endemic. In the context of the Global Malaria Eradication Programme (1955–1968) and up to 1987, 24 countries were certified as malaria-free. Since then, an additional 9 countries have reported (periods of) zero locally acquired cases, leading to a further contraction of the world map of malaria endemicity (1). Using the momentum created by the global efforts against malaria of the past decade, some countries in the subtropical and even the tropical belt have reduced their malaria incidence to the extent that they are considering moving towards malaria elimination. The repertoire of antimalarial tools and interventions available today is sufficient to eliminate malaria from countries where transmission is low and unstable, provided health systems have nationwide coverage and are capable of implementing rigorous and responsive surveillance. Supported by the advocacy efforts of the Malaria Elimination Group (2), there is now renewed interest in pushing the boundaries of malaria-free areas of the world even further.

The elimination of malaria from selected countries is stated explicitly in the targets of the Global Malaria Action Plan (3), as follows:

- By 2015, at least 8–10 countries currently in the elimination stage will have achieved zero incidence of locally transmitted infection.

- Beyond 2015, countries currently in the pre-elimination stage will move to elimination.

Current elimination efforts are driven by the ministries of health of malaria-endemic countries. They receive technical support from WHO and its partners, and some are supported by financial awards by the Global Fund, but most funds come from national governments.

Considerable progress has been made in malaria elimination during the past few years. Consistent with the goals of the Global Malaria Action Plan, as of 2009, three countries that were in the elimination phase, Armenia, Egypt and Turkmenistan, have reported no locally acquired cases for more than 3 years, and have moved to the phase of prevention of reintroduction. Six countries (Azerbaijan, Georgia, Kyrgyzstan, Tajikistan, Turkey and Uzbekistan, all in the WHO European Region), had moved from the pre-elimination stage to a nationwide elimination approach by 2009 (**Fig. 5.1**). The types of malaria programmes currently implemented worldwide are shown in **Figure 5.2**.

Figure 5.1   Movement of countries between types of programme between 2008 and 2009

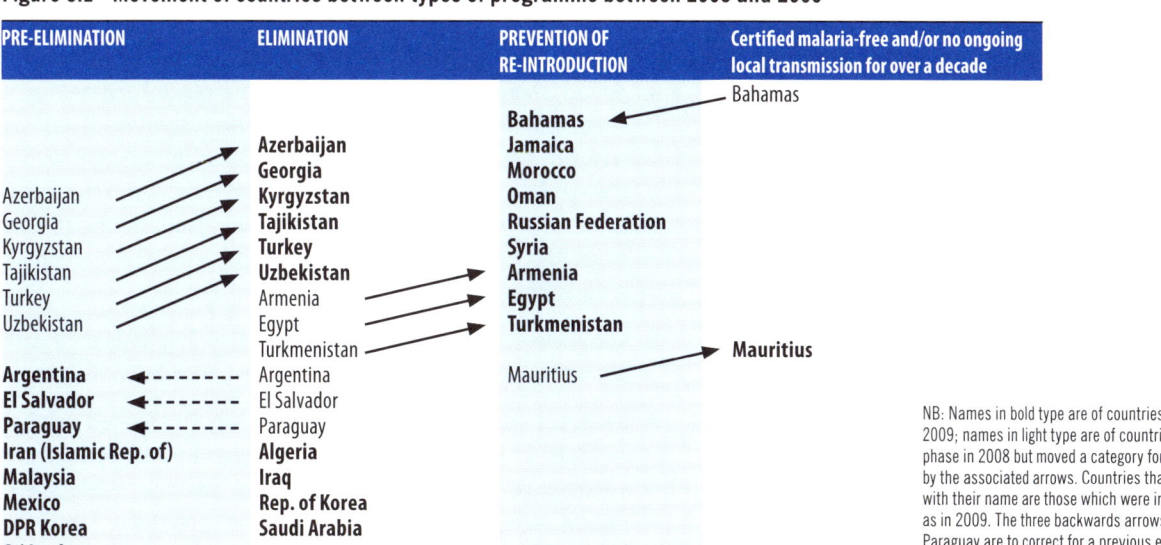

NB: Names in bold type are of countries in the programme phase as of 2009; names in light type are of countries that were in the programme phase in 2008 but moved a category forward or backward as indicated by the associated arrows. Countries that have no arrows associated with their name are those which were in the same category in 2008 as in 2009. The three backwards arrows for Argentina, El Salvador and Paraguay are to correct for a previous error in classification and do not reflect a deterioration of the programme status of these countries.

Figure 5.2   Malaria-free countries and malaria-endemic countries in phases of control*, pre-elimination, elimination and prevention of reintroduction, end 2008

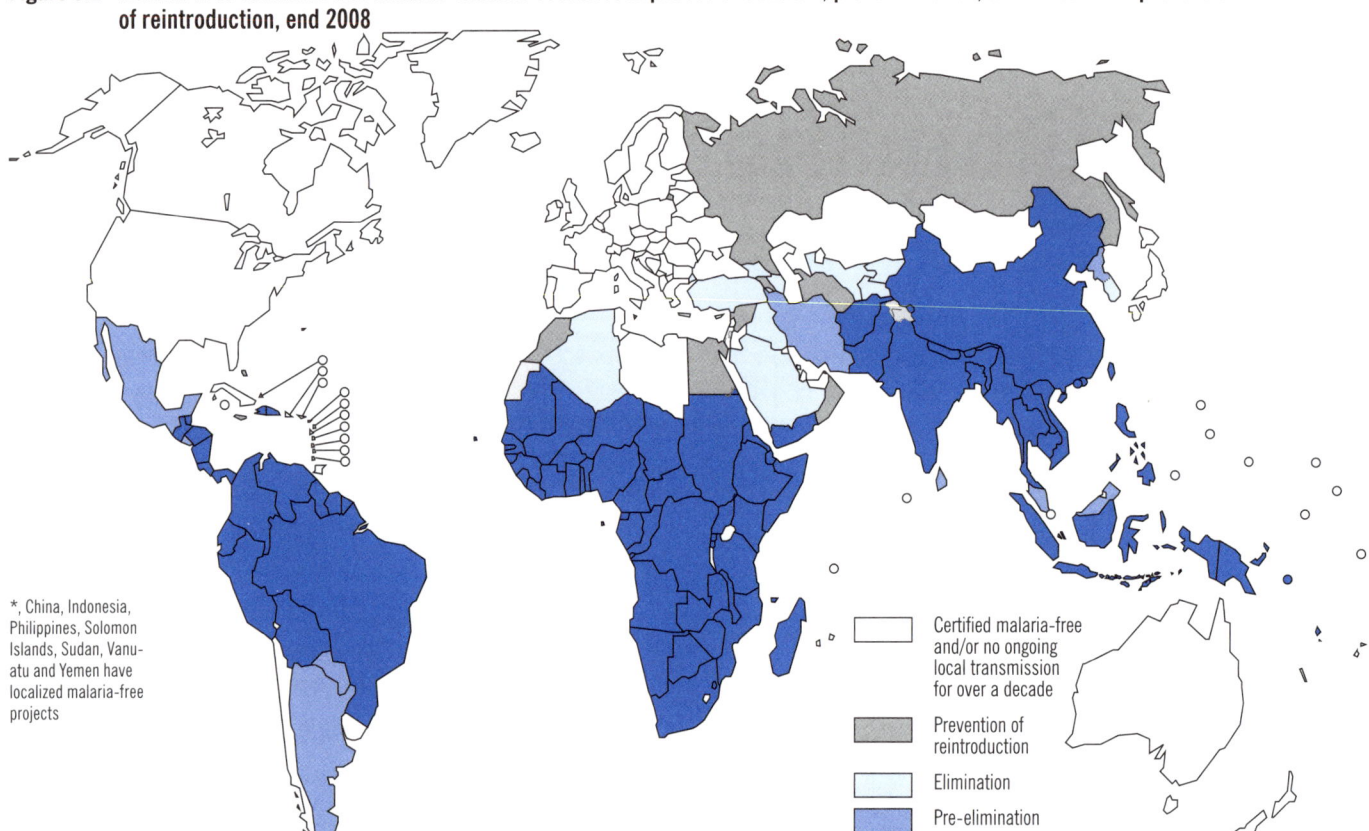

*, China, Indonesia, Philippines, Solomon Islands, Sudan, Vanuatu and Yemen have localized malaria-free projects

- ☐ Certified malaria-free and/or no ongoing local transmission for over a decade
- ■ Prevention of reintroduction
- ■ Elimination
- ■ Pre-elimination
- ■ Control

5.2   Definitions

Malaria control: reducing the malaria disease burden to a level at which it is no longer a public health problem.

Malaria elimination: the interruption of local mosquito-borne malaria transmission; reduction to zero of the incidence of infection caused by human malaria parasites in a defined geographical area as a result of deliberate efforts; continued measures to prevent re-establishment of transmission are required.

Certification of malaria elimination: can be granted by WHO after it has been proven beyond reasonable doubt that the chain of local human malaria transmission by *Anopheles* mosquitoes has been fully interrupted in an entire country for at least 3 consecutive years.

Malaria eradication: permanent reduction to zero of the worldwide incidence of infection caused by a specific agent; applies to a particular malaria parasite species. Intervention measures are no longer needed once eradication has been achieved.

5.3   WHO position on malaria elimination *(4)*

1. With rapid scale-up and sustained efforts, major reductions in malaria morbidity and mortality can be made in all epidemiological situations within a relatively short time. Malaria transmission can be interrupted in low-transmission settings and greatly reduced in many areas of high transmission. Global eradication cannot, however, be expected with existing tools.

2. Failure to sustain malaria control and the resulting resurgence of malaria, as has happened in the past, must be avoided at all costs. Therefore, public and government interest in intensified malaria control and elimination must be sustained, even when the malaria burden has been greatly reduced.

3. Countries in areas of low, unstable transmission should be encouraged to proceed to malaria elimination. Before making this decision, however, they should assess its feasibility and take into account the malaria situation in neighbouring countries. Malaria elimination might require cross-border initiatives and regional support and will require strong political commitment.

4. In areas of high, stable transmission, where a marked reduction in malaria transmission has been achieved, a "consolidation period" should be introduced, in which: *i)* control achievements are sustained, even in the face of limited disease; *ii)* health services adapt to the new clinical and epidemiological situation with a lower case load and reduced levels of immunity; and *iii)* surveillance systems are strengthened to allow rapid response to new cases. This transformation phase precedes a decision to reorient programmes towards elimination.

5. Complete interruption of malaria transmission is likely to require additional, novel tools, especially in high-transmission situations.

6. Because malaria control today relies heavily on a limited number of tools, in particular artemisinin derivatives and pyrethroids, which could be lost to resistance at any time, the development of new tools for vector control and other preventive measures, diagnosis, treatment and surveillance must be a priority.

5.4 Strategies

5.4.1 Progression from malaria control to elimination and certification

Countries may envisage elimination of malaria when the malaria control programme has succeeded in reducing morbidity to a marginal level (e.g. not more than five of every 100 episodes of febrile illness are due to malaria during the high-transmission season). The steps for eliminating malaria from a country or area that has reduced its malaria transmission intensity to low levels are shown in **Figure 5.3**. Not all countries will be able to interrupt malaria transmission with the currently available tools.

"Pre-elimination" consists of the period of reorientation of malaria control programmes between the sustained control and elimination stages, when coverage with good-quality laboratory and clinical services, reporting and surveillance are reinforced, followed by other programme adjustments to halt transmission nationwide.

Elimination programmes are characterized by four programme approaches, supported by large investments of local expertise and resources:

- management of all malaria cases: detection, notification, investigation, classification and supervised treatment;
- prevention of onward transmission from existing cases;
- prevention and early detection of imported malaria infections;
- management of malaria foci: identification, investigation, classification, effective vector control in all foci of transmission, geographical mapping over time.

In elimination programmes, the main indicator is the total number of locally acquired infections.

WHO's classification of countries is based on the type of malaria programme being implemented in the worst-affected endemic areas of the country.

5.4.2 Programme profiles in different phases of elimination

As country programmes are redirected towards an elimination approach, the changing programme goal affects the objectives of the interventions and the geographical units in which interventions are made. This change in profile by programme type is summarized in **Table 5.1**, which also lists the "milestones" at which programme transition may become feasible. These milestones should be adjusted for each country and situation, keeping in mind the resource requirements for notification, investigation and follow-up of every malaria case once the elimination programme is set in motion. The actual programme transitions will thus depend on the workload that programme staff can realistically handle, given local circumstances and infrastructure, the available resources and competing demands on the health services. Countries that are currently implementing elimination programmes made the decision to pursue elimination when they had a low remaining case load, usually < 1000 cases per year nationwide.

5.4.3 Type of intervention in each phase of elimination

The type of intervention and the required quality of operations evolve as country programmes are redirected towards an elimination approach, as shown in **Table 5.2** (5).

Figure 5.3   Programme phases from malaria control to elimination

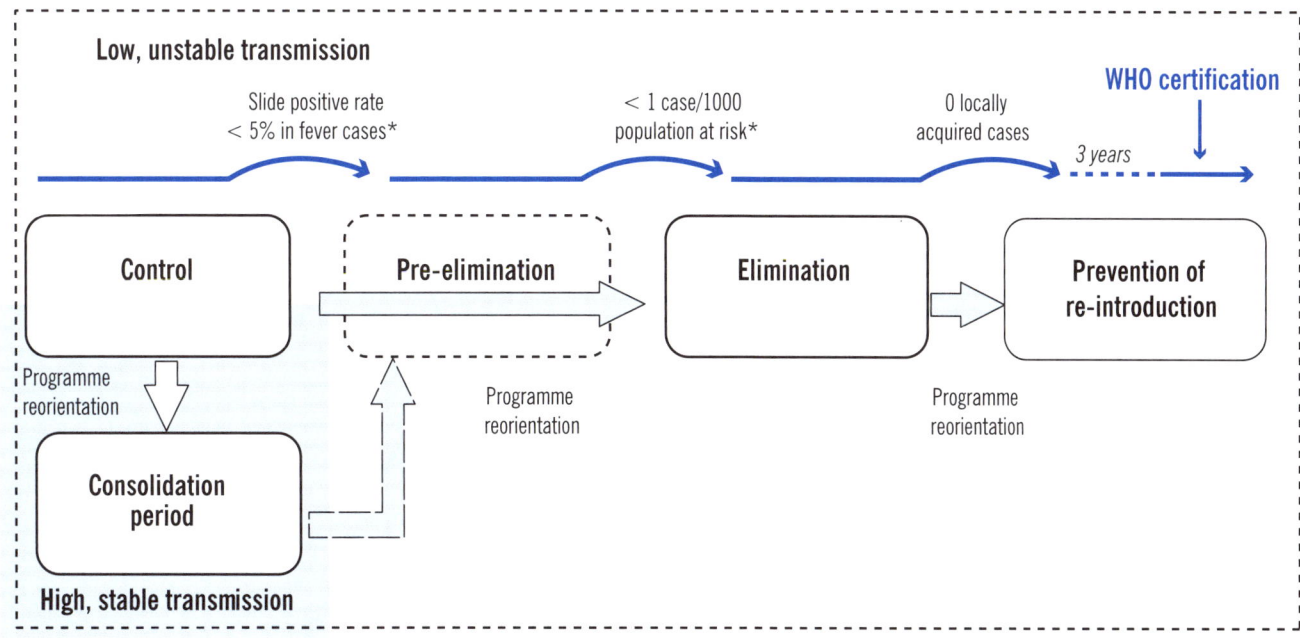

Source: reference (1)
* These milestones are indicative only: in practice, the transitions will depend on the malaria burden that a programme can realistically handle (including case notification and case investigation).

5.5   Progress towards malaria elimination

The parasite species, programme phase, starting year of elimination efforts and last reported cases in countries in pre-elimination, elimination and prevention of reintroduction phases as of 2009 are shown in **Table 5.3**.

5.5.1 Countries that have interrupted transmission and are in the stage of preventing reintroduction of malaria

By 2009, nine countries had interrupted malaria transmission and were implementing intensive programmes to prevent its reintroduction:

- Six countries recently achieved zero cases and aim to maintain this situation: Armenia, Egypt, Morocco, Oman, the Syrian Arab Republic and Turkmenistan.

- Three countries that are generally considered nonendemic, having been malaria-free for well over a decade, experienced outbreaks of locally acquired malaria subsequent to importation of parasites: *P. falciparum* in the Bahamas and Jamaica (certified malaria-free in 1966) and *P. vivax* in the Russian Federation. No deaths were reported in these outbreaks.

The numbers of reported malaria cases in these countries over the past 10 years are shown in **Figure 5.4**.

Table 5.1 Profile by programme type

ITEM	CONTROL PROGRAMME	Pre-elimination programme	Elimination programme	Prevention of reintroduction programme
Main programme goal	Reduce morbidity and mortality	Halt local transmission nationwide	Halt local transmission nationwide	Prevent re-establishment of local transmission
Epidemiological objective	Reduce burden of malaria	Reduce number of active foci to zero	Reduce number of active foci to zero	Prevent introduced cases and indigenous cases secondary to introduced cases
		Reduce number of locally acquired cases to zero	Reduce number of locally acquired cases to zero	
Transmission objective	Reduce transmission intensity	Reduce onward transmission from existing cases	Reduce onward transmission from existing cases	Reduce onward transmission from imported cases
Unit of intervention	Country- or area-wide	Transmission foci	Transmission foci, individual cases (locally acquired and imported)	Recent transmission foci (receptive areas), individual cases (imported cases only)
Indicative milestones for transition to next programme type[a]	SPR <5% in suspected malaria cases	< 1 case per 1000 population at risk per year	Zero locally acquired cases	
Data sources for measuring progress towards reaching milestones	Proxy data: health facility data Confirmatory data: population-based surveys	Proxy data: health facility data, notification reports Confirmatory data: population-based surveys	Notification reports, individual case investigations, genotyping	

Source: reference *(5)*; SPR: slide or rapid diagnostic test positivity rate.

[a]. In practice, the transitions will depend on the malaria burden that a programme can realistically handle, given the local circumstances and available resources and keeping in mind the need to assure notification, investigation and due follow up of all malaria cases.

Figure 5.4 Confirmed locally acquired malaria cases in countries that have interrupted transmission and are preventing the reintroduction of malaria, 1998–2008

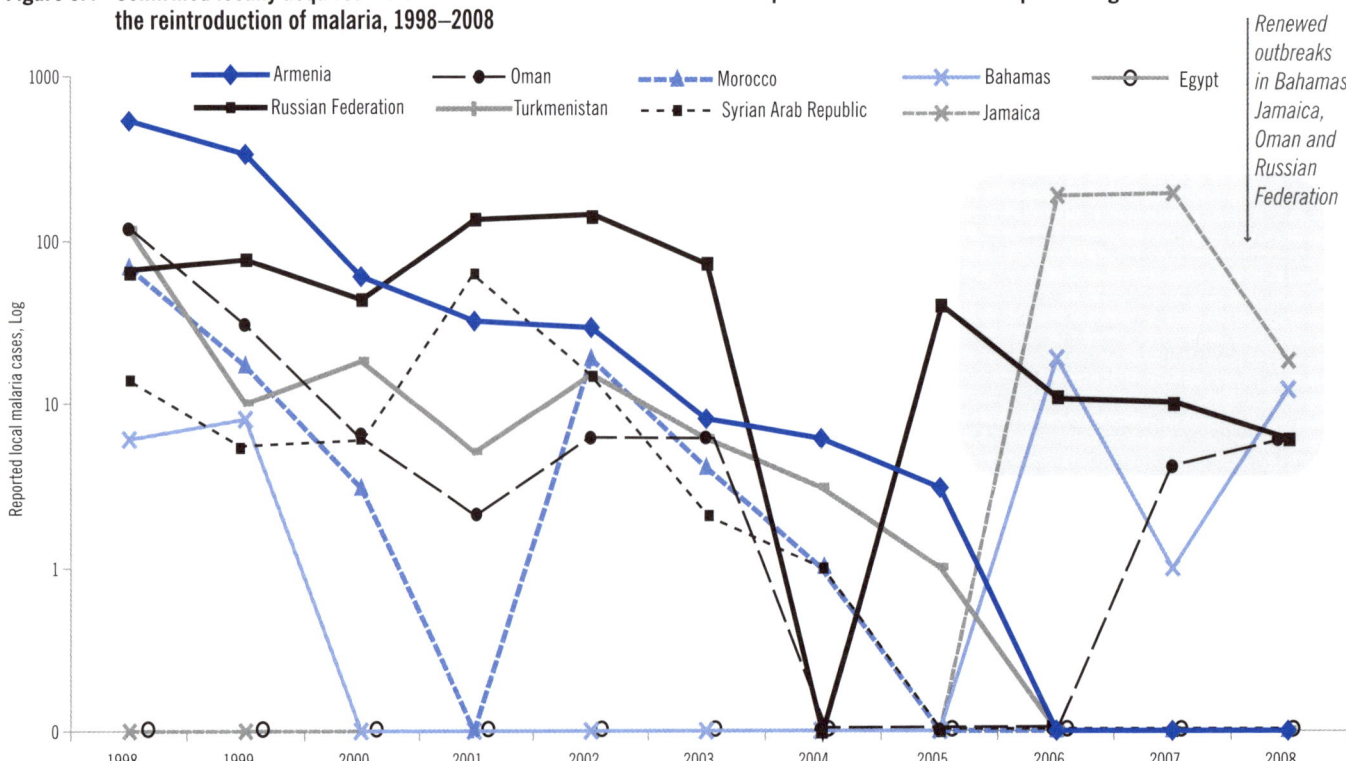

Table 5.2 Interventions by programme type

INTERVENTION	Control programme	Pre-elimination programme[a]	Elimination programme	Prevention of reintroduction programme
Case management	Update drug policy, use of ACT QA/QC of laboratory diagnosis (microscopy/RDT) Clinical diagnosis sometimes acceptable Monitoring antimalarial drug resistance	Drug policy change to: − radical treatment for *P. vivax* − ACT and gametocyte treatment for *P. falciparum* 100% case confirmation by microscopy Microscopy QA/QC Monitoring antimalarial drug resistance	Implementation of new drug policy Routine QA/QC expert microscopy Active case detection Monitoring antimalarial drug resistance	Case management of imported malaria Awareness of drug resistance patterns abroad, to formulate prevention guidelines
Vector control and malaria prevention	Transmission reduction through high population coverage of ITN/LLIN and IRS Entomological surveillance Epidemic preparedness and response IPTp in hyperendemic areas	Geographical reconnaissance Total IRS coverage in foci Integrated vector management and ITN/LLIN as complementary measures in specific situations Epidemic preparedness and response Entomological surveillance	Geographical reconnaissance IRS to reduce transmission in residual active and new active foci Vector control to reduce receptivity in recent foci Outbreak preparedness and response Entomological surveillance Prevention of malaria in travellers	Perfect malaria case detection mechanism Cluster response and prevention Prevention of malaria in travellers, including health education and engagement of travel agencies
Monitoring and evaluation	Improve surveillance and national coverage Country profiles Malaria population surveys (MIS, MICS, DHS)	GIS-based database on cases and vectors Elimination database Central records bank Genotyping, isolate bank Malaria surveys Immediate notification of cases	Case investigation and classification Foci investigation and classification Routine genotyping Malaria surveys Immediate notification of cases Meteorological monitoring	Vigilance Case investigation *P. falciparum* outbreak notification in accordance with IHR Annual reporting to WHO on maintenance of malaria-free status
Health systems issues	Access to treatment Access to diagnostics Health system strengthening (coverage, private-public sectors, QA, health information system)	Engaging private sector Control of OTC sale of anti-malarial medicines Availability of qualified staff	Full cooperation of private sector No OTC sale of antimalarial medicines Free-of-charge diagnosis and treatment for all malaria cases	Integration of malaria programme staff into other health and vector control programmes
Programmatic issues	Programme management, coordination Procurement, supply management Resource mobilization Regional initiative Pharmacovigilance Adherence to the "Three ones" principles Integration with other health programmes for delivery of interventions, e.g. ITN/LLIN, IPTp Domestic/external funding	Elimination programme development Legislation Regional initiative Mobilization of domestic funding Establish malaria elimination committee Reorientation of health facility staff	Implementation of elimination programme Implementation of updated drug policy, vector control, active detection of cases Malaria elimination committee: − manage malaria elimination database − repository of information − periodic review − oversigh Reorientation of health facility staff	WHO certification process
Interventions throughout all programmes	Case management Integrated vector management, including monitoring of insecticide resistance Geographical information collection Human resources development Health education, public relations, advocacy Operational research Technical and operational coordination, including intra- and intersectoral collaboration, both within the country and with neighbouring countries Monitoring and evaluation Independent assessment of reaching milestones Resource mobilization Health systems strengthening			

[a]. The pre-elimination programme is a reorientation phase. The interventions mentioned in this column are introduced during this programme reorientation, to be fully operational at the start of the elimination programme.

ACT: artemisinin-based combination therapy; DHS: Demographic and Health Surveys; GIS: geographic information system; IHR: International Health Regulations (2005); IPTp: intermittent preventive treatment in pregnancy; IRS: indoor residual spraying; ITN: insecticide-treated mosquito net; IVM: integrated vector management; LLIN: long-lasting insecticidal net; MICS: Multiple Indicator Cluster Surveys; MIS: Malaria Indicator Survey; OTC: over-the-counter; QA: quality assurance; QC: quality control; RDT: rapid diagnostic test.
Source: reference *(5)*

Table 5.3 Programme phases for pre-elimination, elimination and prevention of re-introduction

COUNTRY	Current /most recent local *Plasmodium* species	Programme phase in 2009	Start of elimination programme phase*	Last local *P.falciparum* case	Last reported indigenous case
Argentina	*vivax*	pre-elimination			ongoing
Dem. People's Rep. of Korea	*vivax*	pre-elimination			ongoing
El Salvador	both	pre-elimination		ongoing	ongoing
Iran (Islamic Republic of)	both	pre-elimination	2004	ongoing	ongoing
Malaysia	both	pre-elimination		ongoing	ongoing
Mexico	both	pre-elimination		ongoing	ongoing
Paraguay	*vivax*	pre-elimination			ongoing
Sri Lanka	both	pre-elimination		ongoing	ongoing
Algeria	*vivax*	elimination			ongoing
Azerbaijan	*vivax*	elimination	2007	before 1960s	ongoing
Georgia	*vivax*	elimination	2007	before 1960s	ongoing
Iraq	*vivax*	elimination	2005	1987	ongoing
Kyrgyzstan	*vivax*	elimination	2006	before 1960s	ongoing
Republic of Korea	*vivax*	elimination			ongoing
Saudi Arabia	both	elimination	2003	ongoing	ongoing
Tajikistan	both	elimination	2005 (*P.f.*); 2008 (*P.v.*)	ongoing	ongoing
Turkey	*vivax*	elimination	2008	before 1960s	ongoing
Uzbekistan	*vivax*	elimination	2008	before 1960s	ongoing
Armenia	*vivax*	prev. of re-introduction	2006	before 1960s	2005
Bahamas	*falciparum*	prev. of re-introduction		ongoing	ongoing
Egypt	*vivax*	prev. of re-introduction	1997	1997	1997**
Jamaica	*falciparum*	prev. of re-introduction	certified in 1966	ongoing	ongoing
Morocco	*vivax*	prev. of re-introduction	1997	1974	2004
Oman	both	prev. of re-introduction	1991	2003	2003, then local transmission in 2007–2008
Russian Federation	*vivax*	prev. of re-introduction	2005	before 1960s	ongoing
Syrian Arab Republic	*vivax*	prev. of re-introduction	1999	1960s	2004
Turkmenistan	*vivax*	prev. of re-introduction	2005	before 1960s	2005

* Source: reference 4
** Concern has been raised about the accuracy of the surveillance system

Many other countries, such as Australia, Singapore, Tunisia, the United Arab Emirates and the United States of America, were once endemic, have eliminated malaria, and continue to successfully prevent re-establishment of transmission. This is despite having areas with abundant malaria vectors and suitable climate conditions, which make them receptive to the resumption of transmission, and continued importation of parasites from abroad.

5.5.2 Countries in the elimination phase

In 2009, 10 countries were implementing nationwide malaria elimination programmes: Algeria, Azerbaijan, Georgia, Iraq, Kyrgyzstan, the Republic of Korea, Saudi Arabia, Tajikistan, Turkey and Uzbekistan. Only two countries in the elimination phase have remaining foci of active *P. falciparum* transmission: Saudi Arabia and Tajikistan. All others have only *P. vivax*.

As described in **Box 5.1** and shown in **Figure 5.5**, a majority of the 10 "elimination countries" had already eliminated malaria once before. These were countries in the WHO European Region in the Caucasus and Central Asia, and the Republic of Korea.

During the period 1998–2008, the annual number of reported local cases was reduced 100-fold or more in nearly all the elimina-

tion countries (**Fig. 5.6**). The exception was the Republic of Korea, which showed a more sustained transmission pattern. Together, the 10 elimination countries reported just 1672 locally acquired malaria infections in 2008, and 1730 imported cases. Over 60% of the local cases were reported by the Republic of Korea, followed by Tajikistan (19%) and Turkey (10%). None of the elimination countries has reported deaths due to local malaria transmission since 1998, but imported cases continue to result in occasional deaths; e.g. Turkey reported three deaths from imported malaria in 2008.

Since the *World Malaria Report 2008*, a large shift in types of country programme has occurred in the WHO European Region, where only 589 locally acquired malaria cases were reported in 2008, down from > 90 000 in 1995. All the malaria-affected countries of the Region have moved forward one programme phase (Fig. 5.1):

- All six endemic countries (Azerbaijan, Georgia, Kyrgyzstan, Tajikistan, Turkey and Uzbekistan) have moved from pre-elimination to elimination; their national strategies on malaria have been revised to reflect the new elimination challenges.

- The two countries with elimination programmes (Armenia and Turkmenistan) have reported no indigenous cases since 2005 and have moved to the stage of prevention of reintroduction. Turkmenistan has initiated the process for certification of malaria-free status.

BOX 5.1

Historical perspective of "elimination countries"

As can be seen in Figure 5.5, which shows the numbers of reported malaria cases between 1982 (6) and 2008, six of the 10 elimination countries had already eliminated malaria once before: countries in the WHO European Region in the Caucasus and Central Asia, and the Republic of Korea.

The endemic areas in the 10 elimination countries, with the exception of southwestern Saudi Arabia, are all located in the Paleartic ecozone[a], which also includes Europe, northern Africa and the northern part of China. Historically, this region was characterized by widespread malaria endemicity, but malaria here was sensitive to overall development and control efforts and was greatly reduced from the mid-nineteenth century. The incidence diminished further with the advent of DDT in the 1940s and the Global Malaria Eradication Programme in the 1950s and 1960s. *P. falciparum* was eliminated from most of the countries in this ecozone by the middle of the past century and now survives only in Afghanistan and Tajikistan.

By 1975, the WHO European Region, including the former Union of Soviet Socialist Republics but excepting Turkey, was considered malaria-free (7), even though sporadic cases continued to be reported in Azerbaijan and Tajikistan. An upsurge of imported cases, followed by the re-establishment of local transmission, occurred in the Caucasus and the Central Asian republics and to a lesser extent in Russia in the late 1980s and early 1990s, related to the war in Afghanistan and the dissolution of the Union of Soviet Socialist Republics. The reappearance of *P. falciparum* in Tajikistan was first noted in the mid-1990s; falciparum transmission peaked in 2001 at 826 cases nationwide, dropping to two in 2008. It is likely that this species will soon be eliminated from the WHO European Region. When that happens, the geographical spread of *P. falciparum* parasites of the "palearctic strain" will once again be limited to northern Afghanistan.

P. vivax malaria was highly prevalent throughout the Republic of Korea in the first half of the twentieth century but disappeared in the 1960s and 1970s due to malaria eradication efforts; the last two indigenous cases were reported in 1984 (8). The Korean peninsula was subsequently considered non-endemic for malaria, until the 1990s, when malaria re-emerged near the Demilitarized Zone, followed by a protracted outbreak in this area, disproportionally affecting the northern part of the peninsula. In 2008, the Republic of Korea reported the highest number of local cases of the 10 elimination countries.

In Africa north of the Sahara, intensive malaria control and eradication efforts, dating back to the 1940s and 1950s, have led to the elimination of transmission from Egypt, the Libyan Arab Jamahiriya, Morocco and Tunisia and have greatly reduced the risk areas in Algeria. The risk for transmission in Algeria is now limited to small foci in oases, with isolated *P. falciparum* transmission reported in the southernmost areas, which are along the route of trans-Saharan migration and susceptible to importation of parasites. Algeria reported 12 530 cases of malaria in 1968, which was brought down to 90 cases in 1976 (9). Over the next 10 years, the annual number of reported local malaria cases remained in the range 30–70, climbing to 100–200 cases annually in 1988–1998 (6) and returning to 30 or fewer annually thereafter.

Malaria was nearly eliminated from Iraq during implementation of the the Global Malaria Eradication Programme, when the reported numbers fell from 320 926 cases and 760 deaths in 1955 (10) to 2234 cases in 1962 (9). The number of reported cases increased to over 14 000 in 1970 and 1975 (9) but was brought down to some 2000 cases annually in the mid-1980s (6). *P. falciparum* was eliminated in 1987. The first Gulf war resulted in a malaria epidemic, with over 98 000 cases reported annually in 1994 and 1995 (6). Reported local transmission of *P. vivax* malaria is currently limited to foci in the northern governorate of Erbil. Six locally acquired cases were reported in 2008.

The incidence of malaria in Turkey had been reduced from 13 759 reported cases annually in 1955 (10) to only 1263 cases in 1970 (9). The annual number of reported cases remained at that low level until 1975, when it rebounded to 9828, with 37 320 cases the following year and a peak of 115 385 cases in 1977 (9), linked to agricultural development and insecticide resistance in the Çukurova and Amikova plains of southern Turkey, coupled with insufficient coverage by the surveillance system during 1970–1975. The epidemic was steadily controlled, and the country reported only 8675 cases in 1990. A further peak of cases occurred in relation to the first Gulf war and the influx of refugees from Iraq: 84 345 and 82 096 cases were reported in 1994 and 1995. By 1998, Turkey still reported 36 780 local malaria cases. Finally, in 2006, the reported number of cases dropped to below the level achieved in 1970. In 2008, only 166 locally acquired cases were reported in eastern areas bordering the Syrian Arab Republic and Iraq.

Saudi Arabia is the only elimination country that maintained a steady high malaria burden over the past decades, peaking most recently at 36 139 reported confirmed local cases in 1998. The remaining endemic areas border highly endemic areas of Yemen and are part of the Afrotropical ecozone, which also includes Africa south of the Sahara. Over the past decade, Saudi Arabia has greatly reduced the number of locally acquired cases through intensive control, including cross-border cooperation with Yemen. Only 61 local cases were reported in 2008.

---

a. The world's eight ecozones ("zoogeographic regions") are separated from one another by geological features that formed barriers to plant and animal migration (e.g. oceans, high mountain ranges, broad deserts), resulting in the development of plant and animal species (including *Anopheles* species and *Plasmodium* strains) in relative isolation over long periods.

Figure 5.5 Confirmed malaria cases (local and imported) in elimination countries, 1982–2008

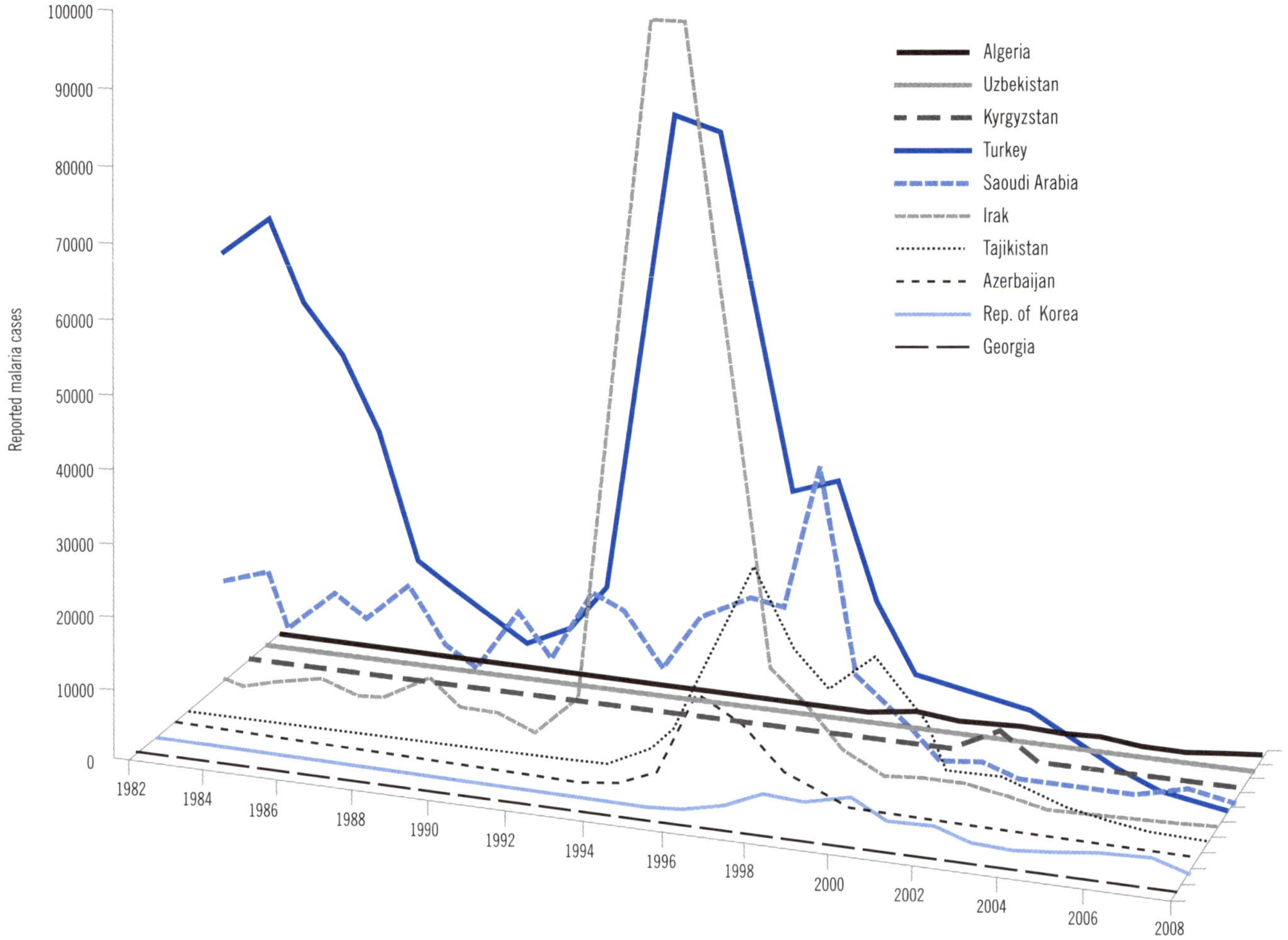

Figure 5.6 Locally acquired confirmed cases, elimination countries, 1998–2008

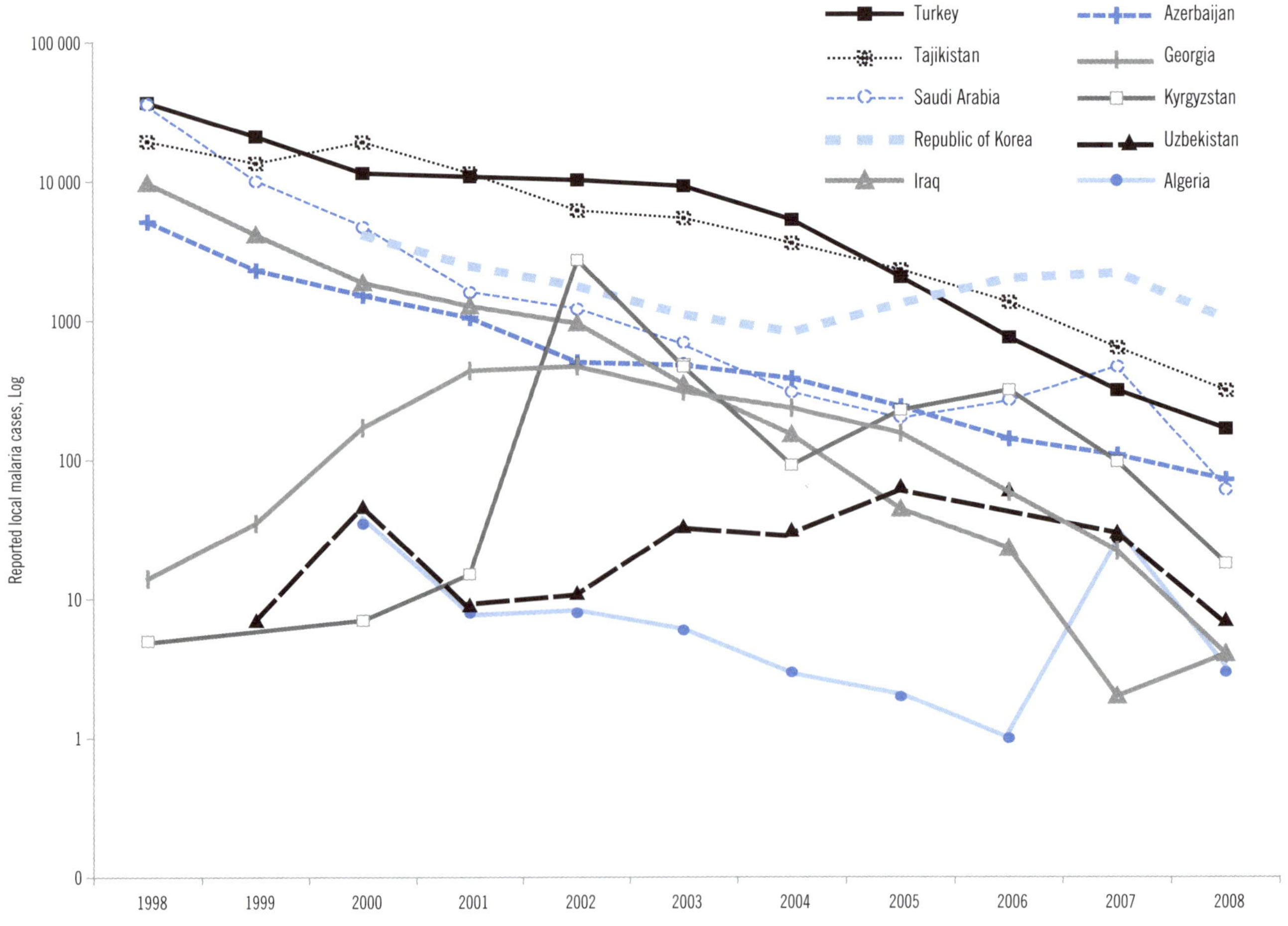

With increased cross-border cooperation, the Region aims for the elimination of malaria by 2015.

In 2008, three countries in the WHO Region of the Americas (El Salvador, Mexico and Paraguay) were considered to be implementing elimination programmes. As of 2009, these countries had been reclassified as in 'pre-elimination' to reflect more accurately the fact that the elimination approach is not yet fully being implemented countrywide in all affected areas. This change in classification does not reflect a deterioration of the programme status of these countries.

5.5.3 Pre-elimination group of countries

As of 2009, eight countries were in the pre-elimination programme phase and are reorientating their programmes to increase emphasis on the quality of surveillance, reporting and information systems:

Argentina, Democratic People's Republic of Korea, El Salvador, Islamic Republic of Iran, Malaysia, Mexico, Paraguay and Sri Lanka.

As described in **Box 5.2** and shown in **Figure 5.7**, of the eight pre-elimination countries, four (Argentina, Democratic People's Republic of Korea, Paraguay and Sri Lanka) had nearly eliminated malaria once before.

The eight pre-elimination countries reported a total of 29 245 confirmed malaria cases in the last year for which data are available, with 96% of cases reported by just four countries: the Islamic Republic of Iran (39%), Malaysia (25%), the Democratic People's Republic of Korea (24%) and Mexico (8%). Sri Lanka had a protracted increase in case load between 1986 and 2000. With the exception of Sri Lanka, none of the pre-elimination countries has reported deaths from malaria during the past decade. In Sri Lanka, local malaria deaths decreased from 115 in 1998 to 2 in 2004; no deaths from malaria have been reported since then.

5.5.4 Countries aspiring to pre-elimination

Swaziland and a number of smaller African island states and territories that were until recently moderately to highly endemic aspire to join the group of "pre-elimination countries" in the coming years. Typically, relatively large parts of the territories of these countries are still affected by malaria. Intense vector control programmes (LLINs and IRS) have been implemented in recent years, with massive external funding, leading to 10-fold or greater reductions in the malaria case load, down to several thousand suspected cases annually. Eventual malaria elimination in these countries will be "ambitious and challenging" (12).

Cape Verde presents a different scenario: the country took part in the malaria eradication campaign of the 1950s and 1960s, when it greatly reduced its original level of endemicity. Rebound epidemics occurred after favourable rains in the late 1970s and 1980s but were successfully controlled. At present, only one of the nine inhabited islands (São Tiago) is considered to have malaria transmission, with seasonal transmission linked to rainfall, resulting over the 12-year period (1996–2007) in a total of 798 malaria cases, of which 608 (75%) were locally acquired. The programme incorporates many aspects of the elimination approach and is reorienting its national strategy towards elimination.

BOX 5.2

Historical perspective of "pre-elimination countries"

The endemic areas in the eight pre-elimination countries are located in the Indo-Malay ecozone (Islamic Republic of Iran, Malaysia and Sri Lanka), the Neotropic ecozone (Argentina, El Salvador, Mexico and Paraguay) and the Palaearctic ecozone (Democratic People's Republic of Korea). Of the eight, only the Islamic Republic of Iran and Malaysia still have a considerable burden of *P. falciparum*, representing 12% and 30% of the total case loads reported in 2008, respectively. Argentina and the Democratic People's Republic of Korea have exclusively *P. vivax*, and the others have almost exclusively *P. vivax*.

Four of the current pre-elimination countries had already approached success in elimination in the second half of the twentieth century. Sri Lanka reported only 31 cases nationwide in 1963 (9); the Democratic People's Republic of Korea was considered malaria-free in the 1980s; in Paraguay, intensive surveillance operations resulted in fewer than 50 reported locally acquired cases (all *P. vivax*) in 1982; and Argentina's reported malaria burden peaked at 5351 cases in 1959 (10) but was brought down to only 41 local cases in 1970 (11).

Figure 5.7 shows that the largest numbers of malaria cases in this group were reported in recent decades in the Democratic People's Republic of Korea and Sri Lanka, which had all but eliminated malaria earlier.

El Salvador, the Islamic Republic of Iran, Malaysia and Mexico have seen more gradual decreases in the numbers of cases over the years, accelerated by implementation of the Global Malaria Control Strategy and the Roll Back Malaria programme in the early and late 1990s, respectively. The remaining endemic areas in these countries are located in regions that have relatively more favourable climate conditions for malaria transmission, combined with more difficult access by central health services and/or cross-border migration from neighbouring endemic countries. As shown in **Figure 5.8,** the remaining foci in these countries are more tenacious, resulting in a relatively flat profile in recent years.

Table 5.4   Within country localized "malaria free" initiatives

COUNTRY	WHO REGION	REGION OR SUB-NATIONAL LEVEL
China	Western Pacific	Hainan
Indonesia	South-East Asia	Java, Bali
Philippines	Western Pacific	Province by province
Solomon Islands	Western Pacific	Temotu
Sudan	Eastern Mediterranean	Khartoum, Gezira
Vanuatu	Western Pacific	Tafea
Yemen	Eastern Mediterranean	Socotra

Figure 5.7 Reported malaria cases in pre-elimination countries, 1982–2008

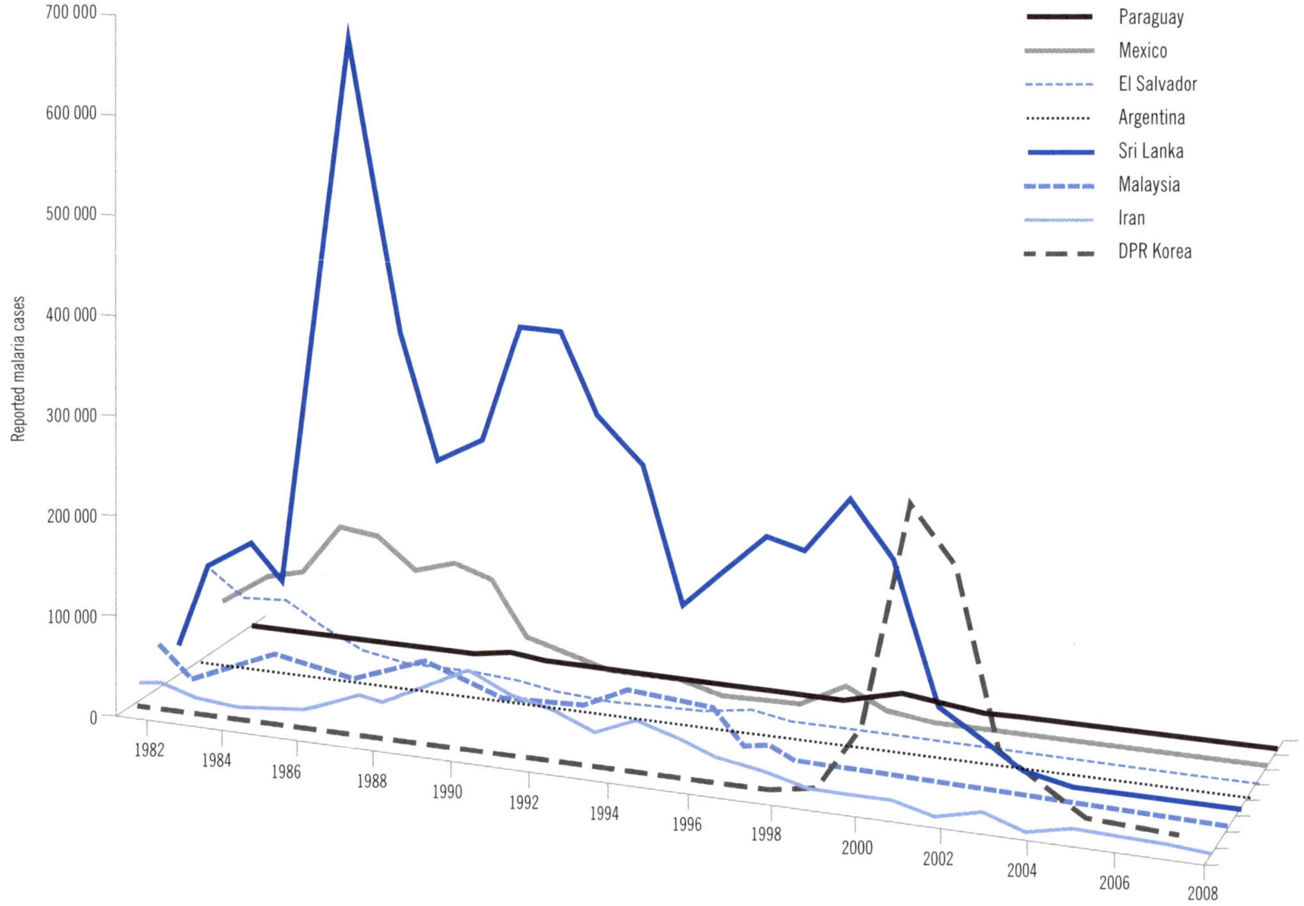

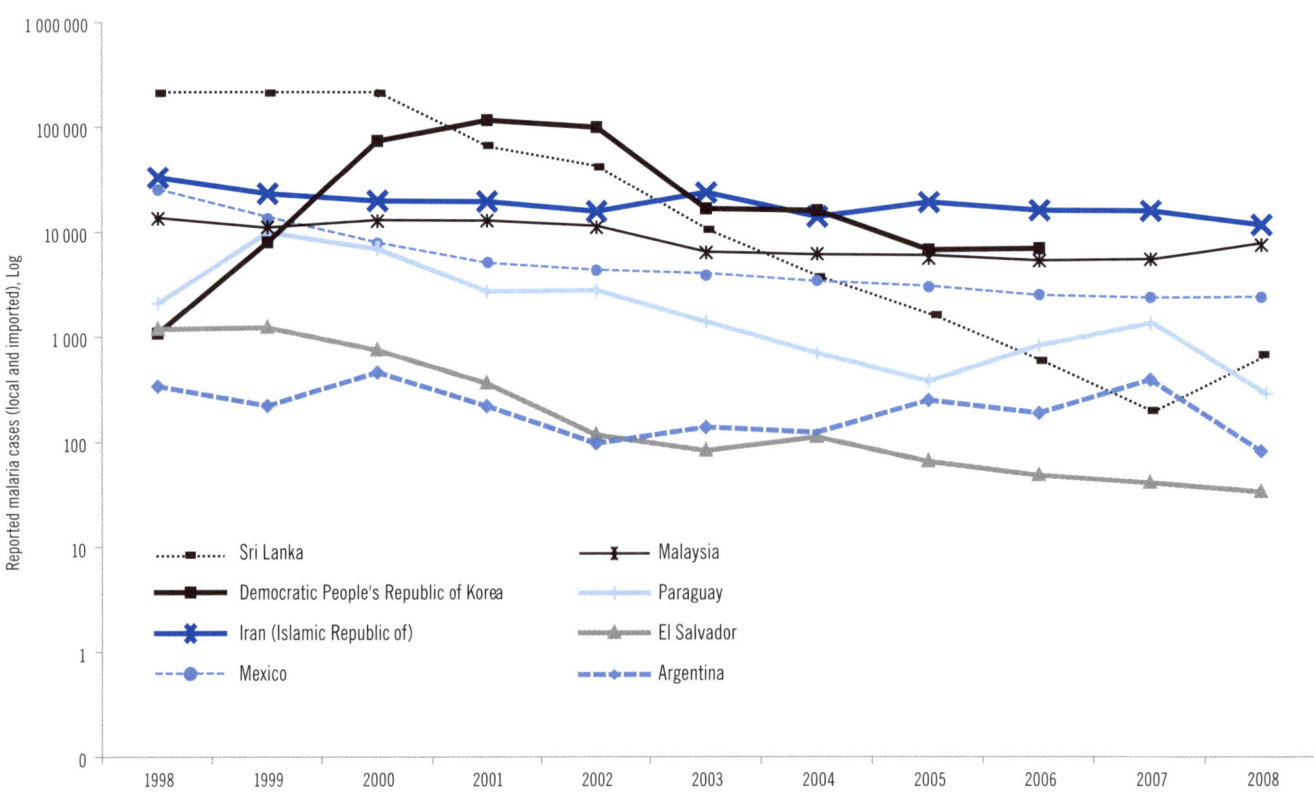

Figure 5.8 Total confirmed malaria cases (local and imported), pre-elimination countries in which trends have been stable, 1998–2008

5.5.5 Countries implementing projects in "malaria-free zones"

Seven malaria-endemic countries are implementing local projects aimed at achieving "malaria-free zones", while the remainder of the country is in the control phase. The term "malaria-free" is in this context not well-defined: while some countries are trying to eliminate the last locally acquired malaria infections in well-defined areas, for instance to encourage tourism (Socotra, Yemen), others in this group are trying to reduce mortality and morbidity due to malaria to a certain level (e.g. Khartoum, Sudan) (13).

The countries that have declared 'malaria-free' projects are listed in **Table 5.4**.

5.6 WHO certification

When a country has had zero locally acquired malaria cases for at least three consecutive years, the government can ask WHO to certify the achievement of elimination. Certification requires proving beyond reasonable doubt that the chain of local human malaria transmission by *Anopheles* mosquitoes has been fully interrupted in the entire country.

The burden of proof of elimination falls on the country requesting certification. This implies that all the available evidence has been evaluated and has been found to be consistent with the assertion that malaria elimination has been achieved and that good-quality surveillance systems are in place that would be capable of detecting local transmission if it were occurring.

The general principles of certification are:

- Certification is for a country as a whole and for all four human malaria species.

- Inspection and evaluation are carried out by a team led by WHO, which then recommends certification, if appropriate.

- The WHO Secretariat shares the final report with WHO and non-WHO experts on malaria elimination for critical review.

- The final decision rests with the WHO Director-General.

- Certification is published in the *Weekly Epidemiological Record*.

Details of the aspects to be covered by the evaluation teams are provided elsewhere (14). Certification of malaria elimination is based on an assessment of the current situation and the likelihood that elimination can be maintained. Countries are requested to continue reporting annually to WHO on the maintenance of their malaria-free status.

Between 1961 and 1987, 24 countries (see **Table 5.5**) were certified as malaria-free by WHO and entered in the *WHO Official Register* of areas where malaria eradication has been achieved (15–17).

Of the certified countries and areas Jamaica, Mauritius and northern Venezuela (Bolivarian Republic of) were unable to maintain the absence of local transmission. Malaria elimination in Mauritius was certified in 1973, but transmission was reintroduced in 1978 and lasted 20 years. Mauritius now has comprehensive surveillance mechanisms, however, and has not reported a local case since 1998; it is once again considered free from local malaria transmission.

In addition to the countries entered in the *WHO Official Register*, the Maldives and Tunisia succeeded in eliminating malaria in 1984 and 1979, respectively. The United Arab Emirates reported its last locally acquired malaria case in 1997, and elimination was certified in January 2007 (17). A further six countries have reported (periods of) zero cases in recent years: Armenia, Egypt, Morocco, Oman, Syrian Arab Republic and Turkmenistan. Procedures for certification are under way with Morocco and have been initiated with Turkmenistan.

Table 5.5   Countries entered into the *WHO Official register* of areas where malaria eradication has been achieved, covering the period 1961–1987

COUNTRY/TERRITORY	DATE OF REGISTRATION
Venezuela, Bolivarian Rep. of (northern)	June 1961
Grenada and Carriacou	November 1962
Saint Lucia	December 1962
Hungary	March 1964
Spain	September 1964
Bulgaria	July 1965
China, Province of Taiwan	November 1965
Trinidad and Tobago	December 1965
Dominica	April 1966
Jamaica	November 1966
Cyprus	October 1967
Poland	October 1967
Romania	October 1967
Italy	November 1970
Netherlands	November 1970
United States of America and its outlying areas of Puerto Rico and the Virgin Islands	November 1970
Cuba	November 1973
Mauritius	November 1973
Portugal	November 1973
Yugoslavia	November 1973
Reunion	March 1979
Australia	May 1981
Singapore	November 1982
Brunei Darussalam	August 1987

Sources: *references 14–16*

References

1. Mendis K et al. From malaria control to eradication: the WHO perspective. *Tropical Medicine and International Health,* 2009, 14:802–809.

2. Feachem RGA, Malaria Elimination Group. *Shrinking the malaria map—a guide for policy makers.* San Francisco, California, Global Health Group, 2009.

3. Roll Back Malaria Partnership. *Global malaria action plan.* Geneva, World Health Organization, 2008 http://www.rollbackmalaria.org/gmap/index.html.

4. World Health Organization. *Global malaria control and elimination: report of a technical review.* Geneva, World Health Organization, 2008. http://apps.who.int/malaria/docs/elimination/MalariaControlEliminationMeeting.pdf

5. World Health Organization. *Malaria elimination. A field manual for low and moderate endemic countries.* Geneva, World Health Organization, 2007. http://apps.who.int/malaria/docs/elimination/MalariaElimination_BD.pdf

6. World Health Organization. Malaria 1982–1997. *Weekly Epidemiological Record,* 1999, 74 :265–272. http://www.who.int/docstore/wer/pdf/1999/wer7432.pdf.

7. World Health Organization. Information on the world malaria situation January–December 1975. *Weekly Epidemiological Record,* 1977, 52:21–36. http://whqlibdoc.who.int/wer/WHO_WER_1977/WER1977_52_21-36%20(N%C2%B03).pdf.

8. Chai JY. Re-emerging *Plasmodium vivax* malaria in the Republic of Korea. *Korean Journal of Parasitology,* 1999, 37:129-143.

9. Malaria 1962–1981. *World Health Statistics Annual 1983.* Geneva, World Health Organization. 1983:791–795.

10. World Health Organization. Malaria, 1955–1964. *Epidemiological and Vital Statistics Report,* 1966, 19:89–99.

11. World Health Organization. Status of malaria eradication during the year 1970. *Weekly Epidemiological Record,* 1971, 46 :293–305. http://whqlibdoc.who.int/wer/WHO_WER_1971/WER1971_46_293-308%20(N%C2%B030).pdf.

12. *Swaziland proposal to Global Fund to fight AIDS, Tuberculosis and Malaria, Eighth call for proposals—HIV and AIDS, tuberculosis and malaria.* Mababane, 2008. http://www.theglobalfund.org/grantdocuments/8SWZM_1759_0_full.pdf.

13. Government of Sudan, WHO Regional Office for the Eastern Mediterranean. *Documentation of Khartoum and Gezira malaria free initiative.* http://www.emro.who.int/RBM/documents/sudan-mfi.pdf.

14. World Health Organization. *Informal consultation on malaria elimination: setting up the WHO agenda.* Geneva, World Health Organization, 2006 (WHO/HTM/MAL/2006.1114). http://apps.who.int/malaria/docs/malariaeliminationagenda.pdf.

15. World Health Organization. Status of malaria eradication during the six months ended 30 June 1965. *Weekly Epidemiological Record,* 1966, 41:173–174. http://whqlibdoc.who.int/wer/WHO_WER_1966/WER1966_41_157-180%20(N%C2%B013).pdf.

16. World Health Organization. World malaria situation 1982. *World Health Statistics Quarterly,* 1984, 37:130-161.

17. World Health Organization. Malaria eradication. *Weekly Epidemiological Record,* 1989, 64:19–20. http://whqlibdoc.who.int/wer/WHO_WER_1989/WER1989_64_13-20%20(N%C2%B03).pdf.

18. World Health Organization. United Arab Emirates certified malaria–free. *Weekly Epidemiological Record,* 2007, 82:30. http://www.who.int/wer/2007/wer8204.pdf.

Chapter 6.
Financing malaria control

The three major sources of funds for malaria control programmes are national government spending, external assistance from donors and household or private "out-of-pocket" expenditure. In the Global Malaria Action Plan *(1)*, it is estimated that these sources comprised 34%, 47% and 19%, respectively, of total spending on malaria globally in 2007. This Report does not address household expenditures but focuses on external funding for malaria and national government spending. It considers the following issues: *i)* trends in international and domestic financing for malaria and their relation to estimated resource requirements; *ii)* how funds disbursed from external agencies have been allocated to different geographical regions, countries and programmes; and *iii)* the relation between external financing, programme implementation and disease trends.

6.1   Sources of information

The methods for obtaining information on malaria financing varied according to the type of information considered: commitments, disbursements or expenditures (see **Box 6.1** for definitions of these terms).

BOX 6.1

> ### Types of financial information
>
> **PLEDGE** – A non-binding announcement of intentions to contribute a certain amount of funds.
>
> **COMMITMENT** – A firm obligation expressed in writing and backed by the availability of the necessary funds for a particular project, programme or sector.
>
> **DISBURSEMENT** – The placement of resources at the disposal of a government or implementing agency.
>
> **EXPENDITURE** – The use of funds to pay for commodities, buildings, equipment, services or salaries.

6.1.1 Commitments

Information on commitments to malaria programmes was obtained from two sources: records of funding agencies on malaria grants awarded (Global Fund, United States President's Malaria Initiative, UNITAID, World Bank[1]), and information supplied by malaria-endemic countries, particularly to obtain host government contributions. Information on commitments is available up to 2008 or 2009.

Commitments represent a firm agreement by a funding agency to provide funds according to a prescribed plan. This may be a budget approved by a national government or a grant agreement between a funding agency and a programme implementer. Commitments provide an indication of the funding priority given to malaria, to particular countries or programmes. Information on commitments can often be obtained for the most recent financial year but do not always translate into programme expenditures, as there may be delays in disbursement of funds or problems in programme implementation which lead to reprogramming of resources. Hence, in analysing what funds have been used for malaria control, it is usually preferable to examine disbursements or actual expenditures, which give a more accurate picture of the extent to which recipients have benefited.

6.1.2 Disbursements

Information on disbursements was obtained from three sources : the database on global health financing maintained by the Institute of Health Metrics and Evaluation *(2, 3)*; records of disbursements by funding agencies, notably the Global Fund and the United States President's Malaria Initiative; information supplied by malaria-endemic countries to WHO annually on host government expenditures and breakdowns of expenditures by type; and information recorded by the Global Fund Enhanced Financial Reporting system on breakdowns of Global Fund expenditures. The various data sources have different levels of completeness. The most comprehensive dataset on disbursements is that maintained by the Institute for Health Metrics and Evaluation, which provides information on the disbursements of 27 agencies that provide funding for malaria; this was supplemented with additional information on disbursements supplied by individual donor agencies. Information on disbursements is available up to 2007.

---

1   World Bank financing for malaria is usually mediated through a credit from the International Development Association, which is an interest-free loan, with repayments starting after 10 years and maturing at 35 or 40 years. An annual service charge of 0.75% applies.

Information on disbursements or expenditures usually lags behind that on budgets or commitments by a minimum of 1 year, because a programme needs time to make such disbursements or expenditures and to compile data. It is sometimes difficult to distinguish between disbursements and expenditures; e.g. transfer of money by a principal recipient of a Global Fund grant to subrecipients may be recorded as an expenditure, although it is yet to be translated into goods and services that benefit target populations. Also, some funds disbursed may not be spent during the year the disbursement was made. In such cases, actual spending may be much less than the disbursements reported by donors. Information on disbursements is, however, generally more complete than that available for expenditures, and was hence central to most of the analyses presented here.

6.1.3 Other health spending

The funds reported as being available for malaria control are usually for specific interventions, such as the purchase and distribution of ITNs, RDTs or medicines. They do not include government funding or external assistance for the support of health systems, because it is difficult to assign specific amounts to malaria, even though malaria programmes clearly benefit from such support. In addition, much external assistance is provided through multilateral channels as technical support or through nongovernmental organizations, and is not always captured by the sources of information examined. Hence, it is possible that the funds available for malaria are greater than those recorded here. Nevertheless, the analysis presented gives an indication of the overall levels of funding for malaria in relation to resource requirements and how these have changed over time.

6.2 Resource requirements and trends in international and domestic financing

6.2.1 Resource requirement

The Global Malaria Action Plan estimated that between US$ 5.0 billion and US$ 6.2 billion will be required per year between 2009 and 2015 to scale-up and sustain the control and elimination of malaria globally (**Table 6.1**).

6.2.2 Commitments by external agencies

Figure 6.1 shows the financial commitments to malaria control by the four largest sources of external funds for malaria. It shows a fivefold increase in commitments for malaria control, from approximately US$ 0.3 billion per year in 2003 to US$ 1.7 billion in 2009, with a particularly large increase in 2009.

6.2.3 Disbursements by external agencies to malaria endemic countries

International disbursements for malaria to malaria-endemic countries increased from US$ 35 million in 2000 to US$ 652 million in 2007[2], an 18-fold increase. The Global Fund accounted for US$,1.3 billion or 62% of all external funds disbursed to malaria-endemic countries between 2000 and 2007 (**Fig. 6.2**). The United States Agency for International Development (including the President's Malaria Initiative) was second to the Global Fund as a source of funds between 2000 and 2007, increasing its malaria funding to countries by a factor of 37, from US$ 6 million in 2000 to US$ 226 million in 2007. The United Kingdom Department for International Development was third, increasing its contributions from US$ 2 million in 2000 to US$ 29 million in 2007. Note that Global Fund disbursements for malaria, at US$ 1.3 billion, represent only 48% of the US$ 2.6 billion

Table 6.1 Annual global resource requirements (US$ millions) for malaria control

REQUIREMENT	2009	2010	2015	2020	2025
Prevention					
Long-lasting insecticidal nets and insecticide-treated nets	2091	2091	1689	1807	1035
Indoor residual spraying	1632	1883	2026	2047	1531
Intermittent preventive treatment in pregnancy IPTp	6	8	9	9	10
Subtotal	3729	3982	3724	3863	2576
Case management					
Rapid diagnostic tests RDTs	679	975	368	109	43
Artemisinin-based combination therapies ACTs	257	356	164	1087	41
Chloroquine and primaquine	5	5	2	1	–
Severe case management	27	23	16	9	4
Programme support	638	839	764	787	714
Total	5335	6180	5038	5856	3378

---

2 Another US$ 200 million were disbursed in 2007 but were either directed to research or to regional programmes and are difficult to assign to individual countries or programme implementation. In particular, the disbursement of the Bill and Melinda Gates Foundation for malaria was US$ 160 million in 2007, but much of this contribution was for research and is not represented in country contributions.

3 If government budgets or expenditure appeared to include external assistance, the external assistance was excluded.

committed for malaria by the Fund between 2003 and 2007; some of the commitments are withheld during initial grant negotiations and again at Phase 2 review when poorly performing grants are reduced. This illustrates that information on commitments to malaria may not provide an accurate picture of funds immediately available for malaria control.

Figure 6.1 Funding commitments of the Global Fund, UNITAID, the US President's Malaria Initiative and the World Bank, 2003–2009

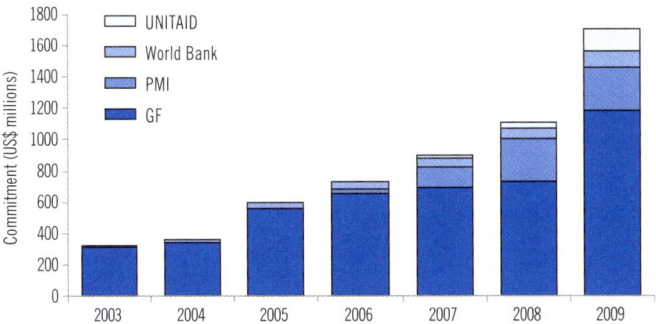

PMI: US President's Malaria Initiative; GF: Global Fund;

Annual commitments for World Bank-funded projects were calculated from the planned disbursements described in project appraisal documents, or, if these were not available, by assuming a constant flow of funds throughout the life of a project, with funding starting 6 months after board approval. Commitments of the PMI were allocated to calendar years proportionally according to the number of months of a financial year falling in each calendar year. Annual commitments of the Global Fund were calculated on the assumption of a project life span of 5 years and a constant flow of funds throughout that period. Commitments of UNITAID were distributed evenly to calender years according to the expected project length.

Figure 6.2 Disbursements to malaria-endemic countries 2000–2007

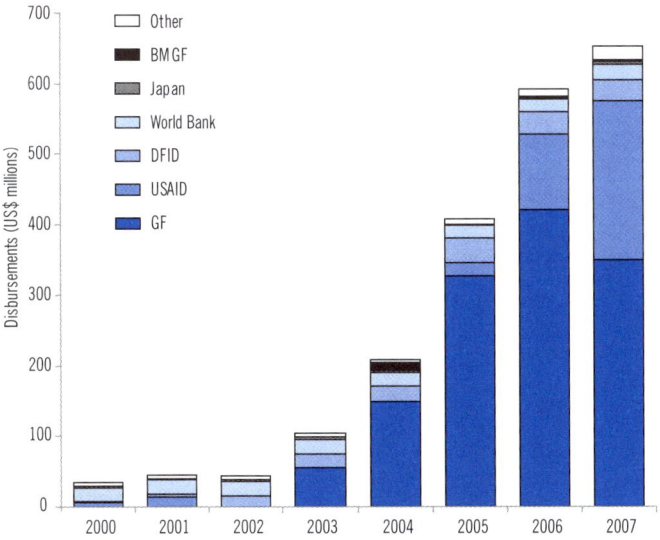

Source: *Institute of Health Metrics and Evaluation database with amendments to the President's Malaria Initiative and World Bank disbursements*

BMGF: Bill and Melinda Gates Foundation; DFID: Department for International Development (United Kingdom); USAID, United States Agency for International Development; GF: Global Fund to fight AIDS, Tuberculosis and Malaria

---

4 Kiszewski et al. (2007) (4) estimated that US$ 3.5–5.6 billion would be required per year between 2006 and 2015 but used a slightly different basis for calculation, e.g. without budgeting for the use of RDTs for diagnosing malaria in children under 5 years of age in Africa.

5 In the Global Malaria Action Plan *(1)*, it was estimated that government and household financing had been approximately equal to external financing in 2007.

6.2.4 Domestic financing in malaria-endemic countries

Information on domestic financing for malaria is insufficiently complete to allow a comprehensive analysis of trends. An important issue, however, is whether government financing for malaria remains stable in the presence of large quantities of external financing, or whether it is reduced or increases. The analysis was restricted to 31 countries that provided information on government financing for malaria for at least 5 of the past 9 years and included data for 2007 or 2008. When possible, government expenditure was used; if this information was not available, government budgets for malaria were used[3]. **Figure 6.3** shows the changes in domestic financing for malaria in these countries, averaged for each WHO region, each country being given equal weight. Although the trends among these counties might not be generalizable, they represent the only information currently available. The evidence that external financing for malaria displaces government financing is mixed: domestic financing for malaria increased in a range of countries in all regions, but a potential downwards trend between 2007 and 2008 was seen in two regions, and there was a steady decrease between 2005 and 2008 in the South-East Asia Region. Better information on domestic financing for malaria would allow a more accurate, complete picture of global malaria financing.

6.2.5 Commitments in relation to projected requirements

While the increase in external assistance for malaria has been unprecedented, the total funds available for malaria control are still lower than the annual amount estimated in the Global Malaria Action Plan to be necessary for successful control of malaria globally: more than US$ 5 billion per year[4]. Even if the high level of malaria commitments for 2009 (US$ 1.7 billion) is translated into disbursements and programme expenditures and complemented by equal levels of government and private sector funding[5], the total funds available for malaria control would be in the region of US$ 3.4 billion, or only 70% of projected requirements.

Figure 6.3 Trends in governmental expenditures for malaria, 2004–2008

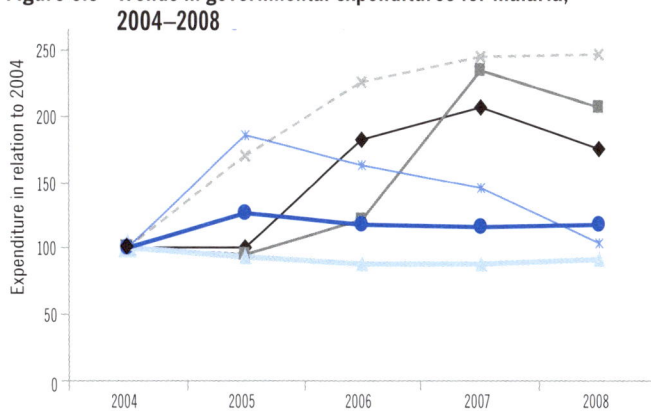

Source: National malaria programme reports to WHO

AFR, African Region; EMR, Eastern Mediterranean Region; EUR, European Region; RA, Region of the Americas; SEAR, South-East Asia Region; WPR, Western Pacific Region – Government financing for malaria in each region is indexed at 100 in 2004; subsequent values represent the percentage of the 2004 value, i.e. 250 for the Region of the Americas in 2008 indicates that government spending in 2008 value was 250% of the 2004 value or an increase of 150%.

6.3 Allocation of disbursed funds from external agencies to regions, countries and programmes

6.3.1 Disbursements by external agencies, by WHO region

The Global Fund was the dominant source of external finance in all regions between 2000 and 2007, except for the South-East Asia Region, where World Bank funding accounted for 55% of disbursements by external agencies (**Fig. 6.4**). The Global Fund accounted for 96% of disbursements in the European Region, 88% in the Eastern Mediterranean Region and 92% in the Region of the Americas. In the African Region, Global Fund support represented 60% of external support, with 22% from the United States Agency for International Development, 9% from the United Kingdom Department for International Development, 3% from the World Bank and 1% from the Japan International Cooperation Agency.

Between 2000 and 2007, disbursements by external agencies for malaria increased by a factor of 40 in the WHO African Region, 30 in the Eastern Mediterranean Region (since 2003), 18 in the European Region, 14 in the Western Pacific Region and 14 in the Region of the Americas. Only the South-East Asia Region registered no substantial increase in external assistance, with 2007 levels only 1.4 times those of 2000. This was partly due to the conclusion of a major World Bank project in India in 2005, which was not replaced until 2008. Even if the new World Bank vector-borne disease control project is included, however, the increase in funding to the South-East Asia Region is the least of all regions.

Figure 6.4   Disbursements by external agencies for malaria by WHO Region

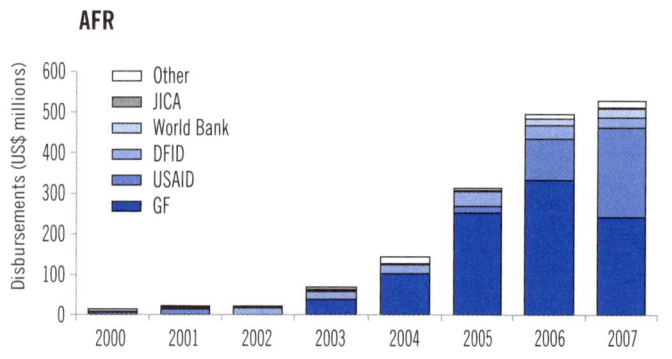

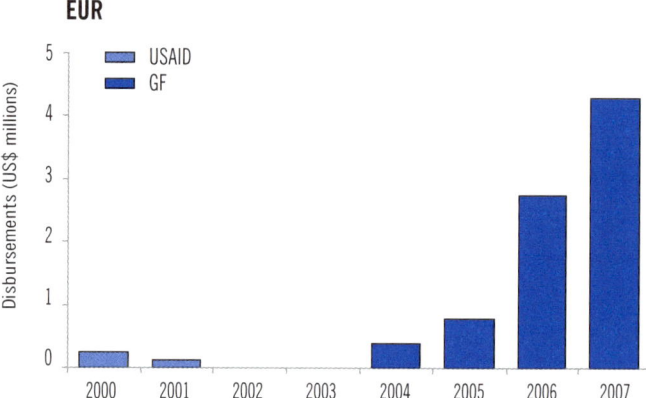

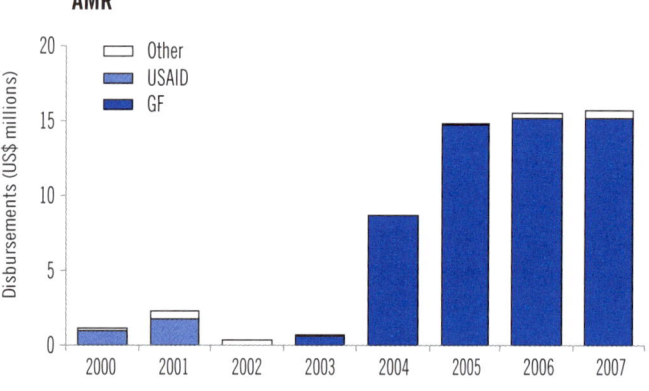

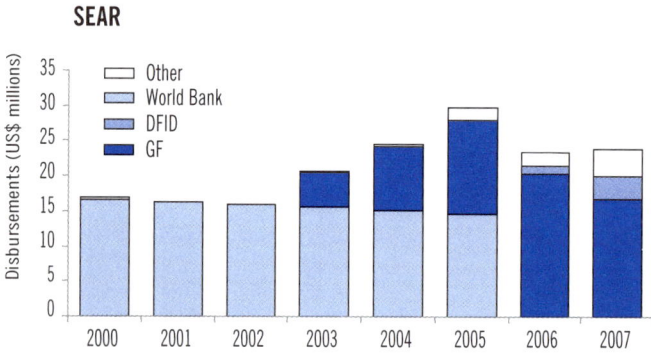

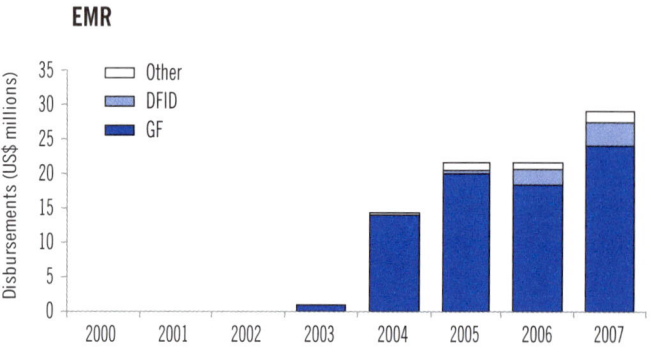

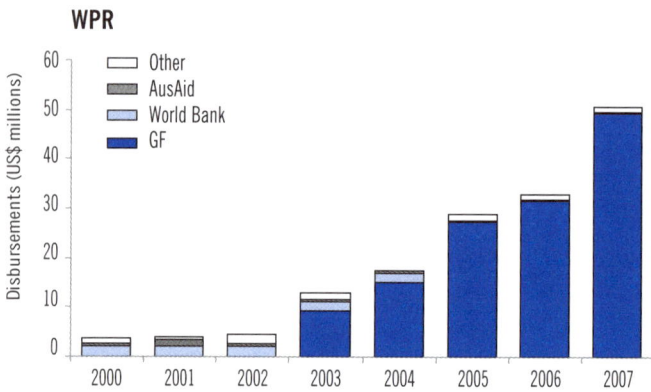

Source: Institute for Health Metrics and Evaluation database, with amendments to the disbursements of the United States President's Malaria Initiative and the World Bank

AFR, African Region; RA, Region of the Americas; EMR, Eastern Mediterranean Region; EUR, European Region; SEAR, South-East Asia Region; WPR, Western Pacific Region; JICA, Japan International Cooperation Agency; USAID, United States Agency for International Development; DFID, Department for International Development (United Kingdom); GFATM, Global Fund to fight AIDS, Tuberculosis and Malaria

Figure 6.5 Disbursements from external agencies 2000–2007, in relation to three measures of malaria burden

a) *Funding per person at risk of malaria*

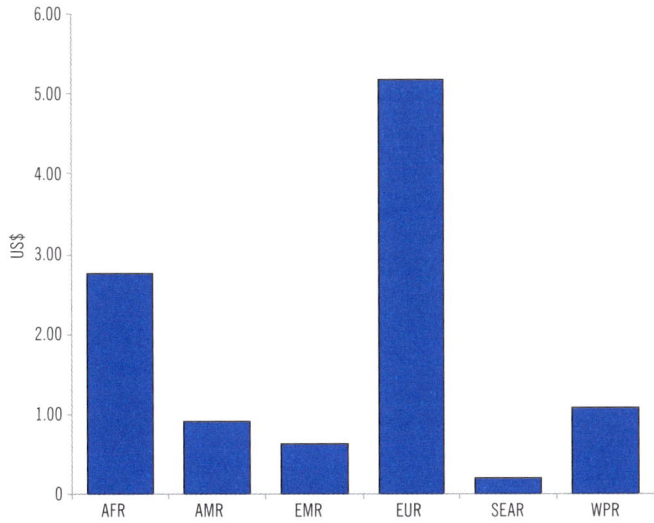

b) *Funding per case of malaria*

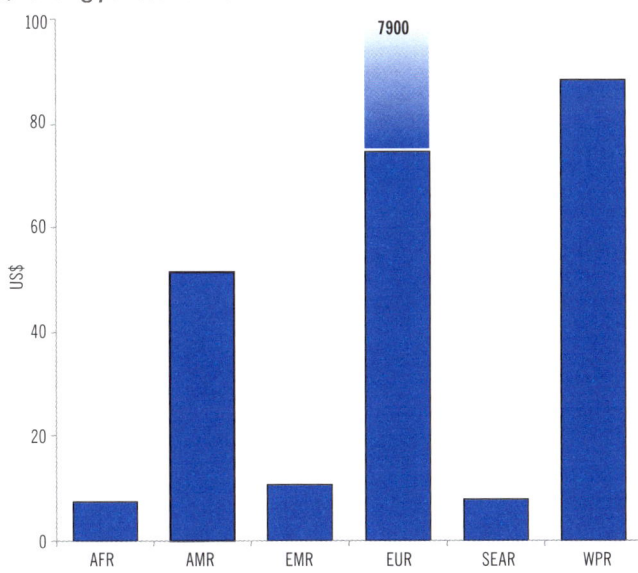

c) *Funding per death from malaria*

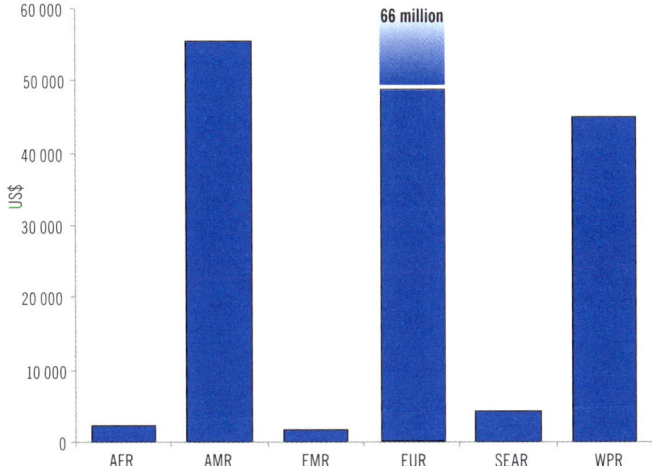

Source: Institute for Health Metrics and Evaluation database with amendments to the disbursements of the United States President's Malaria Initiative and the World Bank
AFR: African Region; AMR: Region of the Americas; EMR: Eastern Mediterranean Region; EUR: European Region; SEAR: South-East Asia Region; WPR: Western Pacific Region

6.3.2 Disbursements by external agencies in relation to epidemiological need

Figure 6.5 shows external assistance in relation to three measures of malaria burden: population at risk for malaria,[6] estimated number of cases of malaria and estimated number of deaths from malaria. Such an analysis of funding in relation to need does not take into account domestic sources of funds, the overall level of development of malaria programmes in countries, purchasing power, the types of interventions needed in different epidemiological settings or their cost. Nevertheless, it can give some insight into the extent to which external assistance flows to countries with high disease burdens.

For many countries, the population at risk is the most useful measure, as it defines the number of people to be protected by vector control programmes, such as with ITNs or IRS. When implemented, vector control programmes are expected to account for the majority of a malaria programme's spending and hence can provide a guide to the levels of resource needs (1). In countries with low disease burdens, where much of the population is classified as at low risk, however, the primary methods of control may be case detection and treatment, surveillance and epidemic prevention. In these countries, the number of malaria cases may be a better guide to resource need.

Populations at risk for malaria in the European Region received the most assistance, at US$ 5.18 per person, followed by the African Region, at US$ 2.76. The lower levels of assistance to other regions are partly due to the large numbers of people living in areas of relatively low risk (fewer than one case per 1000 per year). Figure 6.5 also shows disbursements in relation to the estimated numbers of cases and deaths due to malaria and suggests that larger amounts are received by malaria-endemic countries in the European, Western Pacific and the Americas regions. The African Region receives less external assistance in relation to the estimated numbers of cases or deaths due to malaria.

6.3.3 Disbursements by country

The number of countries receiving external assistance for malaria increased from 29 in 2000 to 76 in 2007 (out of a total of 108 malaria-endemic countries in 2007), the largest increase being in Africa (see **Fig. 6.6**). Only two malaria endemic sub-Saharan countries, Botswana and Chad, did not receive external assistance.

The number of agencies funding malaria control also increased between 2000 and 2007, from 14 to 22, with the largest increase in the African Region (from 12 to 19 agencies). In 2007, 15 countries in the Region received funds from a single external agency;[7] seven

---

6 Populations at low risk for malaria (living in areas with fewer than one case reported per 1000 per year) are given half the weight of populations at high risk (those living in areas with one or more case reported per 1000 per year). This procedure was followed in order that countries with only populations at low risk for malaria could be included in the analysis and also to take into account the greater need for malaria programmes and funds in countries with larger proportions of their population at high risk for malaria. The weighting is quite arbitrary, but similar results are obtained if populations at low risk are weighted as 0 or 1.

---

7 In 13 countries, the Global Fund was the sole external source of funds, the exceptions being the Congo (from Spain) and Liberia (from the United States).

Table 6.2 External assistance disbursed to malaria-endemic countries, 2000–2007 (US$ millions)

AFR	Total	% in region	AMR	Total	% in region	EUR	Total	% in region
Kenya	182	11%	Haiti	10	16%	Tajikistan	3.2	37%
UR Tanzania	155	10%	Guatemala	9	16%	Uzbekistan	2.0	23%
Ethiopia	151	9%	Honduras	8	13%	Georgia	1.7	20%
Uganda	123	8%	Peru	8	13%	Kyrgyzstan	1.7	20%
Mozambique	95	6%	Bolivia (Pluri. State of)	7	12%	Azerbaijan	–	0%
Zambia	88	6%	Nicaragua	5	8%	Turkey	–	0%
Rwanda	79	5%	Colombia	4	7%	TOTAL	8.6	100%
Nigeria	79	5%	Suriname	4	6%			
Angola	68	4%	Ecuador	2	3%			
Malawi	63	4%	Venezuela (Bol. Rep. of)	2	3%			
Madagascar	63	4%	Guyana	1	2%			
DR Congo	62	4%	Brazil	0	0%			
Senegal	56	3%	Argentina	–	0%	SEAR	Total	% in region
Ghana	51	3%	Belize	–	0%	India	108	63%
Niger	28	2%	Costa Rica	–	0%	Indonesia	19	11%
Benin	28	2%	Dominican Republic	–	0%	Myanmar	11	6%
Burundi	23	1%	El Salvador	–	0%	Bangladesh	8	5%
Cameroon	22	1%	French Guiana	–	0%	Timor-Leste	7	4%
Eritrea	20	1%	Mexico	–	0%	Nepal	7	4%
Mali	20	1%	Panama	–	0%	Sri Lanka	6	4%
Liberia	19	1%	Paraguay	–	0%	Thailand	5	3%
Zimbabwe	17	1%	TOTAL	59	100%	Bhutan	1	1%
Gambia	15	1%				Dem. People's Rep. Korea	–	0%
Burkina Faso	14	1%				TOTAL	172	100%
Togo	13	1%						
Gabon	12	1%						
Namibia	11	1%						
Central African Republic	11	1%						
Sierra Leone	8	1%	EMR	Total	% in region	WPR	Total	% in region
Guinea	8	0%	Sudan	44	50%	Philippines	37	24%
Equatorial Guinea	5	0%	Somalia	21	24%	Lao People's Dem. Rep.	35	22%
Côte d'Ivoire	4	0%	Yemen	8	9%	China	27	18%
South Africa	3	0%	Afghanistan	7	8%	Viet Nam	18	11%
Mauritania	3	0%	Pakistan	6	7%	Cambodia	18	11%
Sao Tome and Principe	3	0%	Djibouti	2	2%	Papua New Guinea	12	8%
Guinea-Bissau	2	0%	Islamic Republic of Iran	–	0%	Solomon Islands	6	4%
Comoros	2	0%	Iraq	–	0%	Vanuatu	3	2%
Swaziland	1	0%	Saudi Arabia	–	0%	Malaysia	–	0%
Congo	0	0%	TOTAL	88	100%	Rep. of Korea	–	0%
Cape Verde	0	0%				TOTAL	155	100%
Botswana	–	0%						
Chad	–	0%						
TOTAL	1 606	100%						

Source: Institute for Health Metrics and Evaluation database with amendments to disbursements from the United States President's Malaria Initiative and the World Bank
0% indicates that the country received less than US$ 0.5 million, while a dash indicates that the country received no external assistance.

Figure 6.6 Numbers of countries receiving external assistance for malaria control

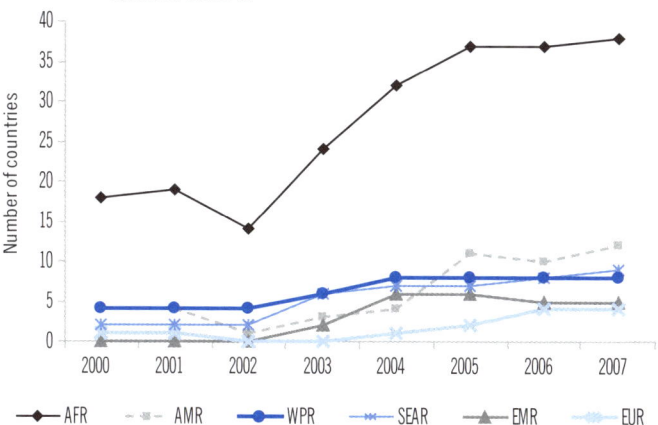

Source: Institute for Health Metrics and Evaluation database with amendments to the disbursements of the United States President's Malaria Initiative and the World Bank

AFR, African Region; AMR, Region of the Americas; EMR, Eastern Mediterranean Region; EUR, European Region; SEAR, South-East Asia Region; WPR, Western Pacific Region

countries from five or more external agencies (United Republic of Tanzania, 11; Kenya, 7; Mozambique, 6; Zambia, 6; Angola, 5; Nigeria, 5; and Uganda, 5). Ten countries accounted for 54% of disbursements between 2000 and 2007 (**Table 6.2**); all except India were in the African Region. The latest commitments for malaria in round 8 of the Global Fund and from the United States President's Malaria Initiative are likely to change this pattern.

Figure 6.7 shows malaria disbursements by external agencies per person at risk for malaria in relation to the size of the population at risk. It suggests that smaller countries (such as Sao Tome and Principe, Suriname and Vanuatu) receive more funds per capita than larger countries (such as China, India and Pakistan). Some countries receive more external assistance than others with equivalent populations at risk (e.g. Gambia, Kenya and Malawi). Other countries, such as Cape Verde, Congo and Brazil, are outliers from the overall trend and appear to have lower levels of external funding even after their size is taken into account. The pattern of funding whereby smaller countries receive higher per capita amounts may be appropriate if malaria programmes for smaller populations have proportionally higher fixed costs; however, programmes in smaller countries may also have lower costs for distribution of commodities such as ITNs, ACTs and diagnostics. An obstacle to increasing funding in larger countries is affordability; if all countries had received US$ 5 per capita (as received by the top 25% of countries) during the period analysed,

Figure 6.7 Relation between funds disbursed per person at risk for malaria and number of people at risk

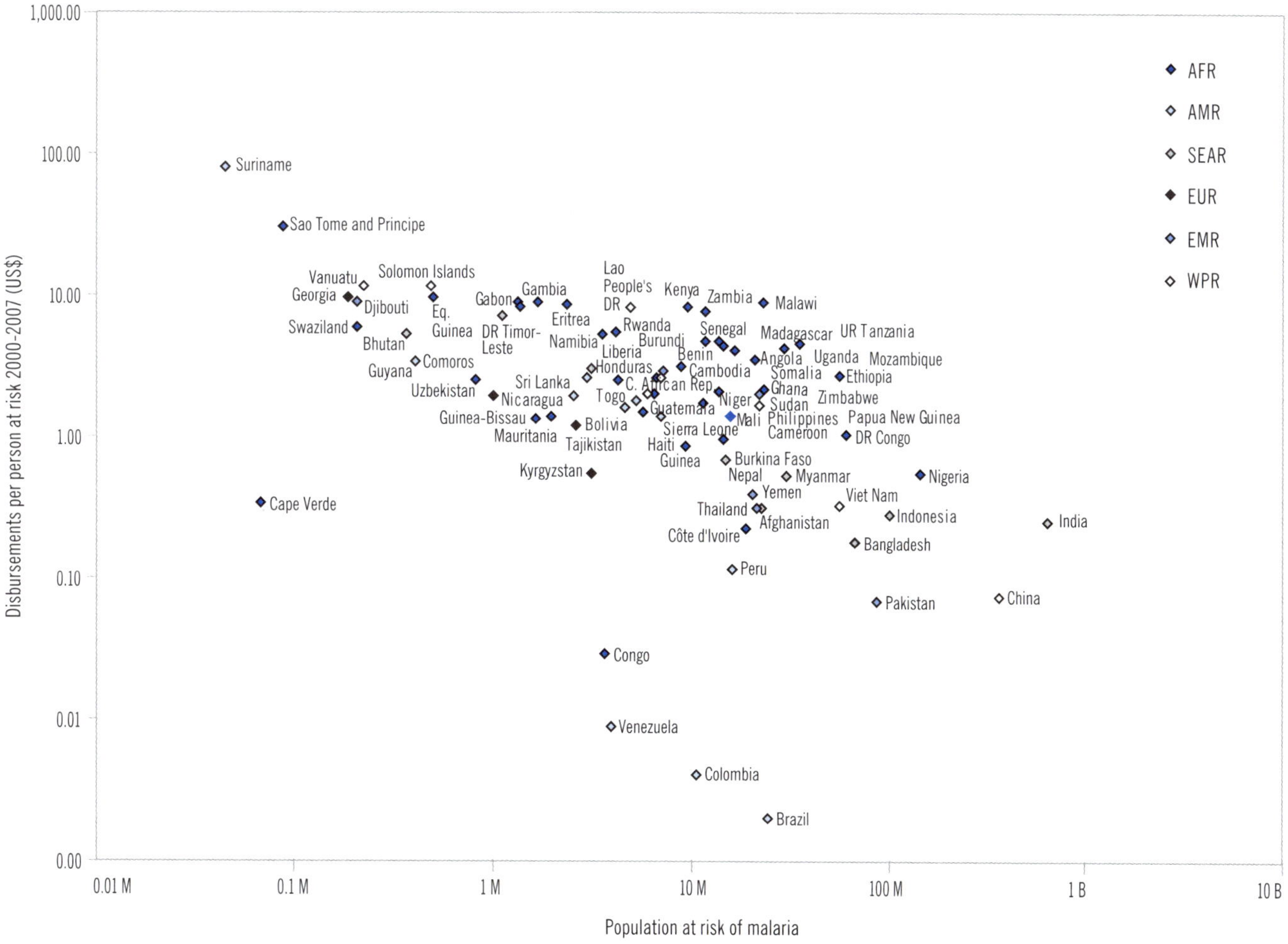

Source: Disbursements: Institute for Health Metrics and Evaluation database with amendments to disbursements from the United States President's Malaria Initiative and the World Bank; populations at risk: reports from malaria-endemic countries to WHO

AFR, African Region; RA, Region of the Americas; SEAR, South-East Asia Region; EUR, European Region; EMR, Eastern Mediterranean Region; WPR, Western Pacific Region

Figure 6.8 Uses of funds from different sources

a) *GFATM*

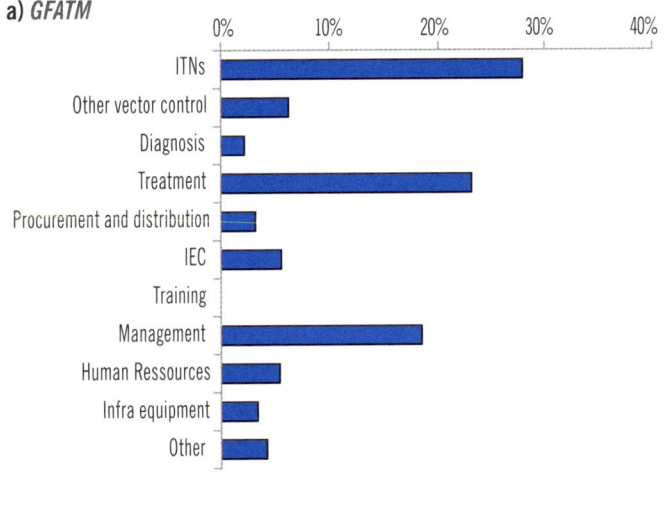

b) *Government*

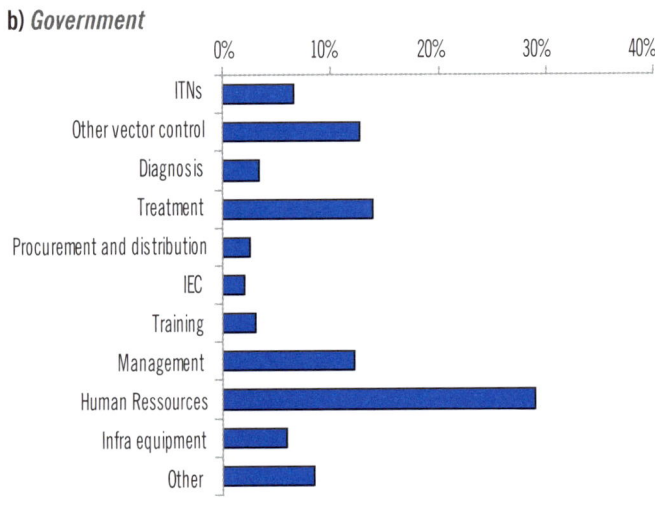

c) *PMI*

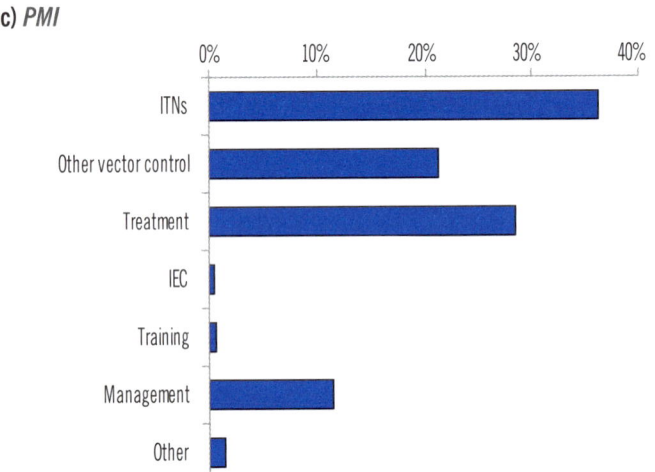

Sources: GFATM (Global Fund to fight AIDS, Tuberculosis and Malaria): Enhanced financial reporting system; Government, annual reports from malaria-endemic countries to WHO; PMI (United States President's Malaria Initiative): Third annual report, 2009 (6)

ITN, insecticide-treated net; IEC, information, education and communication

the amount required for malaria programmes would be more than US$ 2 billion per year, or three times current disbursements to endemic countries.

Very large countries such as China and India appear to be particularly disadvantaged with respect to receipt of external assistance for malaria control, as noted previously by Snow et al. *(5)*. Part of the reason for the apparently low levels of disbursements in very large countries might be that the populations at risk are estimated less precisely and may be overestimated. Populations at risk in large countries are defined within comparatively large administrative units (the median population size of a district in India is 1.5 million), in which the entire population may be classified as being at high risk, even if malaria is confined to a limited area. In smaller countries, where the administrative units are smaller (the median population of a district in Suriname is 22 000), areas with malaria transmission can be delineated more precisely. Therefore, while the observation that large countries receive less external financing is a concern, the imprecision in defining populations at risk in such countries should be taken into account, as should other factors that determine the need for external financing, such as the availability of domestic funds.

6.3.4 Expenditures by programme

Funds from different agencies are used in different ways. **Figure 6.8** gives a breakdown of government expenditure in 28 countries for which there were reports of how government financing for malaria was used in 2008. Each country is weighted equally. The breakdown of expenditures for any one country depends on factors that include the epidemiological situation, the level of external financing, the level of support from subnational administrative bodies and the level of health system development. The graph conceals wide variation among countries (e.g. countries in the South-East Asia Region appear to devote more resources to antimalarial medicines) but illustrates how government financing frequently covers the fixed costs of operating malaria programmes, including human resources and programme management (such as information systems, planning workshops and supervision). Figure 6.8 also shows that funds supplied by the Global Fund and the United States President's Malaria Initiative are often used to finance variable costs, such as the provision of commodities and their distribution.

The ratio of expenditures for vector control programmes to case management programmes is 1.11 for government financing, 1.34 for the Global Fund and 1.99 for the United States President's Malaria Initiative. The differences in ratios between funding sources may be due partly to differences in country representation, as the President's Malaria Initiative is limited to Africa. The projected ratio of funds required for vector control to case management in the Global Malaria Action Plan was 3.8 in 2009 and 2.9 in 2010, suggesting that more spending on vector control programmes is required.

6.4 Relations between external financing, programme implementation and disease trends

6.4.1 Disbursements and programme implementation

Figure 6.9 shows the numbers of nets procured between 2004 and 2008 per person at risk for malaria versus the amount of external assistance disbursed per head in the African Region between 2003 and 2007. It suggests that some countries that receive higher levels of external assistance per capita (Djibouti, Sao Tome and Principe) have been able to procure more nets per head of population than countries with lower funding ratios (Côte d'Ivoire, Nigeria). It also suggests that some countries have procured more nets per head of population than would be expected given the level of external assistance provided (Congo, Mali), possibly because of use of domestic resources, cost savings (e.g. using volunteers in mass campaigns) or gaps in the data. Other countries appear to have procured fewer nets than expected (Comoros, Swaziland, United Republic of Tanzania), perhaps because external assistance was targeted to other programmes, such as IRS or diagnosis and treatment, less efficient use of funds or gaps in the data on net procurement.

As information on net procurement and deliveries outside Africa is less complete, a similar analysis could not be undertaken. It would be informative to examine procurements of other commodities, such as RDTs and ACTs, but complete databases are not available.

6.4.2 Disbursements and malaria disease trends

Figure 6.10 shows the relation between disbursements by external agencies per capita between 2000 and 2007 and evidence for a decrease in the burden of malaria, as highlighted in Chapter 4 of this Report. Approximately 60% of countries receiving more than US$ 7 per person at risk reported a reduction in the number of cases of malaria since 2000, whereas only 26% of countries receiving US$ 7 or less reported reductions. Although few (10) countries received

Figure 6.10 Relation between external assistance disbursed in 2000–2007 per person at risk for malaria and decrease in malaria cases, 2000–2008

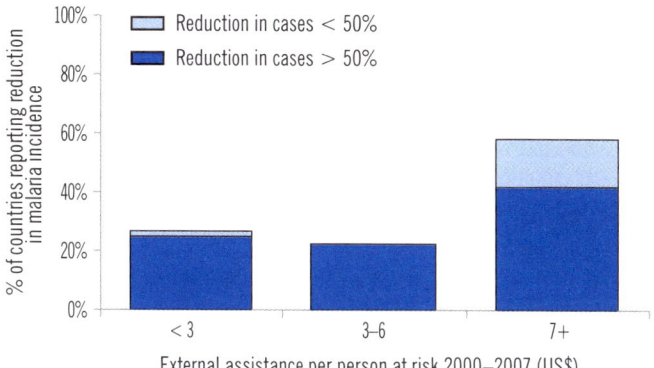

Sources: Disbursements: Institute for Health Metrics and Evaluation database with amendments to disbursements by the United States President's Malaria Initiative and the World Bank; trends in cases: reports from malaria-endemic countries to WHO

Figure 6.9 Relation between disbursements by external agencies for malaria control and nets procured by endemic countries

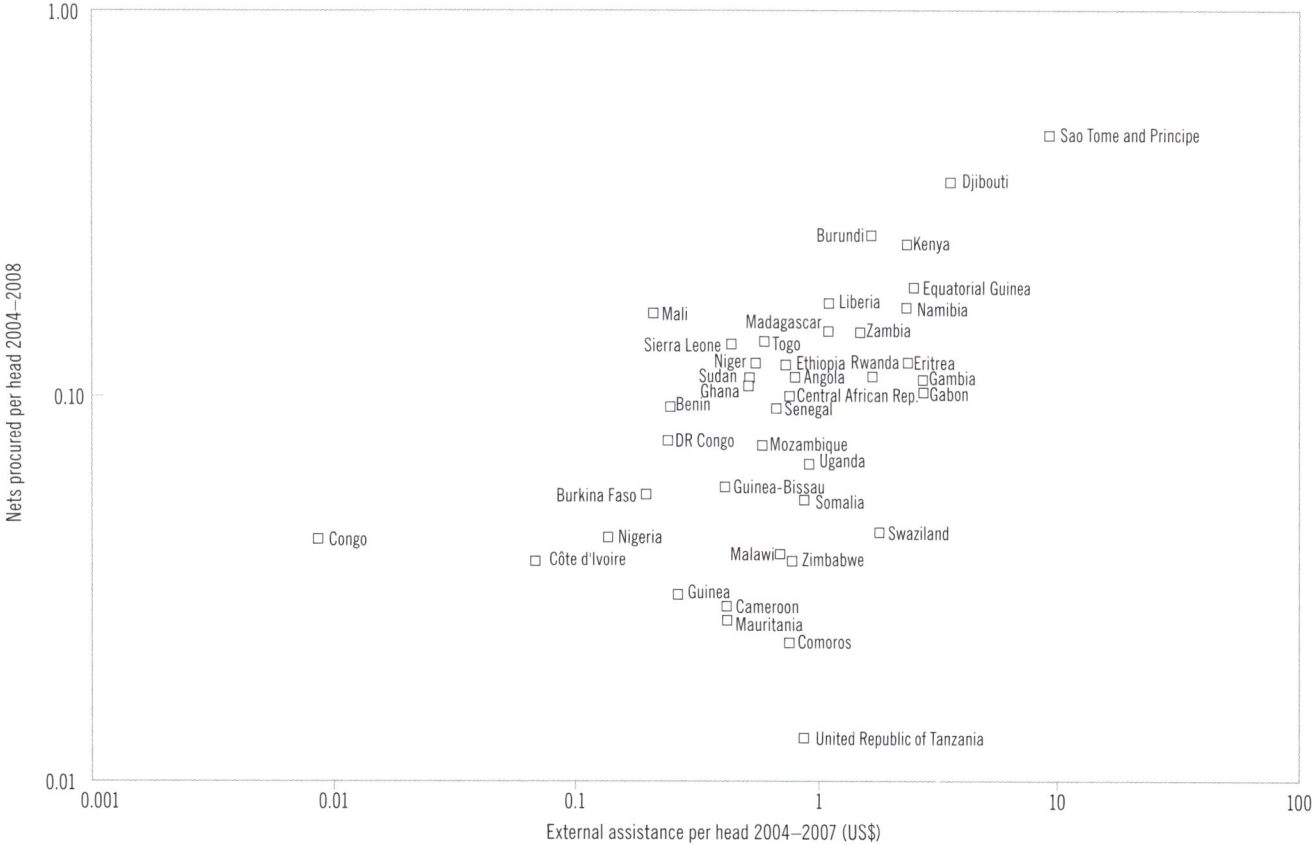

Source: Disbursements: Institute for Health Metrics and Evaluation database with amendments to disbursements by the United States President's Malaria Initiative and the World Bank; nets procured: records of the Alliance for Malaria Prevention, updated March 2009

such a high level of assistance, the observation suggests that high levels of external assistance per person at risk for malaria are associated with decreases in the incidence of malaria.

While success in reducing the incidence of malaria is seen in some countries with high levels of external assistance (Eritrea, Georgia, Sa0 Tome and Principe, Suriname, Solomon Islands and Vanuatu), evidence is lacking for others (e.g. Djibouti, Equatorial Guinea[8] and Gabon), perhaps because control programmes are implemented less than optimally or because of other factors that reduce the impact of malaria control, such as unfavourable climate conditions. It may also be due to deficient surveillance systems that are unable to detect change because of inconsistent reporting or reliance on suspected rather than confirmed cases.

Some countries with less external assistance per capita have reported success in reducing the number of cases of malaria. These tend to be richer countries with better developed malaria programmes, which probably receive more domestic resources per head. Alternatively, some investments in health systems strengthening that affect malaria may not have been captured in this analysis. While high levels of funding may be responsible for decreases in malaria incidence, funding agencies may tend to place funds in countries where success is more likely or has already been demonstrated.

While the increases in funds have been substantial, the current level of financing does not yet meet the estimated requirements for successful control of malaria and for reaching the MDG of more than US$ 5 billion per year.

The limited funds for malaria control appear to be disproportionately focused on smaller countries with lower disease burdens. There is evidence that high levels of external assistance are associated with decreases in malaria incidence, but positive trends are seen primarily in countries with low disease burdens, where success is more easily achieved.

Countries that substantially reduce the burden of malaria cases can face difficulties in justifying continued investment in malaria control. Continued or increased support is, however, critical to protect current achievements and move towards elimination. Financing of malaria programmes is also placed at risk by the global financial crisis. A prolonged recession could force shelving of elimination plans in many countries and jeopardize the fragile progress made in malaria control.

Conclusions

The funds committed to malaria control from international sources have increased substantially, from around US$ 0.3 billion in 2003 to US$ 1.7 billion in 2009. The massive increase is due primarily to the emergence of the Global Fund and greater commitments to malaria control by the United States President's Malaria Initiative, UNITAID, the World Bank and a range of bilateral agencies.

Disbursements to malaria-endemic countries are less than the amounts committed; about US$ 0.65 billion were disbursed to malaria-endemic countries in 2007, the latest year for which comprehensive data are available. Approximately 80% of funds disbursed were targeted to the WHO African Region, which accounts for about 30% of the population at risk and 90% of global cases and deaths. The South-East Asia Region received the least money per person at risk for malaria and saw the smallest increase in disbursements from external financing between 2000 and 2007.

Contributions from national governments are more difficult to establish. Domestic financing for malaria has increased in many countries in all regions, although there may have been decreases between 2007 and 2008 in two regions, and there was a steady decrease in the South-East Asia Region between 2005 and 2008.

References

1. *The global malaria action plan*. Geneva, World Health Organization, Roll Back Malaria, 2008. http://www.rollbackmalaria.org/gmap.

2. Ravishankar N et al. Financing of global health: tracking development assistance for health from 1990 to 2007. *Lancet*, 2009, 373:2113–2124.

3. Health Metrics and Evaluation. Seattle, Washington, University of Washington. www.healthmetricsandevaluation.org.

4. Kiszewski A et al. A global index representing the stability of malaria transmission. *American Journal of Tropical Medicine and Hygiene*, 2004, 70:486–498.

5. Snow RW et al. International funding for malaria control in relation to populations at risk of stable *Plasmodium falciparum* transmission. *PLoS Medicine*, 2008, 5:e142. doi: 10.1371/journal.pmed.0050142.

6. *Working with communities to save lives in Africa. The President's Malaria Initiative, third annual report*. Washington DC, United States Agency for International Development, 2009. www.fightingmalaria.gov/resources/reports/pmi_annual_report09.pdf.

---

8 Large reductions in mortality among children under 5 years were observed on Bioko Island after intensified vector control and improved access to treatment, but such success has not yet been reported elsewhere in Equatorial Guinea.

31 high-burden countries

ANGOLA

Angola had an estimated 3.9 million cases of malaria in 2006. Transmission occurs all year round, with greater seasonality in the south. In 2008, 77% of the 3 432 424 suspected malaria cases were parasitologically tested. No adequate historical data were available to identify changes in the number of confirmed outpatient cases, but inpatient malaria cases and deaths in 2008 have decreased by about 52% and 42%, respectively, from the average of 2001–2006. It is not clear, however, if this is a true decrease, as there was no report on the completeness of data. Implementation of IRS, which began in 2005, continued in selected districts, covering 133 687 households and protecting over 736 000 people at risk (4%). The programme delivered 3.8 million LLINs during 2006 and 2008, adequate to cover 45% of the 16 million people at risk. In the 2006–2007 survey, 33% of households had a mosquito net, but only 18% of children slept under an ITN. The programme delivered over 2 million ACT treatment courses in 2007 and 2.3 million in 2008, enough to treat 69% of reported malaria cases. Funding increased from US$ 16 million in 2004 to over US$ 36 million in 2007, financed by the government, the Global Fund, United Nations agencies, the World Bank, bilateral agencies and others.

I.   EPIDEMIOLOGICAL PROFILE

Population, endemicity and malaria burden

Population (in thousands)	2008	%
All age groups	18 021	
< 5 years	3 170	18
≥ 5 years	14 850	82

Population by malaria endemicity (in thousands)	2008	%
High transmission ≥ 1/1000	18 021	100
Low transmission (0–1/1000)	0	0
Malaria-free (0 cases)	0	0
Rural population	7 795	43

Vector and parasite profiles

Major *Anopheles* species	*gambiae, arabiensis, funestus, coustani, flavicosta, melas, nili, paludis, pharoensis*
Plasmodium species	*falciparum, vivax*

Stratification of burden (reported cases, per 1000)

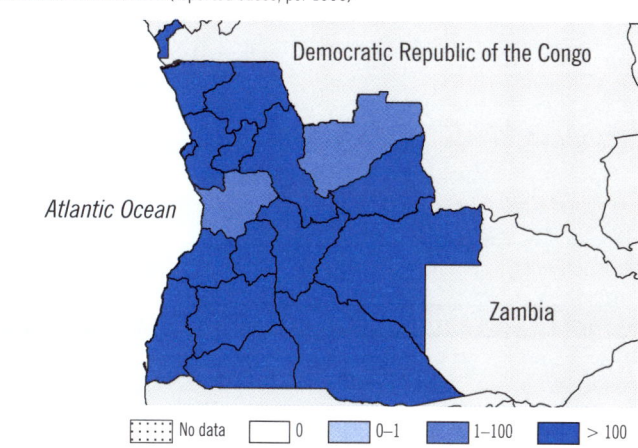

No data | 0 | 0–1 | 1–100 | > 100

Trends in malaria morbidity and mortality

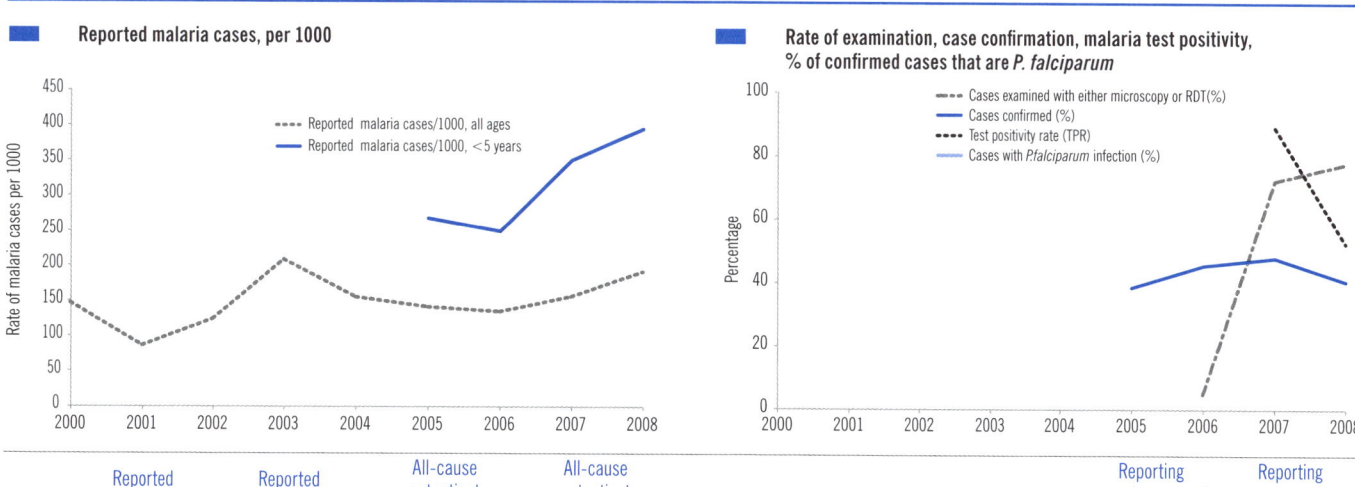

■ Reported malaria cases, per 1000

- - - Reported malaria cases/1000, all ages
— Reported malaria cases/1000, <5 years

■ Rate of examination, case confirmation, malaria test positivity, % of confirmed cases that are *P. falciparum*

- - - Cases examined with either microscopy or RDT(%)
— Cases confirmed (%)
····· Test positivity rate (TPR)
— Cases with *P.falciparum* infection (%)

Year	Reported malaria cases, all ages	Reported malaria cases, < 5 years	All-cause outpatient consultations, all ages	All-cause outpatient consultations, < 5 years	Examined	Positive	*P. falciparum*	Reporting completeness of outpatient health facilities (%)	Reporting completeness of districts (%)
2000	2 080 348		2 585 804						
2001	1 249 767		1 971 655						
2002	1 862 662		2 919 857						
2003	3 246 258		4 293 505						
2004	2 489 170		3 829 317						
2005	2 329 316	815 314	3 608 468			889 572			
2006	2 283 097	770 639	3 833 556		106 801	1 029 198			
2007	2 726 530	1 097 783	4 170 770		1 964 879	1 295 535			
2008	3 432 424	1 246 884	8 617 884	2 710 349	2 659 344	1 377 992			

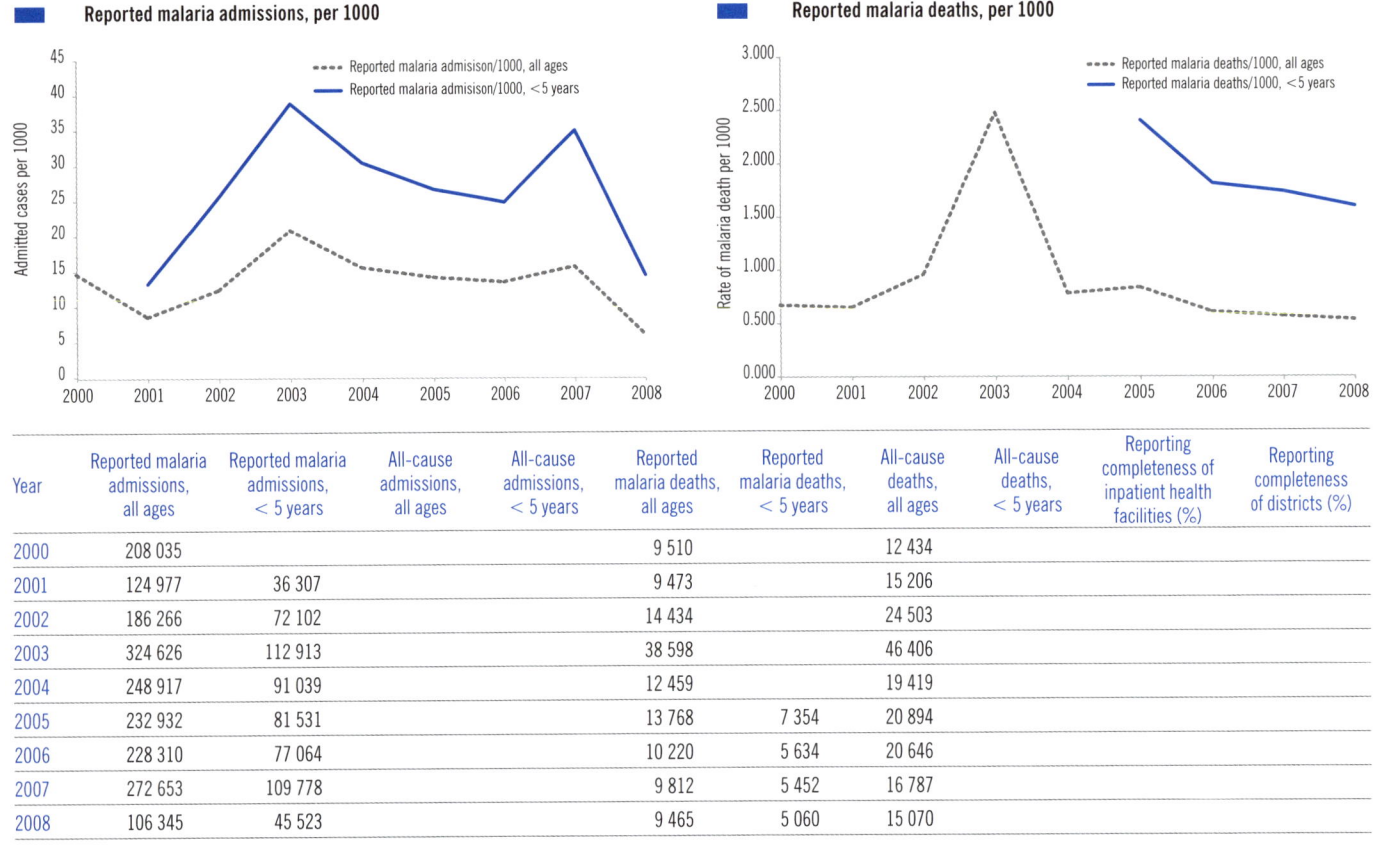

Reported malaria admissions, per 1000

- Reported malaria admission/1000, all ages
- Reported malaria admission/1000, <5 years

Reported malaria deaths, per 1000

- Reported malaria deaths/1000, all ages
- Reported malaria deaths/1000, <5 years

Year	Reported malaria admissions, all ages	Reported malaria admissions, < 5 years	All-cause admissions, all ages	All-cause admissions, < 5 years	Reported malaria deaths, all ages	Reported malaria deaths, < 5 years	All-cause deaths, all ages	All-cause deaths, < 5 years	Reporting completeness of inpatient health facilities (%)	Reporting completeness of districts (%)
2000	208 035				9 510		12 434			
2001	124 977	36 307			9 473		15 206			
2002	186 266	72 102			14 434		24 503			
2003	324 626	112 913			38 598		46 406			
2004	248 917	91 039			12 459		19 419			
2005	232 932	81 531			13 768	7 354	20 894			
2006	228 310	77 064			10 220	5 634	20 646			
2007	272 653	109 778			9 812	5 452	16 787			
2008	106 345	45 523			9 465	5 060	15 070			

II.   INTERVENTION POLICIES AND STRATEGIES

Intervention	WHO-RECOMMENDED POLICIES / STRATEGIES	Yes or No	Year adopted	OPTIONAL POLICIES / STRATEGIES	Yes or No	Year adoped
Insecticide-treated nets (ITN)	Distribution of ITN/LLINs – Free	Yes	2001	Distribution – Antenatal care	Yes	2001
	Targeting all age groups	No	–	Distribution – EPI routine and campaign	Yes	2005
				Targeting children < 5 years and pregnant women	Yes	2000
				ITN distribution is subsidized	Yes	2005
Indoor residual spraying (IRS)	IRS is a primary vector control intervention	Yes	2003	Insecticide-resistance management implemented	Yes	2005
	DDT is used for IRS (public health) only	No	–	Where IRS is conducted, other options are also implemented, e.g. ITN	Yes	2003
				IRS is used for prevention and control of epidemics	Yes	2003
Intermittent preventive treatment (IPT)	IPT used to prevent malaria during pregnancy	Yes	2005			
Case management	Oral artemisinin monotherapies banned (prohibited from registration or removed from the system)	Yes	2004	Parasitological confirmation for patients ≥ 5 years only	No	–
	Parasitological confirmation for patients of all ages	Yes	2001	Malaria diagnosis is free of charge in the public sector	Yes	2002
	ACT is free of charge for < 5 years old in the public sector	Yes	2005	ACT is free of charge for patients ≥ 5 years in the public sector	Yes	2006
	Diagnosis of malaria of inpatients is based on parasitological confirmation	Yes	2005	ACT is delivered at community level through community agents (beyond the health facilities)	No	–
	Pre-referral treatment with quinine or artemether IM or artesunate suppositories	Yes	2004	Uncomplicated malaria cases are admitted	No	–
	Oversight regulation of case management in the private sectors	No	–			
	RDTs used at community level	No	–			

Antimalarial policy	Type of medicine	Year adopted	Study year	Results of therapeutic efficacy tests				Percentiles: 25%	75%
				No. of studies	Median	Minimum	Maximum		
First-line treatment of *P. falciparum* (unconfirmed)	AL	2006	2004-2004	2	1.1	0	2.3	0	2.3
First-line treatment of *P. falciparum* (confirmed)	AL	2006	2004-2004	2	1.1	0	2.3	0	2.3
Treatment failure of *P. falciparum*	QN(7d)	2006							
Treatment of severe malaria	QN(7d)	2006							
Treatment of *P. vivax*	–	–							

III. IMPLEMENTING MALARIA CONTROL

Coverage of ITN: survey data

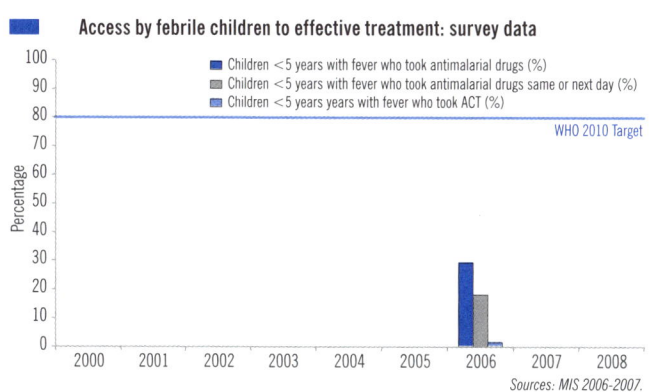

Sources: MIS 2006-2007.

Coverage of IRS and ITN: programme data

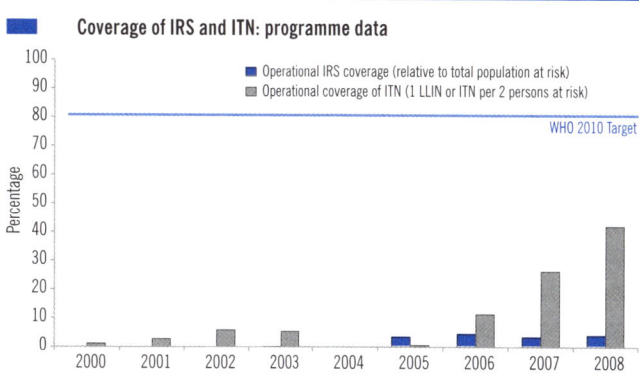

Access by febrile children to effective treatment: survey data

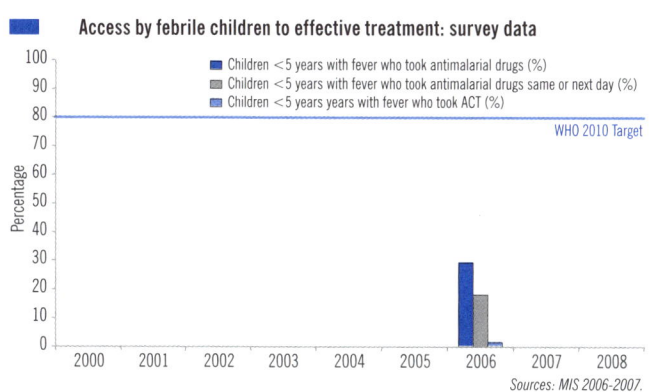

Sources: MIS 2006-2007.

Access to effective treatment: programme data

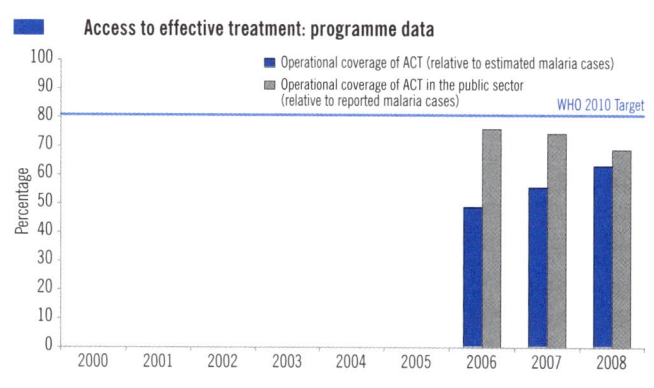

Year	Pregnant women who slept under any net (%)	Pregnant women who slept under an ITN (%)	Children < 5 years with fever (%)	Febrile children < 5 years who sought treatment in HF (%)	Number of households protected by IRS	Number of people protected by IRS	Number of ITNs and/or LLINs	Number of 1st-line treatment courses received	Number of ACT treatment courses received
2000							85 000		
2001							204 600		
2002							450 000		
2003						30 000	430 000		
2004									
2005					100 000	590 000	45 889		
2006		22	–	–	115 000	780 257	984 760	1 700 000	1 736 200
2007			–	–	110 826	612 776	1 495 165	2 031 760	2 031 760
2008			–	–	133 687	736 231	1 471 200	2 363 970	2 363 970

IV. FINANCING MALARIA CONTROL

Governmental and external financing

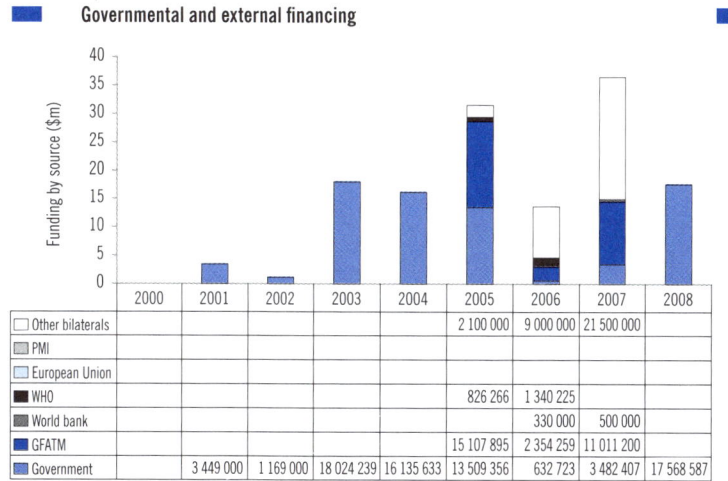

	2000	2001	2002	2003	2004	2005	2006	2007	2008
Other bilaterals						2 100 000	9 000 000	21 500 000	
PMI									
European Union									
WHO						826 266	1 340 225		
World bank							330 000	500 000	
GFATM						15 107 895	2 354 259	11 011 200	
Government		3 449 000	1 169 000	18 024 239	16 135 633	13 509 356	632 723	3 482 407	17 568 587

Breakdown of expenditure by intervention in 2008

No data

V. SOURCE OF INFORMATION

PROGRAMME DATA		SURVEY AND OTHER DATA	
Reported cases	Surveillance data	Insecticide-treated nets (ITN)	MIS 2006-07, MIS 2007
Operational coverage of ITNs, IRS and access to medicines	Programme report	Treatment	MIS 2006-07, MIS 2007
Financial data	Programme report	Use of health services	MICS 2001

BANGLADESH

A total of 50.6 million people are at risk for malaria, and more than 95% of all the malaria cases in the country are reported from 13 highly endemic districts, affecting 11 million people. The three Hill Tract Districts (Bandarban, Khagrachari and Rangamati) and the Cox's Bazar district report more than 80% of all malaria cases and deaths every year, with perennial transmission in two peaks, before (March–May) and after the monsoon (September–November). There is no evidence of a systematic decrease in the number of reported cases between 2001 and 2008, and most reported cases are unconfirmed. Of those that are confirmed, more than 70% are due to *P. falciparum*. A total of 154 malaria deaths were reported in 2008, fewer than had been reported in the previous 8 years. Although IRS is the principal mosquito control method, applied selectively in high-risk areas, no data were made available by the programme. The programme delivered nearly 1.9 million ITNs in 2008, of which two thirds were LLINs. The programme adopted ACT as first-line treatment for malaria in 2004 and delivered 225 270 full treatment courses in 2008, enough to treat all confirmed cases. Total financing for malaria in 2008 was approximately US$ 11 million, the main sources being the Government (US$ 528 000), the Global Fund (US$ 9.6 million), the World Bank (US$ 700 000) and WHO (US$ 220 000).

I.   EPIDEMIOLOGICAL PROFILE

Population, endemicity and malaria burden

Population (in thousands)	2008	%
All age groups	160 000	
< 5 years	16 710	10
≥ 5 years	143 290	90

Population by malaria endemicity (in thousands)	2008	
High transmission ≥ 1/1000	11 649	7
Low transmission (0–1/1000)	42 150	26
Malaria-free (0 cases)	106 201	66
Rural population	116 688	73

Vector and parasite profiles

Major *Anopheles* species	*dirus, minimus, philippinensis, sundaicus*
Plasmodium species	*falciparum, vivax*

Stratification of burden (reported cases, per 1000)

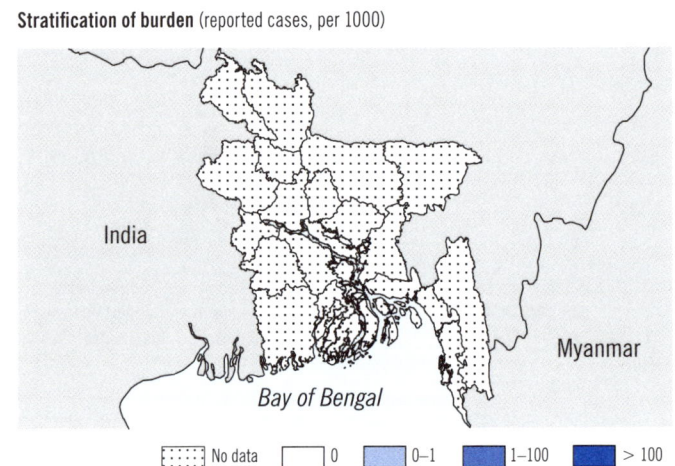

Trends in malaria morbidity and mortality

Reported malaria cases, per 1000

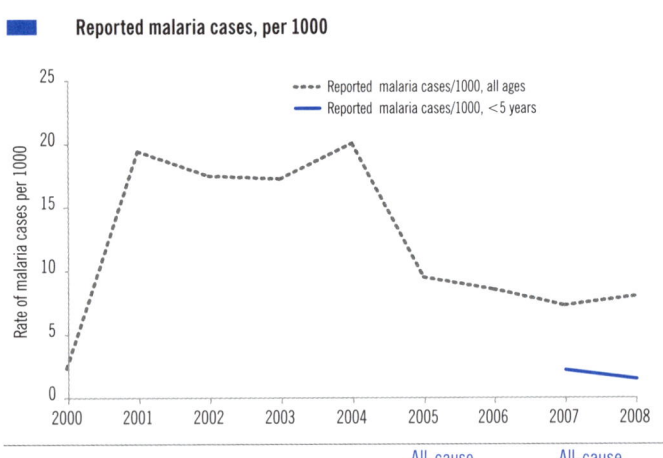

Rate of examination, case confirmation, malaria test positivity, % of confirmed cases that are *P. falciparum*

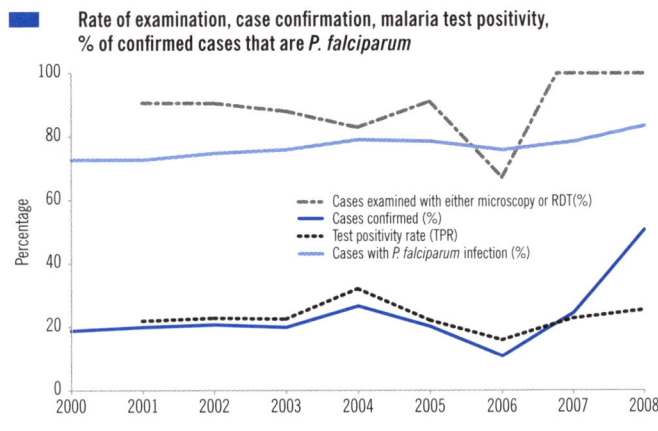

Year	Reported malaria cases, all ages	Reported malaria cases, < 5 years	All-cause outpatient consultations, all ages	All-cause outpatient consultations, < 5 years	Examined	Positive	P. falciparum	Reporting completeness of outpatient health facilities (%)	Reporting completeness of districts (%)
2000	320 011					54 223	39 272		
2001	2 776 477				250 258	54 216	39 274		
2002	2 543 782				275 987	62 269	46 418		
2003	2 554 223				245 258	54 654	41 356		
2004	3 016 262				185 215	58 894	46 402		
2005	1 445 831				220 025	48 121	37 679		
2006	1 320 581				209 991	32 857	24 828		
2007	1 140 424	35 698			270 137	59 857	46 803	100*	100*
2008	1 275 192	23 450			442 506	84 590	70 331	100*	100*

* : This information relates to 13 high endemic districts contributing about 95% of total malaria in the country.

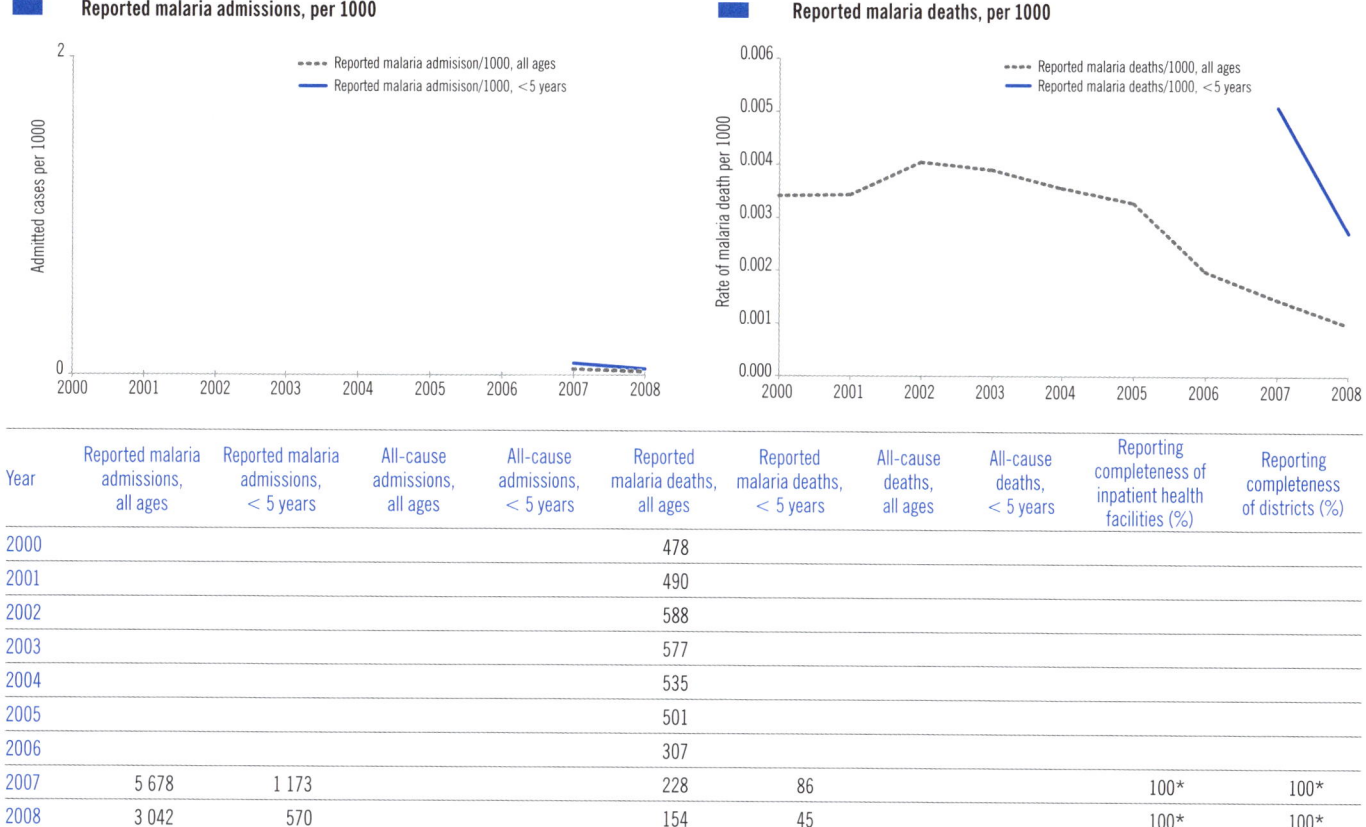

Reported malaria admissions, per 1000

Reported malaria admisison/1000, all ages
Reported malaria admisison/1000, <5 years

Reported malaria deaths, per 1000

Reported malaria deaths/1000, all ages
Reported malaria deaths/1000, <5 years

Year	Reported malaria admissions, all ages	Reported malaria admissions, < 5 years	All-cause admissions, all ages	All-cause admissions, < 5 years	Reported malaria deaths, all ages	Reported malaria deaths, < 5 years	All-cause deaths, all ages	All-cause deaths, < 5 years	Reporting completeness of inpatient health facilities (%)	Reporting completeness of districts (%)
2000					478					
2001					490					
2002					588					
2003					577					
2004					535					
2005					501					
2006					307					
2007	5 678	1 173			228	86			100*	100*
2008	3 042	570			154	45			100*	100*

* : This information relates to 13 high endemic districts contributing about 98% of total malaria in the country

II. INTERVENTION POLICIES AND STRATEGIES

Intervention	WHO-RECOMMENDED POLICIES / STRATEGIES	Yes or No	Year adopted	OPTIONAL POLICIES / STRATEGIES	Yes or No	Year adoped
Insecticide-treated nets (ITN)	Distribution of ITN/LLINs — Free	Yes	2008	Distribution — Antenatal care	No	–
	Targeting all age groups	Yes	2000	Distribution — EPI routine and campaign	No	–
				Targeting children < 5 years and pregnant women	Yes	2000
				ITN distribution is subsidized	No	–
Indoor residual spraying (IRS)	IRS is a primary vector control intervention	No	–	Insecticide-resistance management implemented	No	–
	DDT is used for IRS (public health) only	No	–	Where IRS is conducted, other options are also implemented, e.g. ITN	Yes	2000
				IRS is used for prevention and control of epidemics	Yes	2000
Intermittent preventive treatment (IPT)	IPT used to prevent malaria during pregnancy	No	–			
Case management	Oral artemisinin monotherapies banned (prohibited from registration or removed from the system)	Yes	2004	Parasitological confirmation for patients ≥ 5 years only	No	–
	Parasitological confirmation for patients of all ages	Yes	2009	Malaria diagnosis is free of charge in the public sector	Yes	2000
	ACT is free of charge for < 5 years old in the public sector	Yes	2004	ACT is free of charge for patients ≥ 5 years in the public sector	Yes	2004
	Diagnosis of malaria of inpatients is based on parasitological confirmation	Yes	2000	ACT is delivered at community level through community agents (beyond the health facilities)	Yes	2008
	Pre-referral treatment with quinine or artemether IM or artesunate suppositories	No	–	Uncomplicated malaria cases are admitted	No	–
	Oversight regulation of case management in the private sectors	No	–			
	RDTs used at community level	Yes	2008			

Antimalarial policy	Type of medicine	Year adopted	Results of therapeutic efficacy tests						
			Study year	No. of studies	Median	Minimum	Maximum	Percentiles: 25%	75%
First-line treatment of P. falciparum (unconfirmed)	CQ+PQ	2004							
First-line treatment of P. falciparum (confirmed)	AL	2004	2003–2007	2	0.45	0	0.899	0	0.899
Treatment failure of P. falciparum	QN+D, QN+T, QN+T or D	2004							
Treatment of severe malaria	AM, QN	2004							
Treatment of P. vivax	CQ+PQ(14d)	2004							

III. IMPLEMENTING MALARIA CONTROL

Coverage of ITN: survey data

No data

Coverage of IRS and ITN: programme data

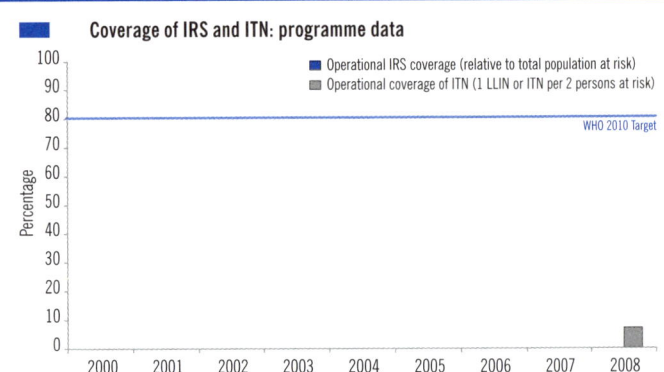

Access by febrile children to effective treatment: survey data

No data

Access to effective treatment: programme data

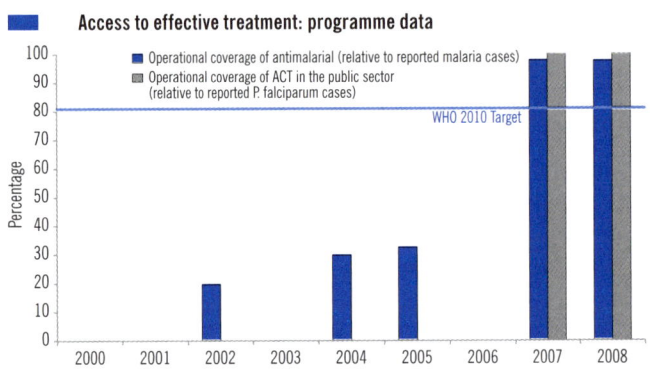

Year	Pregnant women who slept under any net (%)	Pregnant women who slept under an ITN (%)	Children < 5 years with fever (%)	Febrile children < 5 years who sought treatment in HF (%)	Number of households protected by IRS	Number of people protected by IRS	Number of ITNs and/or LLINs	Number of 1st-line treatment courses received	Number of ACT treatment courses received
2000									
2001									
2002									60 000	
2003									
2004									66 615	
2005									78 401	
2006								2 200	
2007									241 398	114 990
2008							1 863 940	164 394	225 270

IV. FINANCING MALARIA CONTROL

Governmental and external financing

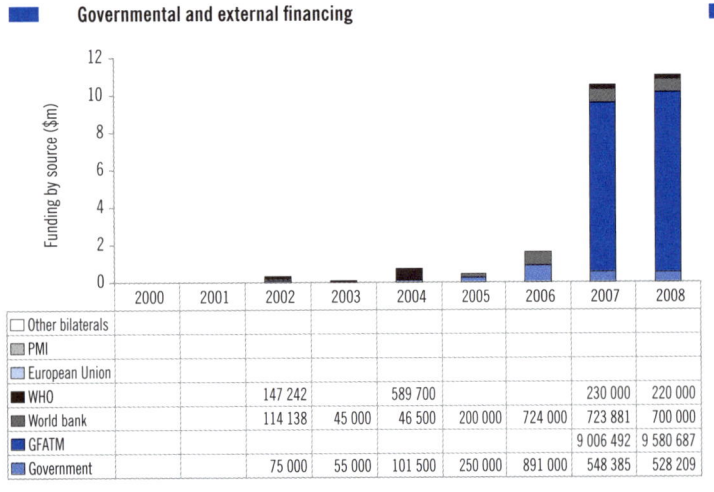

	2000	2001	2002	2003	2004	2005	2006	2007	2008
Other bilaterals									
PMI									
European Union									
WHO			147 242		589 700			230 000	220 000
World bank			114 138	45 000	46 500	200 000	724 000	723 881	700 000
GFATM								9 006 492	9 580 687
Government			75 000	55 000	101 500	250 000	891 000	548 385	528 209

Breakdown of expenditure by intervention in 2008

No data

V. SOURCE OF INFORMATION

PROGRAMME DATA		SURVEY AND OTHER DATA	
Reported cases	Surveillance data	Insecticide-treated nets (ITN)	No surveys
Operational coverage of ITNs, IRS and access to medicines	Programme report	Treatment	No surveys
Financial data	Programme report	Use of health services	DHS 2004

BRAZIL

Transmission occurs mainly in the Amazon region, where 10–15% of the population is at risk, accounting for 60% of reported cases. Brazil accounts for over half the total estimated number of cases in the Region of the Americas. The number of reported cases rose from 388 303 in 2001 to 606 067 in 2005 but decreased to 315 642 in 2008. All reported malaria cases are laboratory confirmed, and approximately 15% of cases in 2008 were due to *P. falciparum*. Although IRS is the principal method of mosquito control, applied in high-risk areas, national data were not made available. Only a limited number of ITNs (10 000) were delivered in 2007. The supply of first-line antimalarial drugs is apparently sufficient to treat all reported cases, and 45 717 ACT doses were distributed in 2008, adequate to treat all *P. falciparum* cases. Funding for malaria control increased to more than US$ 106 million in 2008, provided almost exclusively by the Government.

I. EPIDEMIOLOGICAL PROFILE

Population, endemicity and malaria burden

Population (in thousands)	2008	%
All age groups	191 972	
< 5 years	16 125	8
≥ 5 years	175 846	92

Population by malaria endemicity (in thousands)	2008	%
High transmission ≥ 1/1000	9 262	5
Low transmission (0–1/1000)	7 577	4
Malaria-free (0 cases)	175 133	91
Rural population	27 475	14

Vector and parasite profiles

Major *Anopheles* species	*albimanus, albitarsis, darlingi, nuneztovari*
Plasmodium species	*falciparum, vivax*

Stratification of burden (reported cases, per 1000)

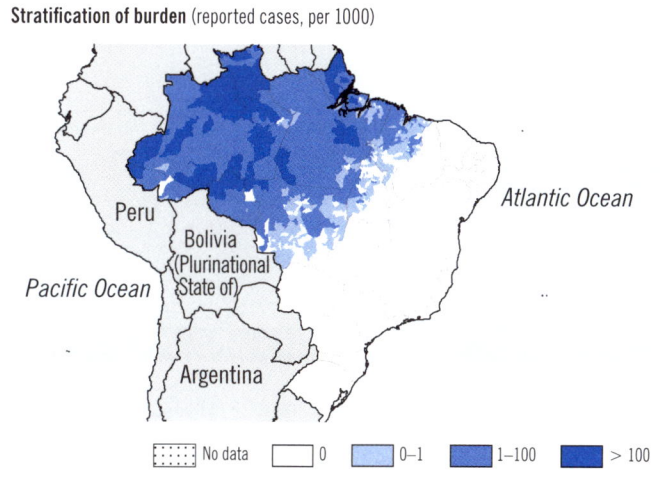

Legend: No data | 0 | 0–1 | 1–100 | > 100

Trends in malaria morbidity and mortality

Reported malaria cases, per 1000

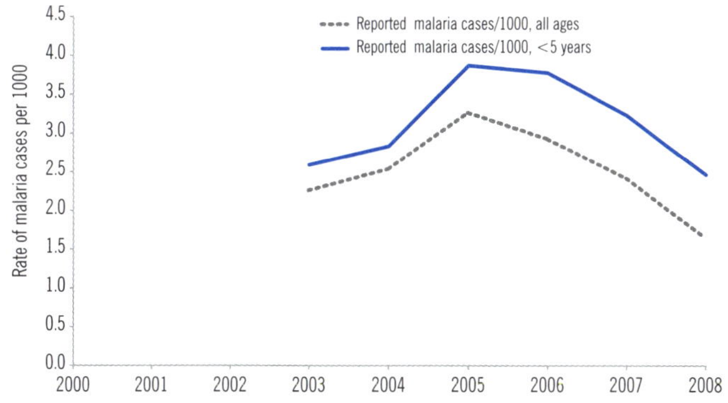

- ---- Reported malaria cases/1000, all ages
- —— Reported malaria cases/1000, < 5 years

Rate of examination, case confirmation, malaria test positivity, % of confirmed cases that are *P. falciparum*

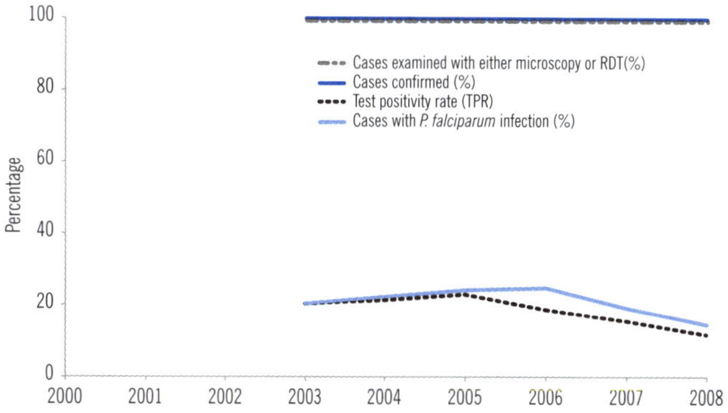

- ---- Cases examined with either microscopy or RDT(%)
- —— Cases confirmed (%)
- ···· Test positivity rate (TPR)
- —— Cases with *P. falciparum* infection (%)

Year	Reported malaria cases, all ages	Reported malaria cases, < 5 years	All-cause outpatient consultations, all ages	All-cause outpatient consultations, < 5 years	Examined	Positive	*P. falciparum*	Reporting completeness of outpatient health facilities (%)	Reporting completeness of districts (%)
2000									
2001									
2002									
2003	408 765	45 704	1969 314 789		2 008 764	408 765	83 765		
2004	464 901	49 688	1997 751 427		2 194 780	464 901	104 376		
2005	606 067	67 180	2192 807 385		2 660 539	606 067	147 150		
2006	549 469	64 358	2404 857 167		2 959 489	549 469	136 868		
2007	458 041	53 718	2699 038 287		2 983 553	458 041	88 249		
2008	315 642	39 826	2935 995 890		2 721 017	315 642	46 289		

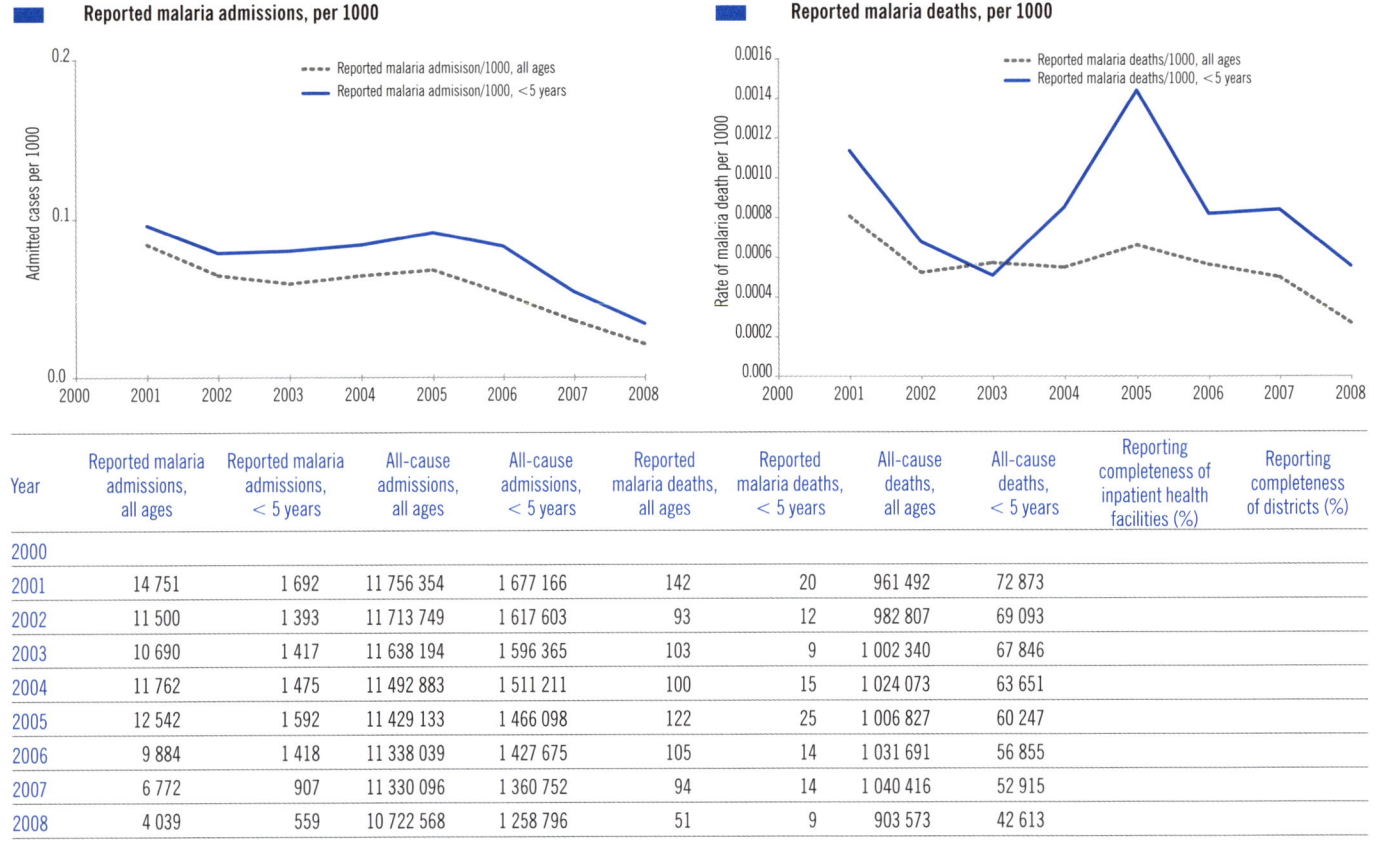

Reported malaria admissions, per 1000

- - - - Reported malaria admission/1000, all ages
——— Reported malaria admission/1000, <5 years

Reported malaria deaths, per 1000

- - - - Reported malaria deaths/1000, all ages
——— Reported malaria deaths/1000, <5 years

Year	Reported malaria admissions, all ages	Reported malaria admissions, < 5 years	All-cause admissions, all ages	All-cause admissions, < 5 years	Reported malaria deaths, all ages	Reported malaria deaths, < 5 years	All-cause deaths, all ages	All-cause deaths, < 5 years	Reporting completeness of inpatient health facilities (%)	Reporting completeness of districts (%)
2000										
2001	14 751	1 692	11 756 354	1 677 166	142	20	961 492	72 873		
2002	11 500	1 393	11 713 749	1 617 603	93	12	982 807	69 093		
2003	10 690	1 417	11 638 194	1 596 365	103	9	1 002 340	67 846		
2004	11 762	1 475	11 492 883	1 511 211	100	15	1 024 073	63 651		
2005	12 542	1 592	11 429 133	1 466 098	122	25	1 006 827	60 247		
2006	9 884	1 418	11 338 039	1 427 675	105	14	1 031 691	56 855		
2007	6 772	907	11 330 096	1 360 752	94	14	1 040 416	52 915		
2008	4 039	559	10 722 568	1 258 796	51	9	903 573	42 613		

II. INTERVENTION POLICIES AND STRATEGIES

Intervention	WHO-RECOMMENDED POLICIES / STRATEGIES	Yes or No	Year adopted	OPTIONAL POLICIES / STRATEGIES	Yes or No	Year adoped
Insecticide-treated nets (ITN)	Distribution of ITN/LLINs — Free	Yes	2007	Distribution — Antenatal care	No	–
	Targeting all age groups	Yes	2007	Distribution — EPI routine and campaign	No	–
				Targeting children < 5 years and pregnant women	No	–
				ITN distribution is subsidized	No	–
Indoor residual spraying (IRS)	IRS is a primary vector control intervention	Yes	1958	Insecticide-resistance management implemented	Yes	2004
	DDT is used for IRS (public health) only	No	–	Where IRS is conducted, other options are also implemented, e.g. ITN	Yes	–
				IRS is used for prevention and control of epidemics	Yes	
Intermittent preventive treatment (IPT)	IPT used to prevent malaria during pregnancy	No	–			
Case management	Oral artemisinin monotherapies banned (prohibited from registration or removed from the system)	Yes	2007	Parasitological confirmation for patients ≥ 5 years only	No	–
	Parasitological confirmation for patients of all ages	Yes	1972	Malaria diagnosis is free of charge in the public sector	Yes	1972
	ACT is free of charge for < 5 years old in the public sector	Yes	2006	ACT is free of charge for patients ≥ 5 years in the public sector	Yes	2006
	Diagnosis of malaria of inpatients is based on parasitological confirmation	Yes	1972	ACT is delivered at community level through community agents (beyond the health facilities)	Yes	2006
	Pre-referral treatment with quinine or artemether IM or artesunate suppositories	No	–	Uncomplicated malaria cases are admitted	Yes	–
	Oversight regulation of case management in the private sectors	No	–			
	RDTs used at community level	Yes	2007			

Antimalarial policy	Type of medicine	Year adopted	Study year	No. of studies	Median	Minimum	Maximum	Percentiles: 25%	75%
					Results of therapeutic efficacy tests				
First-line treatment of *P. falciparum* (unconfirmed)	–	–							
First-line treatment of *P. falciparum* (confirmed)	AL or AS+MQ	2006							
Treatment failure of *P. falciparum*	–	–							
Treatment of severe malaria	QN, AM, AS	2006							
Treatment of *P. vivax*	CQ+PQ(7d)	2006							

III. IMPLEMENTING MALARIA CONTROL

Coverage of ITN: survey data

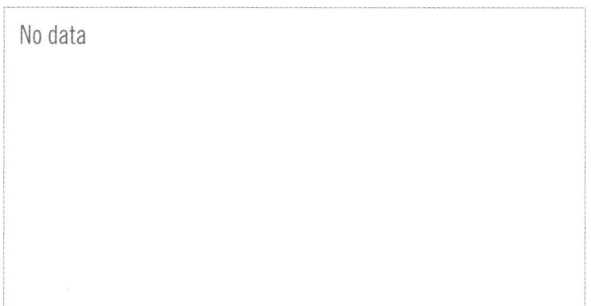

No data

Coverage of IRS and ITN: programme data

No data

Access by febrile children to effective treatment: survey data

No data

Access to effective treatment: programme data

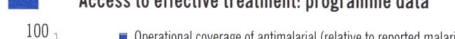
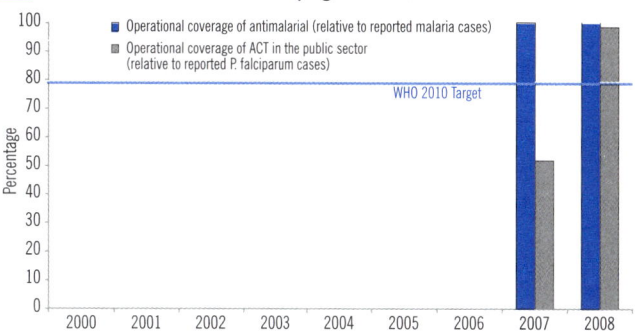

Year	Pregnant women who slept under any net (%)	Pregnant women who slept under an ITN (%)	Children < 5 years with fever (%)	Febrile children < 5 years who sought treatment in HF (%)	Number of households protected by IRS	Number of people protected by IRS	Number of ITNs and/or LLINs	Number of 1st-line treatment courses received	Number of ACT treatment courses received
2000									
2001									
2002									
2003									
2004									
2005									
2006									
2007								10 000	459 513	45 918
2008								347 086	45 717

IV. FINANCING MALARIA CONTROL

Governmental and external financing

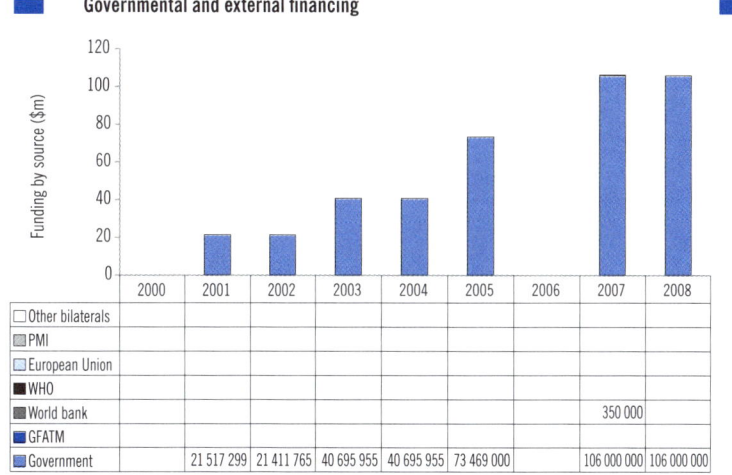

	2000	2001	2002	2003	2004	2005	2006	2007	2008
☐ Other bilaterals									
▨ PMI									
☐ European Union									
■ WHO									
■ World bank								350 000	
■ GFATM									
■ Government		21 517 299	21 411 765	40 695 955	40 695 955	73 469 000		106 000 000	106 000 000

Breakdown of expenditure by intervention in 2008

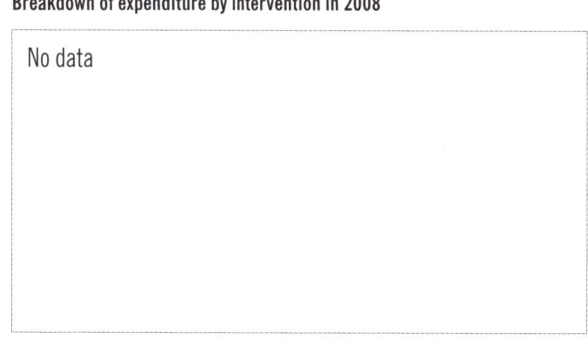

No data

V. SOURCE OF INFORMATION

PROGRAMME DATA		SURVEY AND OTHER DATA	
Reported cases	Surveillance data	Insecticide-treated nets (ITN)	No surveys
Operational coverage of ITNs, IRS and access to medicines	Programme report	Treatment	No surveys
Financial data	Programme report	Use of health services	DHS 1996

BURKINA FASO

Malaria is more intense in the southern third of the country, occurring seasonally between December and April. Almost all cases are caused by *P. falciparum*. Only about 5% of suspected cases are parasitologically tested. The numbers of reported cases and deaths have increased consistently in recent years, but it is not known if this reflects a real increase in malaria burden or improved reporting. The national malaria programme distributed approximately 1 160 747 LLINs during 2006–2008, far below the number needed to protect the 14 million people at risk. IRS is not a national policy. The national malaria control programme reported delivery of about 2.4 million ACT treatment courses in 2008, enough to cover 63% of 3.8 million suspected malaria cases in need of treatment. Funding increased from US$ 3 million in 2004 to over US$ 116 million in 2008, financed mainly by the Global Fund, United Nations agencies and a limited Government budget.

I. EPIDEMIOLOGICAL PROFILE

Population, endemicity and malaria burden

Population (in thousands)	2008	%
All age groups	15 234	
< 5 years	2 934	19
≥ 5 years	12 300	81

Population by malaria endemicity (in thousands)	2008	%
High transmission ≥ 1/1000	15 234	100
Low transmission (0–1/1000)	0	0
Malaria-free (0 cases)	0	0
Rural population	12 257	80

Vector and parasite profiles

Major *Anopheles* species	gambiae, arabiensis, funestus, brochieri, coustani, flavicosta, hancocki, nili, paludis, pharoensis
Plasmodium species	falciparum, vivax

Stratification of burden (reported cases, per 1000)

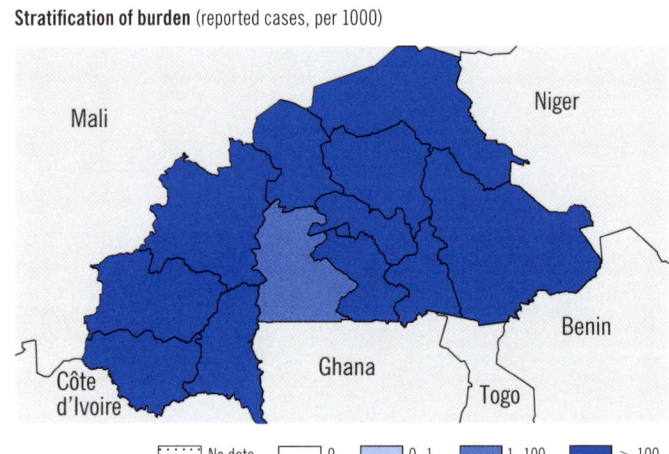

No data | 0 | 0–1 | 1–100 | > 100

Trends in malaria morbidity and mortality

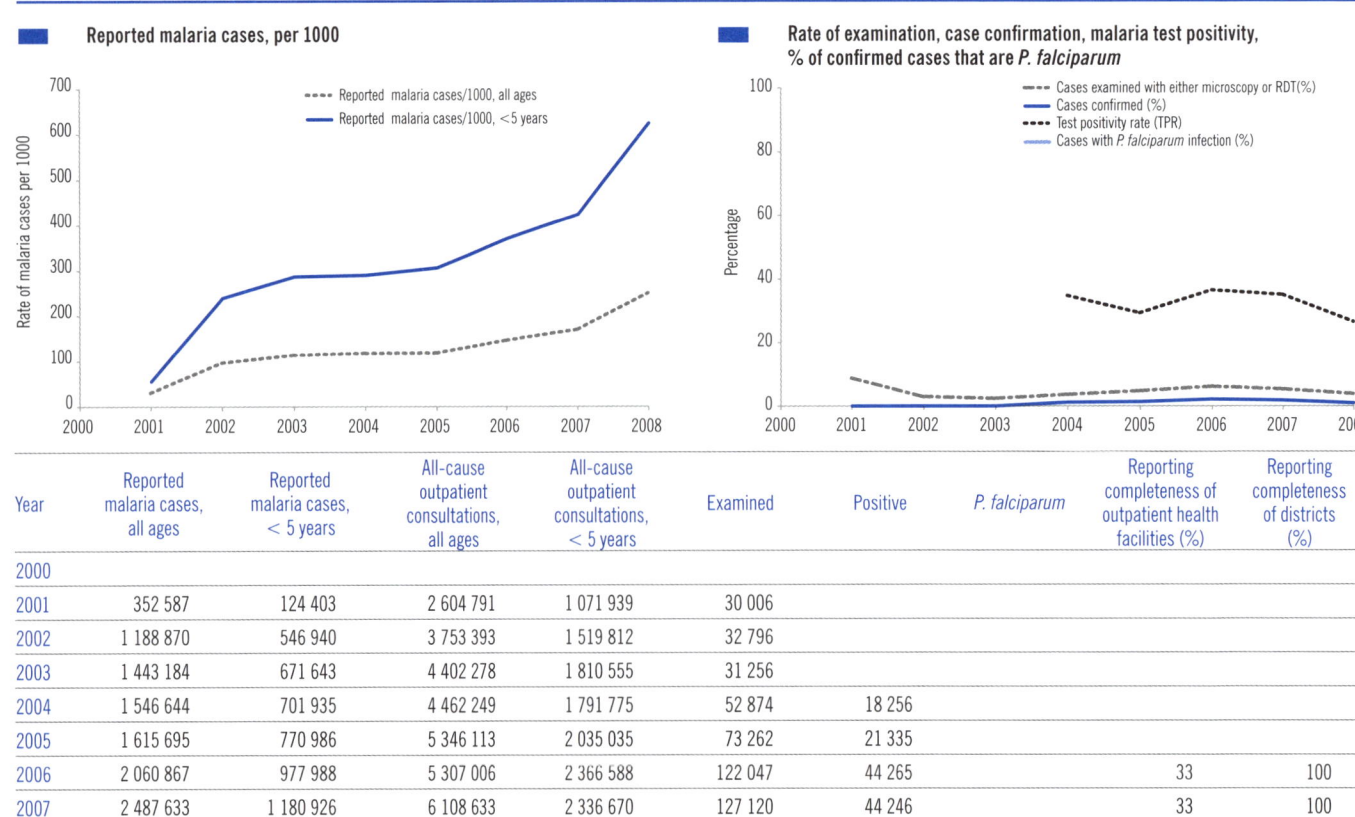

Reported malaria cases, per 1000
- Reported malaria cases/1000, all ages
- Reported malaria cases/1000, <5 years

Rate of examination, case confirmation, malaria test positivity, % of confirmed cases that are *P. falciparum*
- Cases examined with either microscopy or RDT(%)
- Cases confirmed (%)
- Test positivity rate (TPR)
- Cases with *P. falciparum* infection (%)

Year	Reported malaria cases, all ages	Reported malaria cases, < 5 years	All-cause outpatient consultations, all ages	All-cause outpatient consultations, < 5 years	Examined	Positive	*P. falciparum*	Reporting completeness of outpatient health facilities (%)	Reporting completeness of districts (%)
2000									
2001	352 587	124 403	2 604 791	1 071 939	30 006				
2002	1 188 870	546 940	3 753 393	1 519 812	32 796				
2003	1 443 184	671 643	4 402 278	1 810 555	31 256				
2004	1 546 644	701 935	4 462 249	1 791 775	52 874	18 256			
2005	1 615 695	770 986	5 346 113	2 035 035	73 262	21 335			
2006	2 060 867	977 988	5 307 006	2 366 588	122 047	44 265		33	100
2007	2 487 633	1 180 926	6 108 633	2 336 670	127 120	44 246		33	100
2008	3 790 238	1 834 699	7 533 885	2 972 878	138 414	36 514		33	100

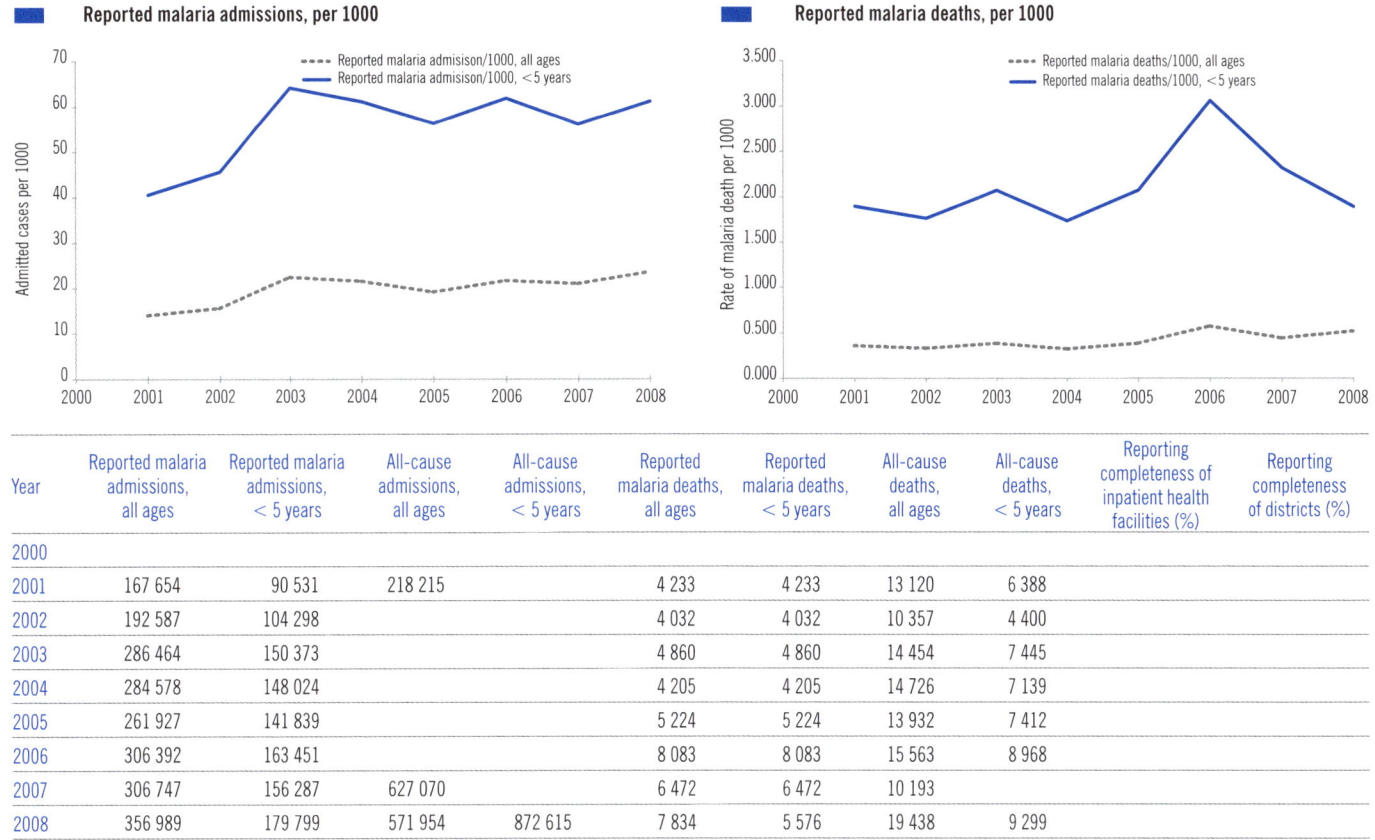

Reported malaria admissions, per 1000

- ····· Reported malaria admisison/1000, all ages
- —— Reported malaria admisison/1000, <5 years

Reported malaria deaths, per 1000

- ····· Reported malaria deaths/1000, all ages
- —— Reported malaria deaths/1000, <5 years

Year	Reported malaria admissions, all ages	Reported malaria admissions, < 5 years	All-cause admissions, all ages	All-cause admissions, < 5 years	Reported malaria deaths, all ages	Reported malaria deaths, < 5 years	All-cause deaths, all ages	All-cause deaths, < 5 years	Reporting completeness of inpatient health facilities (%)	Reporting completeness of districts (%)
2000										
2001	167 654	90 531	218 215		4 233	4 233	13 120	6 388		
2002	192 587	104 298			4 032	4 032	10 357	4 400		
2003	286 464	150 373			4 860	4 860	14 454	7 445		
2004	284 578	148 024			4 205	4 205	14 726	7 139		
2005	261 927	141 839			5 224	5 224	13 932	7 412		
2006	306 392	163 451			8 083	8 083	15 563	8 968		
2007	306 747	156 287	627 070		6 472	6 472	10 193			
2008	356 989	179 799	571 954	872 615	7 834	5 576	19 438	9 299		

II. INTERVENTION POLICIES AND STRATEGIES

Intervention	WHO-RECOMMENDED POLICIES / STRATEGIES	Yes or No	Year adopted	OPTIONAL POLICIES / STRATEGIES	Yes or No	Year adoped
Insecticide-treated nets (ITN)	Distribution of ITN/LLINs – Free	Yes	2007	Distribution – Antenatal care	Yes	2005
	Targeting all age groups	Yes	1998	Distribution – EPI routine and campaign	Yes	2005
				Targeting children < 5 years and pregnant women	Yes	2004
				ITN distribution is subsidized	Yes	2005
Indoor residual spraying (IRS)	IRS is a primary vector control intervention	No	–	Insecticide-resistance management implemented	Yes	1998
	DDT is used for IRS (public health) only	No	–	Where IRS is conducted, other options are also implemented, e.g. ITN	No	–
				IRS is used for prevention and control of epidemics	No	–
Intermittent preventive treatment (IPT)	IPT used to prevent malaria during pregnancy	Yes	2005			
Case management	Oral artemisinin monotherapies banned (prohibited from registration or removed from the system)	Yes	2008	Parasitological confirmation for patients ≥ 5 years only	No	–
	Parasitological confirmation for patients of all ages	Yes	1998	Malaria diagnosis is free of charge in the public sector	No	–
	ACT is free of charge for < 5 years old in the public sector	No	–	ACT is free of charge for patients ≥ 5 years in the public sector	No	–
	Diagnosis of malaria of inpatients is based on parasitological confirmation	No	–	ACT is delivered at community level through community agents (beyond the health facilities)	No	–
	Pre-referral treatment with quinine or artemether IM or artesunate suppositories	Yes	2005	Uncomplicated malaria cases are admitted	No	–
	Oversight regulation of case management in the private sectors	No	–			
	RDTs used at community level	No	–			

Antimalarial policy	Type of medicine	Year adopted	Study year	No. of studies	Median	Minimum	Maximum	Percentiles: 25%	75%
					Results of therapeutic efficacy tests				
First-line treatment of *P. falciparum* (unconfirmed)	AL, AS+AQ	–	2005–2007	3	3.4	1.9	12.3	1.9	12.3
First-line treatment of *P. falciparum* (confirmed)	AL, AS+AQ	–							
Treatment failure of *P. falciparum*	QN(7d)	–							
Treatment of severe malaria	QN(7d)	–							
Treatment of *P. vivax*	–	–							

III. IMPLEMENTING MALARIA CONTROL

Coverage of ITN: survey data

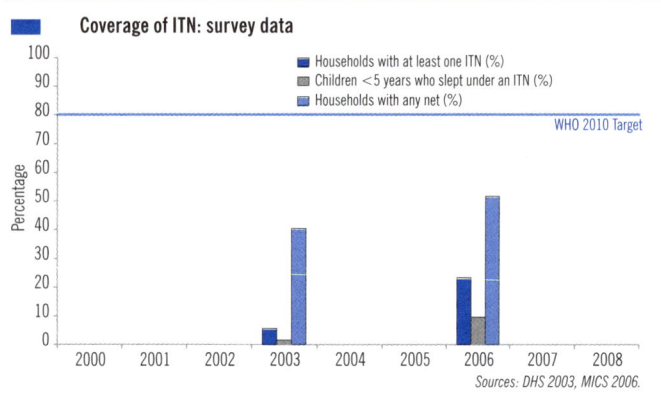

Sources: DHS 2003, MICS 2006.

Coverage of IRS and ITN: programme data

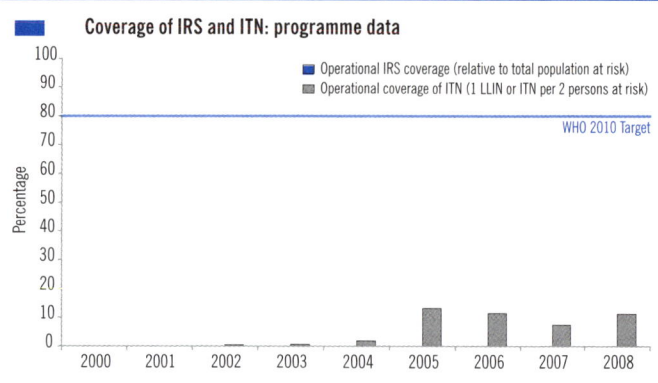

Access by febrile children to effective treatment: survey data

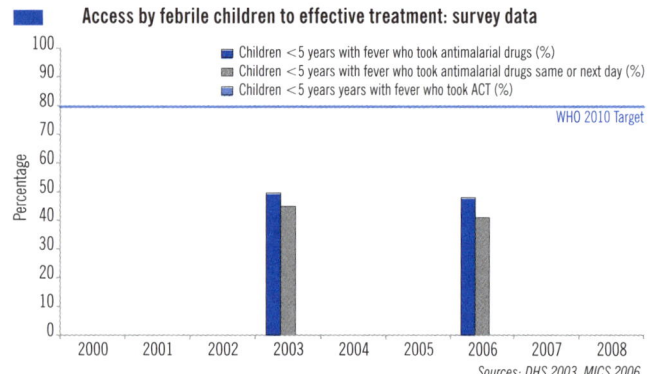

Sources: DHS 2003, MICS 2006.

Access to effective treatment: programme data

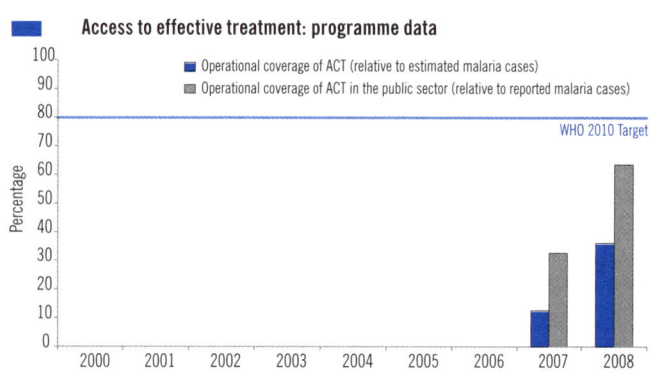

Year	Pregnant women who slept under any net (%)	Pregnant women who slept under an ITN (%)	Children < 5 years with fever (%)	Febrile children < 5 years who sought treatment in HF (%)	Number of households protected by IRS	Number of people protected by IRS	Number of ITNs and/or LLINs	Number of 1st-line treatment courses received	Number of ACT treatment courses received
2000									
2001							5 396	3 643 062	
2002							28 252	5 621 064	
2003	24	3	–	–			41 515	6 084 223	
2004							125 000	5 191 738	
2005							903 000	4 167 908	
2006			–	–			412 200	3 930 296	
2007							24 000	4 981 270	811 507
2008							724 547	2 408 905	2 408 905

IV. FINANCING MALARIA CONTROL

Governmental and external financing

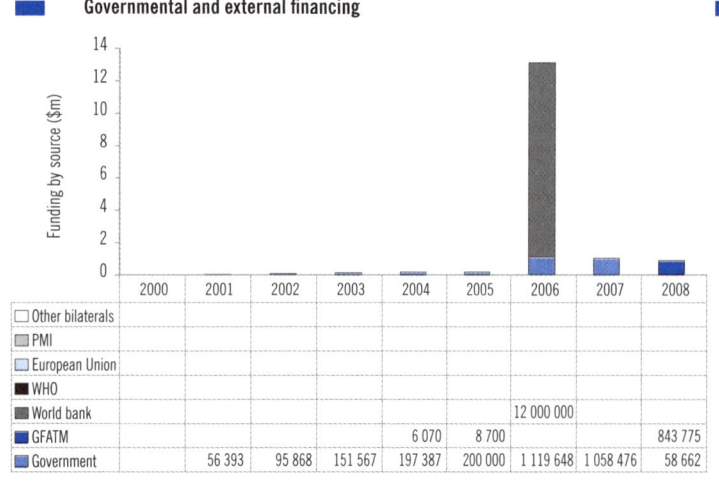

	2000	2001	2002	2003	2004	2005	2006	2007	2008
Other bilaterals									
PMI									
European Union									
WHO									
World bank							12 000 000		
GFATM						6 070	8 700		843 775
Government		56 393	95 868	151 567	197 387	200 000	1 119 648	1 058 476	58 662

Breakdown of expenditure by intervention in 2008

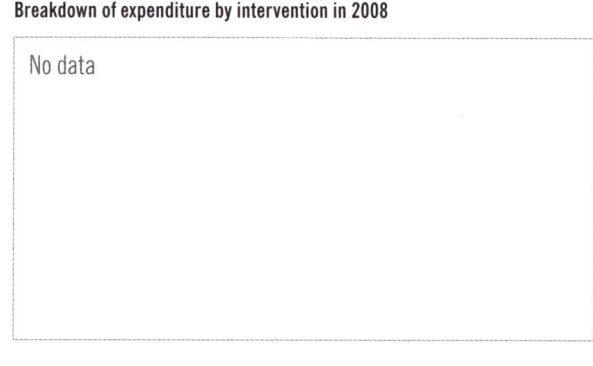

No data

V. SOURCE OF INFORMATION

PROGRAMME DATA		SURVEY AND OTHER DATA	
Reported cases	Surveillance data	Insecticide-treated nets (ITN)	DHS 2003, MICS 2006
Operational coverage of ITNs, IRS and access to medicines	Programme report	Treatment	DHS 2003, MICS 2006
Financial data	Programme report	Use of health services	DHS 2003

CAMBODIA

Approximately 2 million people live in or around forested areas where there is intense malaria transmission. Soldiers, forestry workers and gem miners are at the highest risk. Between 2001 and 2008, the number of reported cases detected in Cambodia fell from 121 612 to 80 644, and the number of reported malaria deaths decreased from 476 to 209. The 2005 demographic and health survey showed that more than 88% of children slept under a mosquito net but less than 5% slept under an ITN. The programme delivered 742 000 ITNs in 2008 (of which 214 973 were LLINs), sufficient to cover 10% of the population living at any risk for malaria, assuming two persons sleeping under each net. Under national treatment policy, artesunate and mefloquine are distributed together in blister packs through the public and private sectors, although resistance to these drugs has been recorded on the Cambodia–Thailand border. National policy promotes the use of RDTs, so that antimalarial treatment is targeted to confirmed cases only. Funding for malaria control appears to have increased appreciably since 2000, with support from the Global Fund in 2007 exceeding US$ 10 million.

I. EPIDEMIOLOGICAL PROFILE

Population, endemicity and malaria burden

Population (in thousands)	2008	%
All age groups	14 562	
< 5 years	1 611	11
≥ 5 years	12 951	89

Population by malaria endemicity (in thousands)	2008	%
High transmission ≥ 1/1000	6 393	44
Low transmission (0–1/1000)	1 369	9
Malaria-free (0 cases)	6 800	47
Rural population	11 425	78

Vector and parasite profiles

Major *Anopheles* species	*minimus, dirus, sundaicus*
Plasmodium species	*falciparum, vivax*

Stratification of burden (reported cases, per 1000)

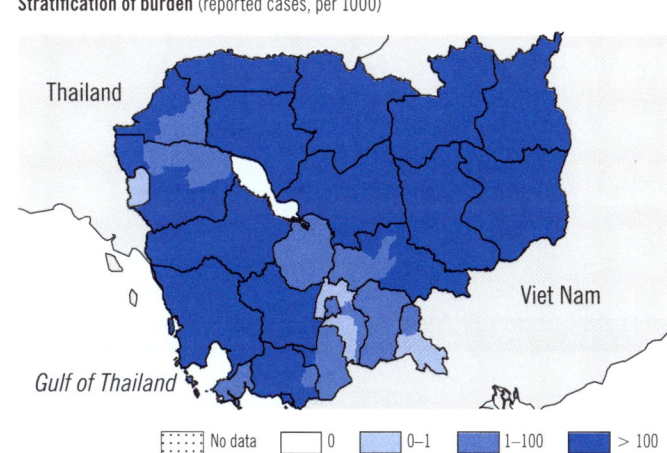

No data | 0 | 0–1 | 1–100 | > 100

Trends in malaria morbidity and mortality

Reported malaria cases, per 1000

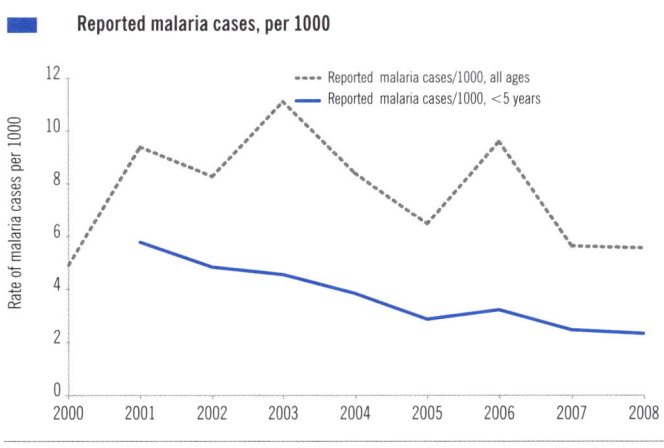

- - - Reported malaria cases/1000, all ages
——— Reported malaria cases/1000, <5 years

Rate of examination, case confirmation, malaria test positivity, % of confirmed cases that are *P. falciparum*

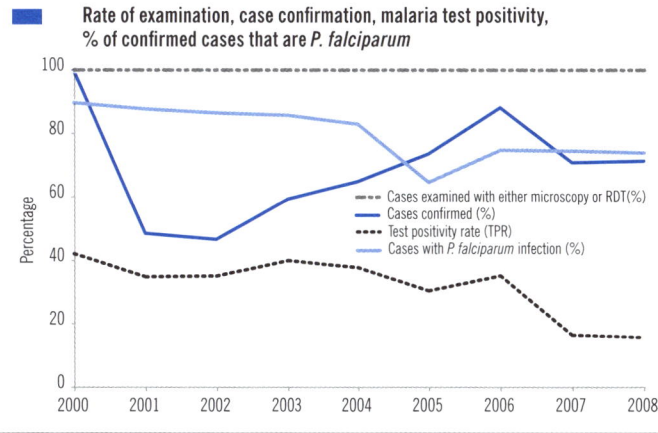

- - - Cases examined with either microscopy or RDT(%)
——— Cases confirmed (%)
······ Test positivity rate (TPR)
——— Cases with *P. falciparum* infection (%)

Year	Reported malaria cases, all ages	Reported malaria cases, < 5 years	All-cause outpatient consultations, all ages	All-cause outpatient consultations, < 5 years	Examined	Positive	*P. falciparum*	Reporting completeness of outpatient health facilities (%)	Reporting completeness of districts (%)
2000	62 442				140 722	62 442	46 150		
2001	121 612	9 854			145 619	53 601	37 105		
2002	109 048	8 057	4 200 432	689 728	133 921	46 902	33 010		
2003	148 743	7 415	4 514 158	747 870	160 354	71 265	36 338		
2004	114 211	6 163	5 302 431	988 026	150 952	59 745	31 129		
2005	89 558	4 566	5 976 718	1 201 908	147 782	49 436	17 482		
2006	134 795	5 135	6 813 409	1 466 784	197 050	78 696	24 779		
2007	80 285	3 965	6 106 629		182 720	42 518	16 518		
2008	80 664	3 811	5 962 415	1 216 139	130 995	42 124	15 095	100	100

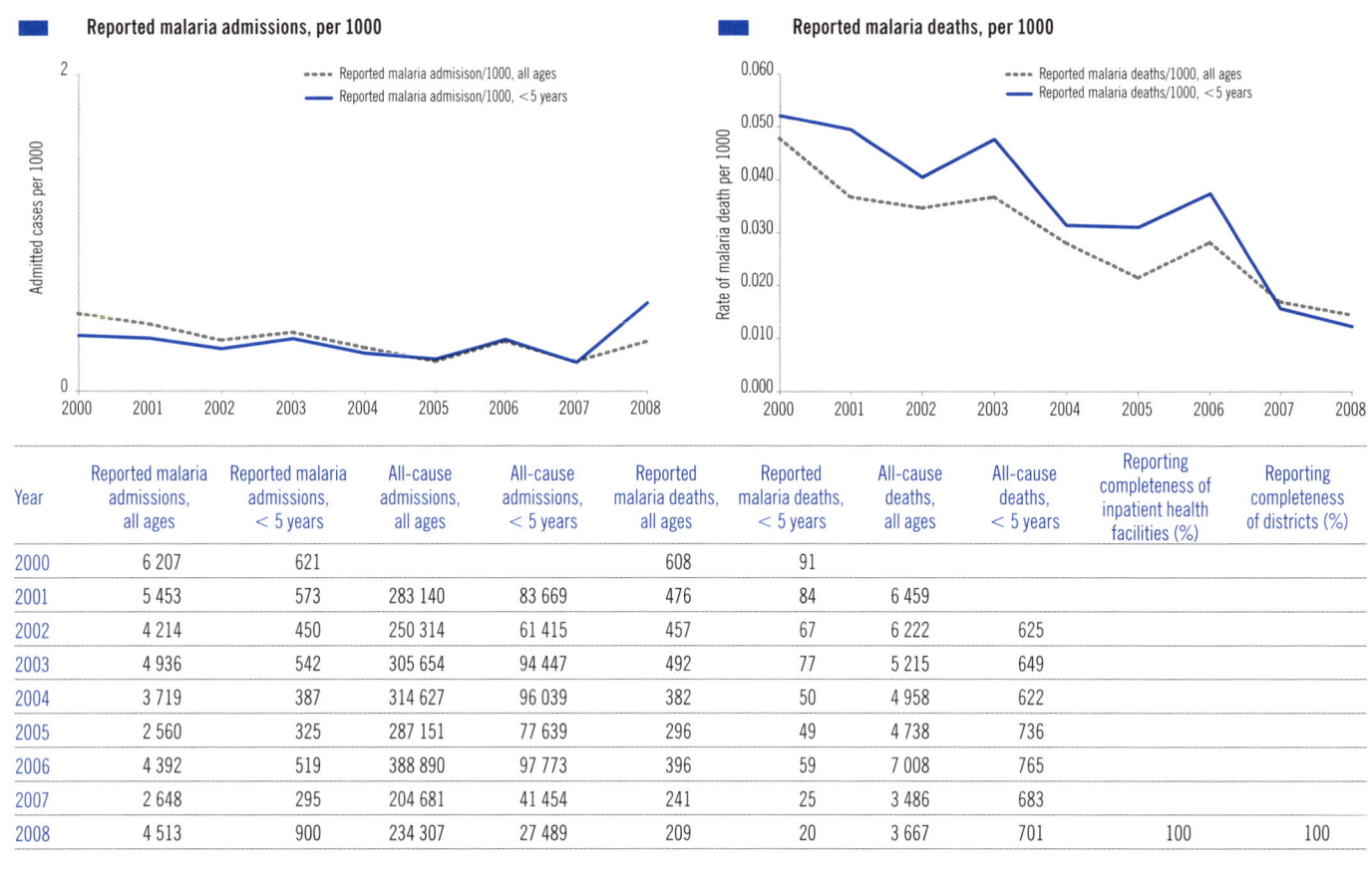

Reported malaria admissions, per 1000
- ---- Reported malaria admisison/1000, all ages
- —— Reported malaria admisison/1000, <5 years

Reported malaria deaths, per 1000
- ---- Reported malaria deaths/1000, all ages
- —— Reported malaria deaths/1000, <5 years

Year	Reported malaria admissions, all ages	Reported malaria admissions, < 5 years	All-cause admissions, all ages	All-cause admissions, < 5 years	Reported malaria deaths, all ages	Reported malaria deaths, < 5 years	All-cause deaths, all ages	All-cause deaths, < 5 years	Reporting completeness of inpatient health facilities (%)	Reporting completeness of districts (%)
2000	6 207	621			608	91				
2001	5 453	573	283 140	83 669	476	84	6 459			
2002	4 214	450	250 314	61 415	457	67	6 222	625		
2003	4 936	542	305 654	94 447	492	77	5 215	649		
2004	3 719	387	314 627	96 039	382	50	4 958	622		
2005	2 560	325	287 151	77 639	296	49	4 738	736		
2006	4 392	519	388 890	97 773	396	59	7 008	765		
2007	2 648	295	204 681	41 454	241	25	3 486	683		
2008	4 513	900	234 307	27 489	209	20	3 667	701	100	100

II. INTERVENTION POLICIES AND STRATEGIES

Intervention	WHO-RECOMMENDED POLICIES / STRATEGIES	Yes or No	Year adopted	OPTIONAL POLICIES/STRATEGIES	Yes or No	Year adoped
Insecticide-treated nets (ITN)	Distribution of ITN/LLINs – Free	Yes	2000	Distribution – Antenatal care	Yes	2006
	Targeting all age groups	Yes	2000	Distribution – EPI routine and campaign	No	–
				Targeting children < 5 years and pregnant women	Yes	2000
				ITN distribution is subsidized	No	–
Indoor residual spraying (IRS)	IRS is a primary vector control intervention	No	–	Insecticide-resistance management implemented	No	–
	DDT is used for IRS (public health) only	No	–	Where IRS is conducted, other options are also implemented, e.g. ITN	No	–
				IRS is used for prevention and control of epidemics	No	–
Intermittent preventive treatment (IPT)	IPT used to prevent malaria during pregnancy	No	–			
Case management	Oral artemisinin monotherapies banned (prohibited from registration or removed from the system)	Yes	2008	Parasitological confirmation for patients ≥ 5 years only	–	–
	Parasitological confirmation for patients of all ages	Yes	2000	Malaria diagnosis is free of charge in the public sector	Yes	–
	ACT is free of charge for < 5 years old in the public sector	Yes	2000	ACT is free of charge for patients ≥ 5 years in the public sector	Yes	2000
	Diagnosis of malaria of inpatients is based on parasitological confirmation	Yes	–	ACT is delivered at community level through community agents (beyond the health facilities)	Yes	2002
	Pre-referral treatment with quinine or artemether IM or artesunate suppositories	Yes	2000	Uncomplicated malaria cases are admitted	Yes	–
	Oversight regulation of case management in the private sectors	–	–			
	RDTs used at community level	Yes	2002			

Antimalarial policy	Type of medicine	Year adopted	Results of therapeutic efficacy tests					
			Study year	No. of studies	Median	Minimum	Maximum	Percentiles: 25% 75%
First-line treatment of *P. falciparum* (unconfirmed)	AS+MQ	2000	2001–2008	26	2.3499	0	14.3	0 7.55
First-line treatment of *P. falciparum* (confirmed)	AS+MQ	2000						
Treatment failure of *P. falciparum*	QN(7d) +T(7d)	2000						
Treatment of severe malaria	AM+MQ	2000						
Treatment of *P. vivax*	CQ	2000						

III. IMPLEMENTING MALARIA CONTROL

Coverage of ITN: survey data

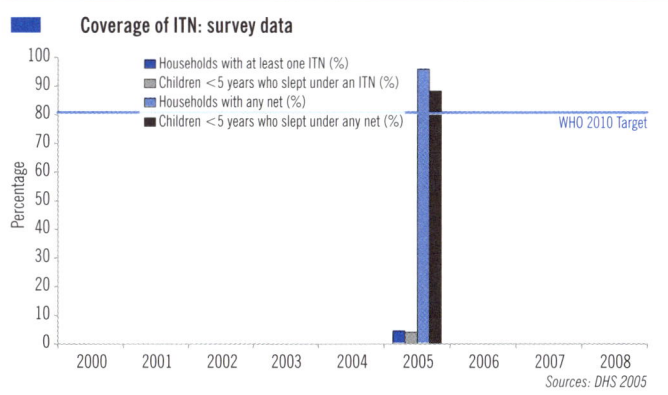

Sources: DHS 2005

Coverage of IRS and ITN: programme data

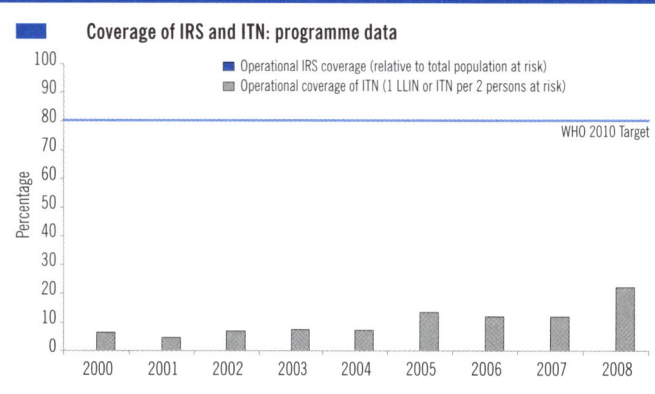

Access by febrile children to effective treatment: survey data

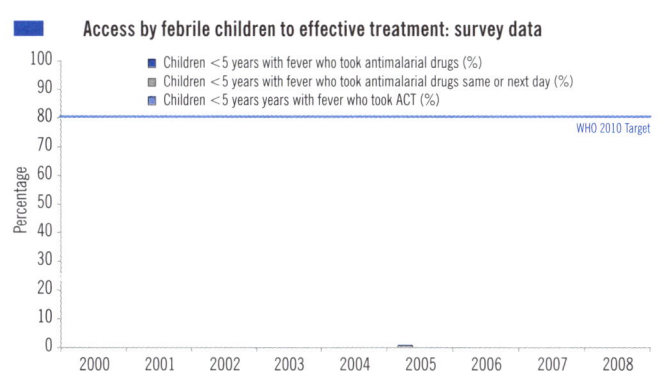

Access to effective treatment: programme data

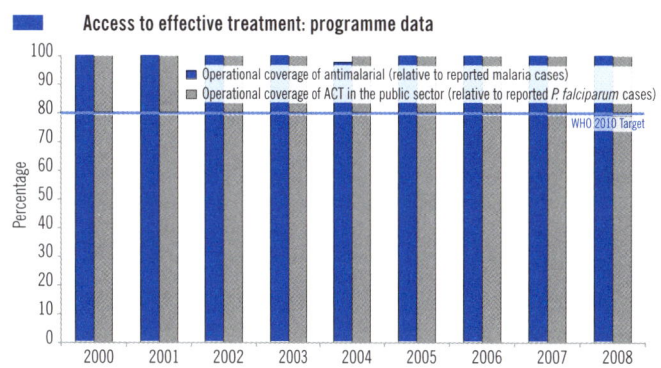

Year	Pregnant women who slept under any net (%)	Pregnant women who slept under an ITN (%)	Children < 5 years with fever (%)	Febrile children < 5 years who sought treatment in HF (%)	Number of households protected by IRS	Number of people protected by IRS	Number of ITNs and/or LLINs	Number of 1st-line treatment courses received	Number of ACT treatment courses received
2000							224 568	216 720	159 987
2001							163 412	127 258	75 678
2002							246 836	169 784	116 184
2003							269 490	127 982	127 382
2004							267 144	89 993	84 421
2005	86	4	–	–			500 318	77 782	75 082
2006							452 316	141 535	112 495
2007							456 581	91 839	150 819
2008							742 748	110 001	81 090

IV. FINANCING MALARIA CONTROL

Governmental and external financing

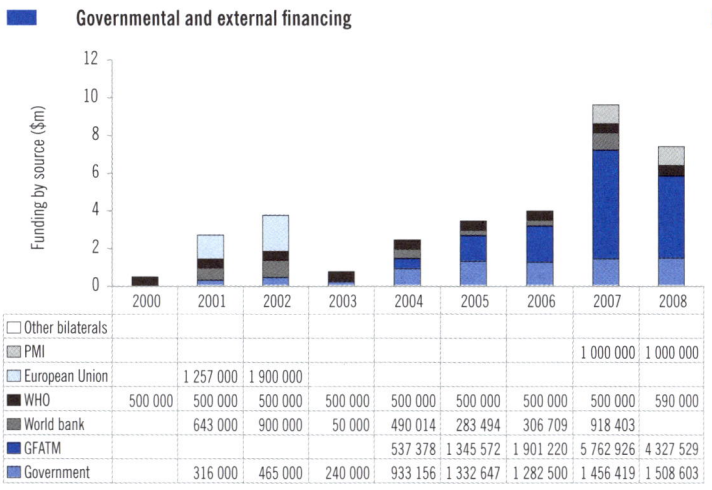

	2000	2001	2002	2003	2004	2005	2006	2007	2008
☐ Other bilaterals									
☐ PMI								1 000 000	1 000 000
☐ European Union		1 257 000	1 900 000						
■ WHO	500 000	500 000	500 000	500 000	500 000	500 000	500 000	500 000	590 000
■ World bank		643 000	900 000	50 000	490 014	283 494	306 709	918 403	
■ GFATM					537 378	1 345 572	1 901 220	5 762 926	4 327 529
■ Government		316 000	465 000	240 000	933 156	1 332 647	1 282 500	1 456 419	1 508 603

Breakdown of expenditure by intervention in 2008

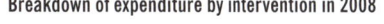
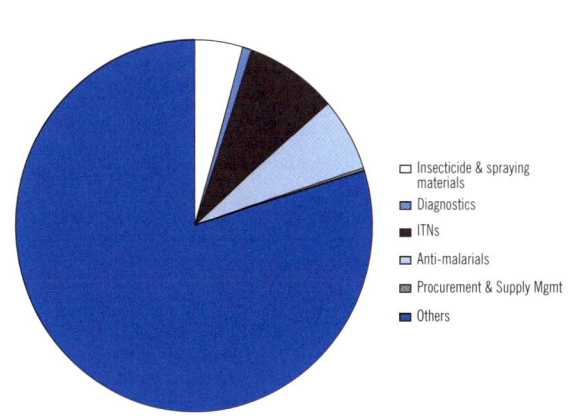

- ☐ Insecticide & spraying materials
- ■ Diagnostics
- ■ ITNs
- ☐ Anti-malarials
- ■ Procurement & Supply Mgmt
- ■ Others

V. SOURCE OF INFORMATION

PROGRAMME DATA		SURVEY AND OTHER DATA	
Reported cases	Surveillance data	Insecticide-treated nets (ITN)	DHS 2005
Operational coverage of ITNs, IRS and access to medicines	Programme report	Treatment	DHS 2005
Financial data	Programme report	Use of health services	DHS 2005

CAMEROON

Cameroon had an estimated 5.6 million malaria cases in 2006. Transmission occurs all year round but is more intense in the south. The number of reported malaria cases jumped from 635 000 in 2006 to nearly 1 650 749 cases in 2008, none of which were confirmed. Similarly, the numbers of malaria inpatient cases and deaths increased six- and fourfold, respectively, perhaps due to improving reporting. The national malaria control programme delivered about 800 000 LLINs in 2008, inadequate to cover the 19.5 million people at risk. The programme delivered 2.56 million ACT treatment courses in 2007 and 1.81 million in 2008, adequate to treat the reported malaria cases in the public sector. In the 2006 multiple indicator cluster survey, 20% of households owned an ITN, only 13% of children slept under an ITN and only 2% of children with fever received an ACT. Funding for malaria control increased from less than US$ 2 million in 2002 to over US$ 26 million in 2008, provided mostly by the Government and the Global Fund.

I. EPIDEMIOLOGICAL PROFILE

Population, endemicity and malaria burden

Population (in thousands)	2008	%
All age groups	19 088	
< 5 years	3 016	16
≥ 5 years	16 072	84

Population by malaria endemicity (in thousands)	2008	%
High transmission ≥ 1/1000	13 537	71
Low transmission (0–1/1000)	5 552	29
Malaria-free (0 cases)	0	0
Rural population	8 248	43

Vector and parasite profiles

Major *Anopheles* species	*gambiae, arabiensis, funestus, brochieri, coustani, flavicosta, hancocki, hargreavesi, melas, moucheti, nili, paludis, pharoensis*
Plasmodium species	*falciparum, vivax*

Stratification of burden (reported cases, per 1000)

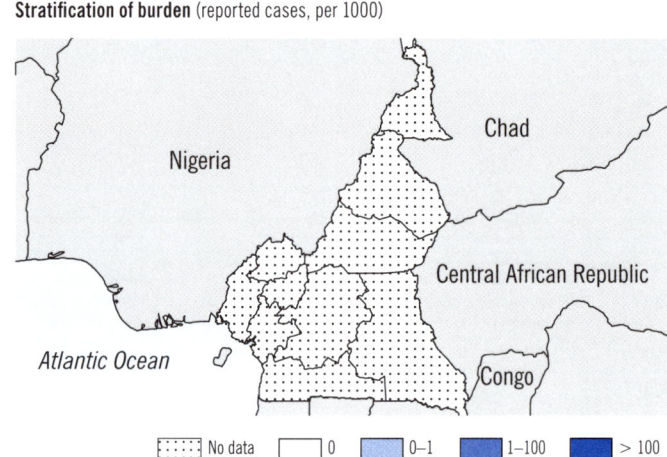

Trends in malaria morbidity and mortality

Reported malaria cases, per 1000

Rate of examination, case confirmation, malaria test positivity, % of confirmed cases that are *P. falciparum*

No data

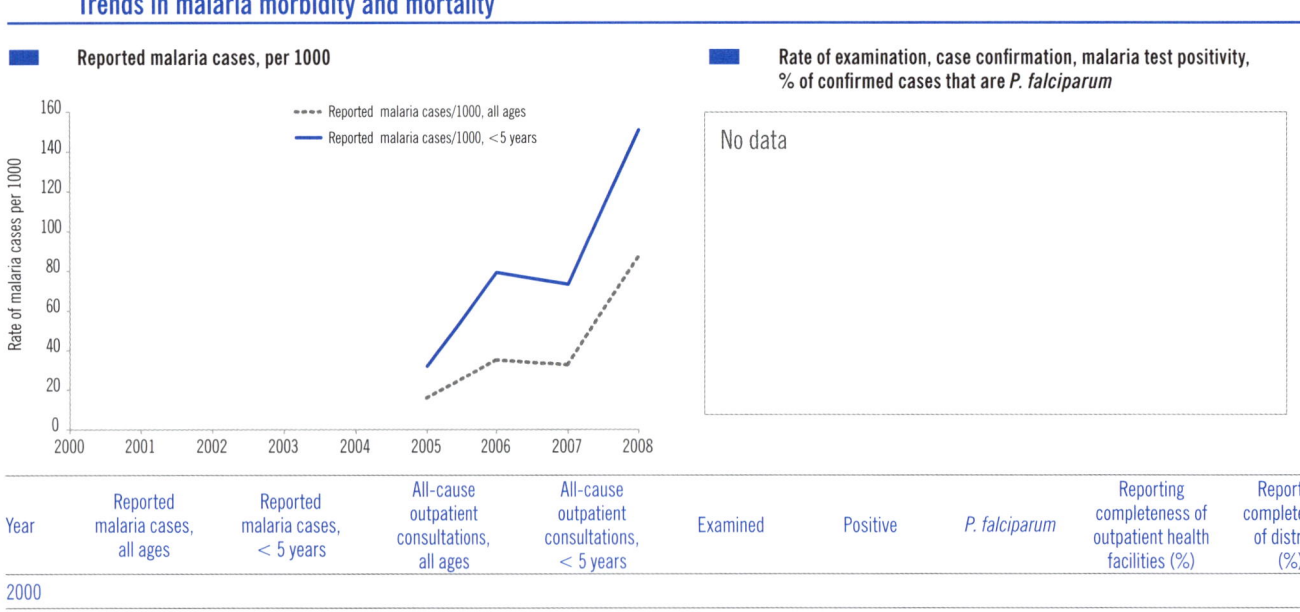

Year	Reported malaria cases, all ages	Reported malaria cases, < 5 years	All-cause outpatient consultations, all ages	All-cause outpatient consultations, < 5 years	Examined	Positive	*P. falciparum*	Reporting completeness of outpatient health facilities (%)	Reporting completeness of districts (%)
2000									
2001									
2002									
2003									
2004									
2005	277 413	89 041	697 665	197 771					
2006	634 507	227 284	1 748 905	462 140					
2007	604 153	214 697	1 668 116	464 190			313 083		
2008	1 650 749	453 811	4 064 854	1 149 790					

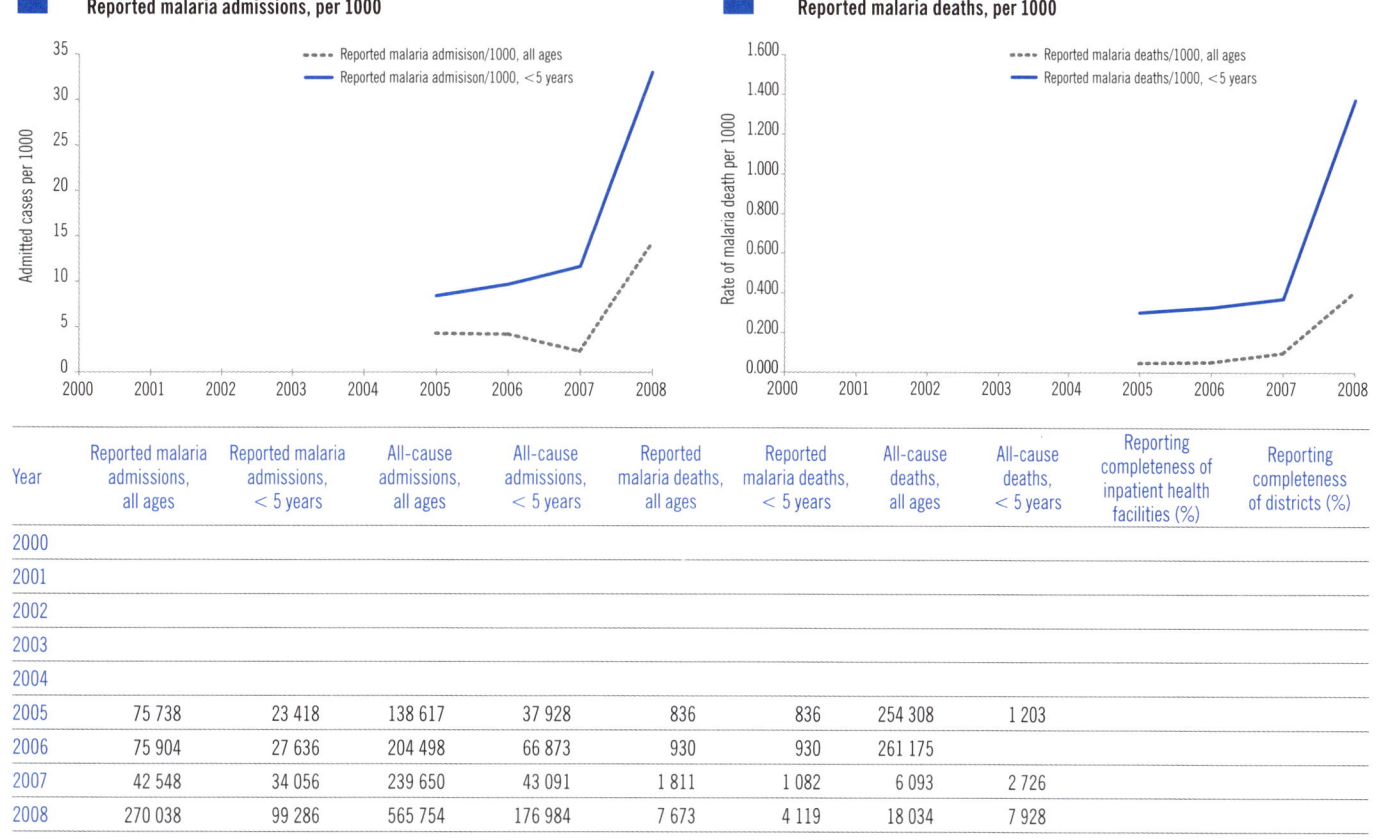

Reported malaria admissions, per 1000

- ···· Reported malaria admission/1000, all ages
- —— Reported malaria admission/1000, <5 years

Reported malaria deaths, per 1000

- ···· Reported malaria deaths/1000, all ages
- —— Reported malaria deaths/1000, <5 years

Year	Reported malaria admissions, all ages	Reported malaria admissions, < 5 years	All-cause admissions, all ages	All-cause admissions, < 5 years	Reported malaria deaths, all ages	Reported malaria deaths, < 5 years	All-cause deaths, all ages	All-cause deaths, < 5 years	Reporting completeness of inpatient health facilities (%)	Reporting completeness of districts (%)
2000										
2001										
2002										
2003										
2004										
2005	75 738	23 418	138 617	37 928	836	836	254 308	1 203		
2006	75 904	27 636	204 498	66 873	930	930	261 175			
2007	42 548	34 056	239 650	43 091	1 811	1 082	6 093	2 726		
2008	270 038	99 286	565 754	176 984	7 673	4 119	18 034	7 928		

II. INTERVENTION POLICIES AND STRATEGIES

Intervention	WHO-RECOMMENDED POLICIES / STRATEGIES	Yes or No	Year adopted	OPTIONAL POLICIES / STRATEGIES	Yes or No	Year adoped
Insecticide-treated nets (ITN)	Distribution of ITN/LLINs — Free	Yes	2003	Distribution — Antenatal care	Yes	2003
	Targeting all age groups	No	—	Distribution — EPI routine and campaign	Yes	2007
				Targeting children < 5 years and pregnant women	Yes	2003
				ITN distribution is subsidized	Yes	2005
Indoor residual spraying (IRS)	IRS is a primary vector control intervention	No	—	Insecticide-resistance management implemented	Yes	2005
	DDT is used for IRS (public health) only	No	—	Where IRS is conducted, other options are also implemented, e.g. ITN	No	—
				IRS is used for prevention and control of epidemics	No	—
Intermittent preventive treatment (IPT)	IPT used to prevent malaria during pregnancy	Yes	2004			
Case management	Oral artemisinin monotherapies banned (prohibited from registration or removed from the system)	Yes	2007	Parasitological confirmation for patients ≥ 5 years only	No	—
	Parasitological confirmation for patients of all ages	No	—	Malaria diagnosis is free of charge in the public sector	No	—
	ACT is free of charge for < 5 years old in the public sector	No	—	ACT is free of charge for patients ≥ 5 years in the public sector	No	—
	Diagnosis of malaria of inpatients is based on parasitological confirmation	Yes	—	ACT is delivered at community level through community agents (beyond the health facilities)	Yes	2008
	Pre-referral treatment with quinine or artemether IM or artesunate suppositories	Yes	—	Uncomplicated malaria cases are admitted	No	—
	Oversight regulation of case management in the private sectors	Yes	—			
	RDTs used at community level	No	—			

					Results of therapeutic efficacy tests					
Antimalarial policy	Type of medicine	Year adopted	Study year	No. of studies	Median	Minimum	Maximum	Percentiles:	25%	75%
First-line treatment of *P. falciparum* (unconfirmed)	AS+AQ	2004								
First-line treatment of *P. falciparum* (confirmed)	AS+AQ	2004								
Treatment failure of *P. falciparum*	QN(7d)	2004								
Treatment of severe malaria	QN(7d)	2004								
Treatment of *P. vivax*	—	—								

III. IMPLEMENTING MALARIA CONTROL

Coverage of ITN: survey data

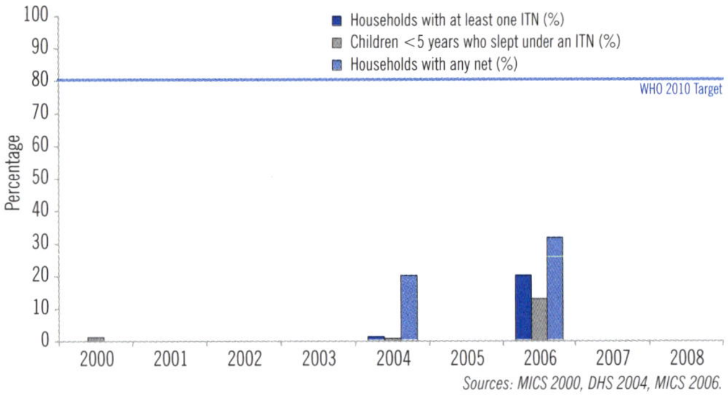

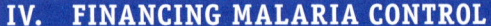

- Households with at least one ITN (%)
- Children <5 years who slept under an ITN (%)
- Households with any net (%)

WHO 2010 Target

Sources: MICS 2000, DHS 2004, MICS 2006.

Coverage of IRS and ITN: programme data

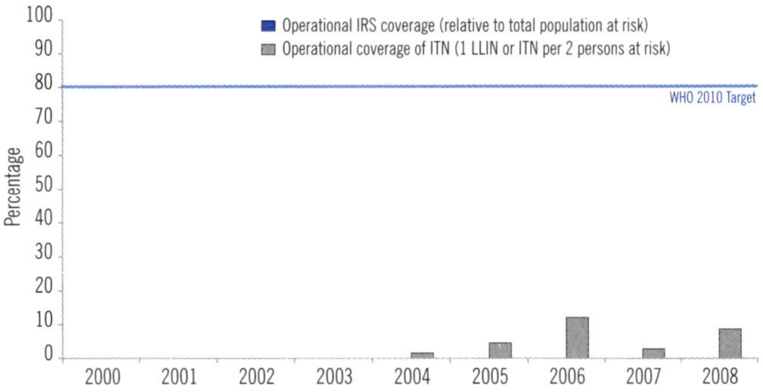

- Operational IRS coverage (relative to total population at risk)
- Operational coverage of ITN (1 LLIN or ITN per 2 persons at risk)

WHO 2010 Target

Access by febrile children to effective treatment: survey data

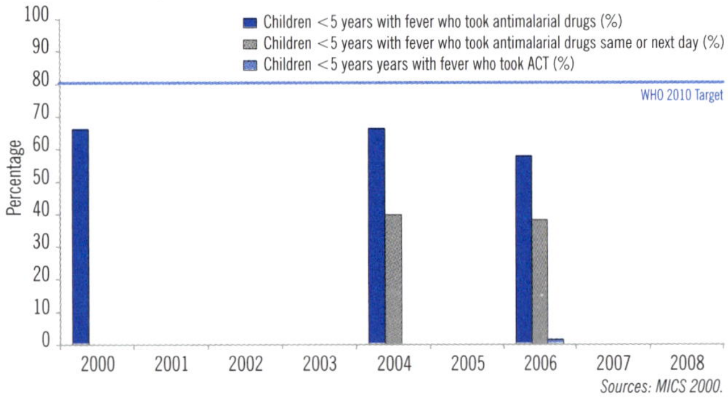

- Children <5 years with fever who took antimalarial drugs (%)
- Children <5 years with fever who took antimalarial drugs same or next day (%)
- Children <5 years years with fever who took ACT (%)

WHO 2010 Target

Sources: MICS 2000.

Access to effective treatment: programme data

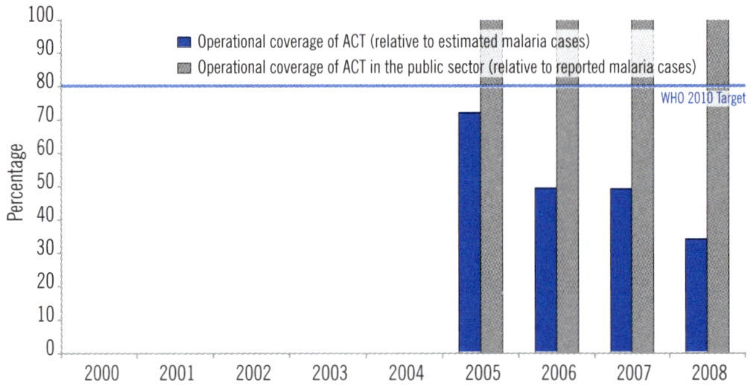

- Operational coverage of ACT (relative to estimated malaria cases)
- Operational coverage of ACT in the public sector (relative to reported malaria cases)

WHO 2010 Target

Year	Pregnant women who slept under any net (%)	Pregnant women who slept under an ITN (%)	Children < 5 years with fever (%)	Febrile children < 5 years who sought treatment in HF (%)	Number of households protected by IRS	Number of people protected by IRS	Number of ITNs and/or LLINs	Number of 1st-line treatment courses received	Number of ACT treatment courses received
2000			–	–					
2001									
2002									
2003									
2004	12	1	–	–			140 443		
2005							404 755	3 583 332	3 583 332
2006			–	–			1 097 510	2 518 305	2 518 305
2007							244 425	2 566 785	2 566 785
2008							802 105	1 814 725	1 814 725

IV. FINANCING MALARIA CONTROL

Governmental and external financing

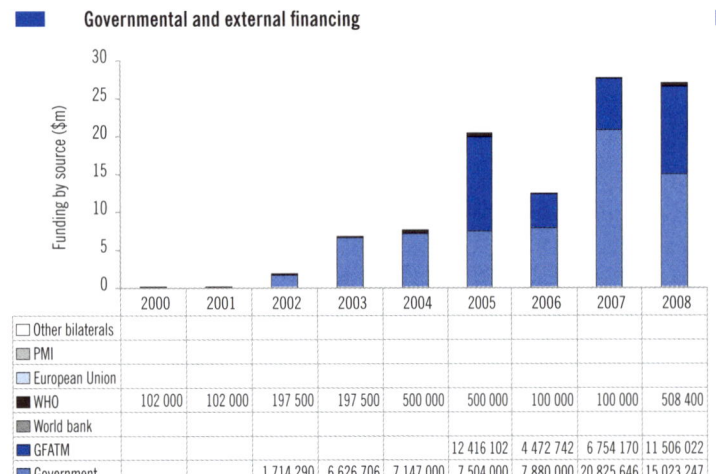

	2000	2001	2002	2003	2004	2005	2006	2007	2008
Other bilaterals									
PMI									
European Union									
WHO	102 000	102 000	197 500	197 500	500 000	500 000	100 000	100 000	508 400
World bank									
GFATM						12 416 102	4 472 742	6 754 170	11 506 022
Government			1 714 290	6 626 706	7 147 000	7 504 000	7 880 000	20 825 646	15 023 247

Breakdown of expenditure by intervention in 2008

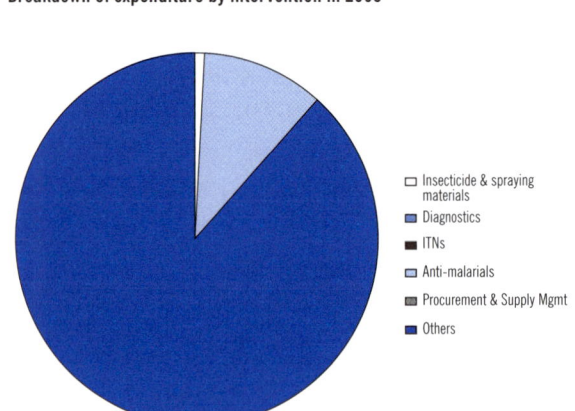

- Insecticide & spraying materials
- Diagnostics
- ITNs
- Anti-malarials
- Procurement & Supply Mgmt
- Others

V. SOURCE OF INFORMATION

PROGRAMME DATA		SURVEY AND OTHER DATA	
Reported cases	Surveillance data	Insecticide-treated nets (ITN)	MICS 2000, DHS 2004, MICS 2006
Operational coverage of ITNs, IRS and access to medicines	Programme report	Treatment	MICS 2000, DHS 2004, MICS 2006
Financial data	Programme report	Use of health services	DHS 2004

CHAD

Malaria transmission is more intense in the south, occurring seasonally between May and December. Almost all cases are caused by *P. falciparum*. Less than 13% of suspected cases are parasitologically tested. The numbers of reported cases remained nearly the same and deaths have increased in recent years, but it is not known if this reflects a real increase in malaria burden or improved reporting. The national malaria programme did not implement major vector control, except for the distribution of 83 000 ITNs in 2007 and 120 000 in 2008, many fewer than are needed to protect the 10 million people at risk. IRS is not a national policy. The number of treatment courses of ACT used in 2006 was far fewer than the estimated number of cases. Malaria control has been funded mainly by the Government, United Nations agencies and bilateral agencies, with no active Global Fund grant.

I. EPIDEMIOLOGICAL PROFILE

Population, endemicity and malaria burden

Population (in thousands)	2008	%
All age groups	10 914	
< 5 years	1 985	18
≥ 5 years	8 928	82

Population by malaria endemicity (in thousands)	2008	%
High transmission ≥ 1/1000	8 731	80
Low transmission (0–1/1000)	2 073	19
Malaria-free (0 cases)	110	1
Rural population	8 009	73

Vector and parasite profiles

Major *Anopheles* species	arabiensis, funestus, arabiensis, coustani, coustani, funestus, nili, pharoensis, pharoensis
Plasmodium species	falciparum, vivax

Stratification of burden (reported cases, per 1000)

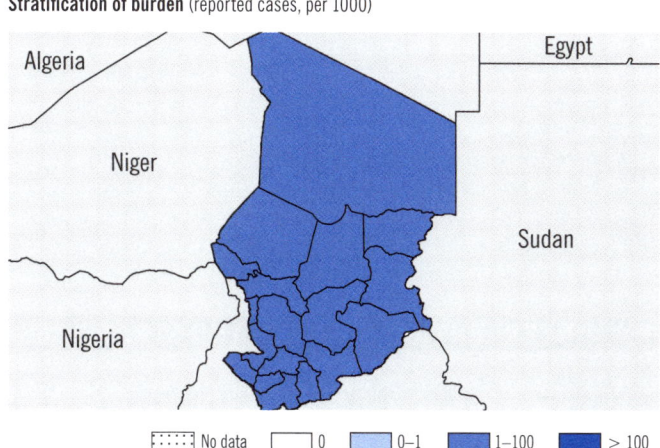

No data   0   0–1   1–100   > 100

Trends in malaria morbidity and mortality

Reported malaria cases, per 1000

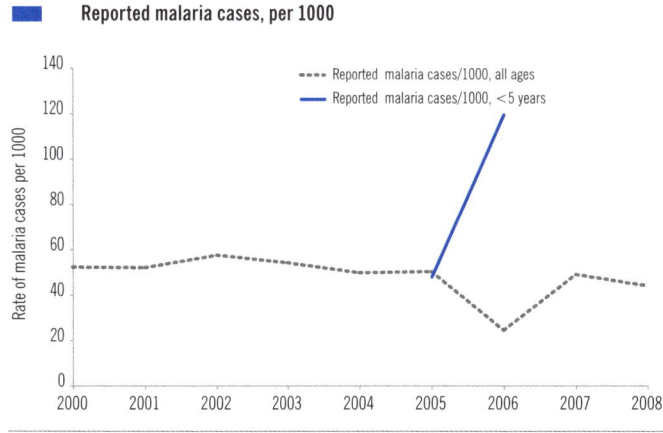

Rate of examination, case confirmation, malaria test positivity, % of confirmed cases that are *P. falciparum*

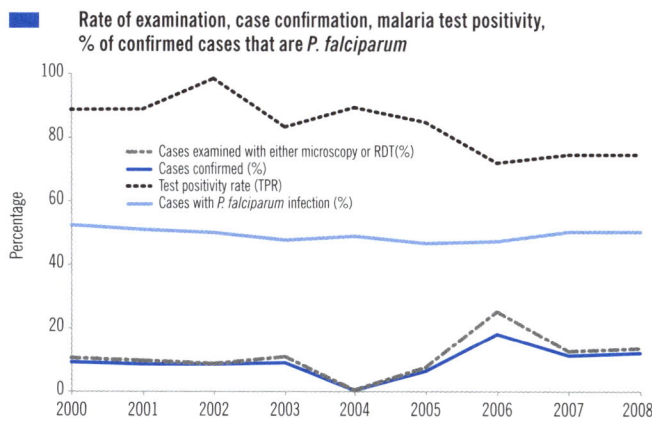

Year	Reported malaria cases, all ages	Reported malaria cases, < 5 years	All-cause outpatient consultations, all ages	All-cause outpatient consultations, < 5 years	Examined	Positive	*P. falciparum*	Reporting completeness of outpatient health facilities (%)	Reporting completeness of districts (%)
2000	437 041		2 040 156		45 283	40 078	20 977		52
2001	451 182		1 980 009		43 180	38 287	19 520		80
2002	517 004		2 084 846		44 689	43 933	21 959		62
2003	505 732		1 953 940		54 381	45 195	21 532		94
2004	481 122		2 002 670		1 525	1 360	665		100
2005	501 846	89 041	1 968 565	197 771	37 439	31 668	14 770		54
2006	251 354	227 284	1 938 177	462 140	62 895	45 155	21 354		83
2007	518 832		2 196 462		64 884	58 288	24 282		83
2008	478 987		2 159 832		64 171	57 644	24 015		90

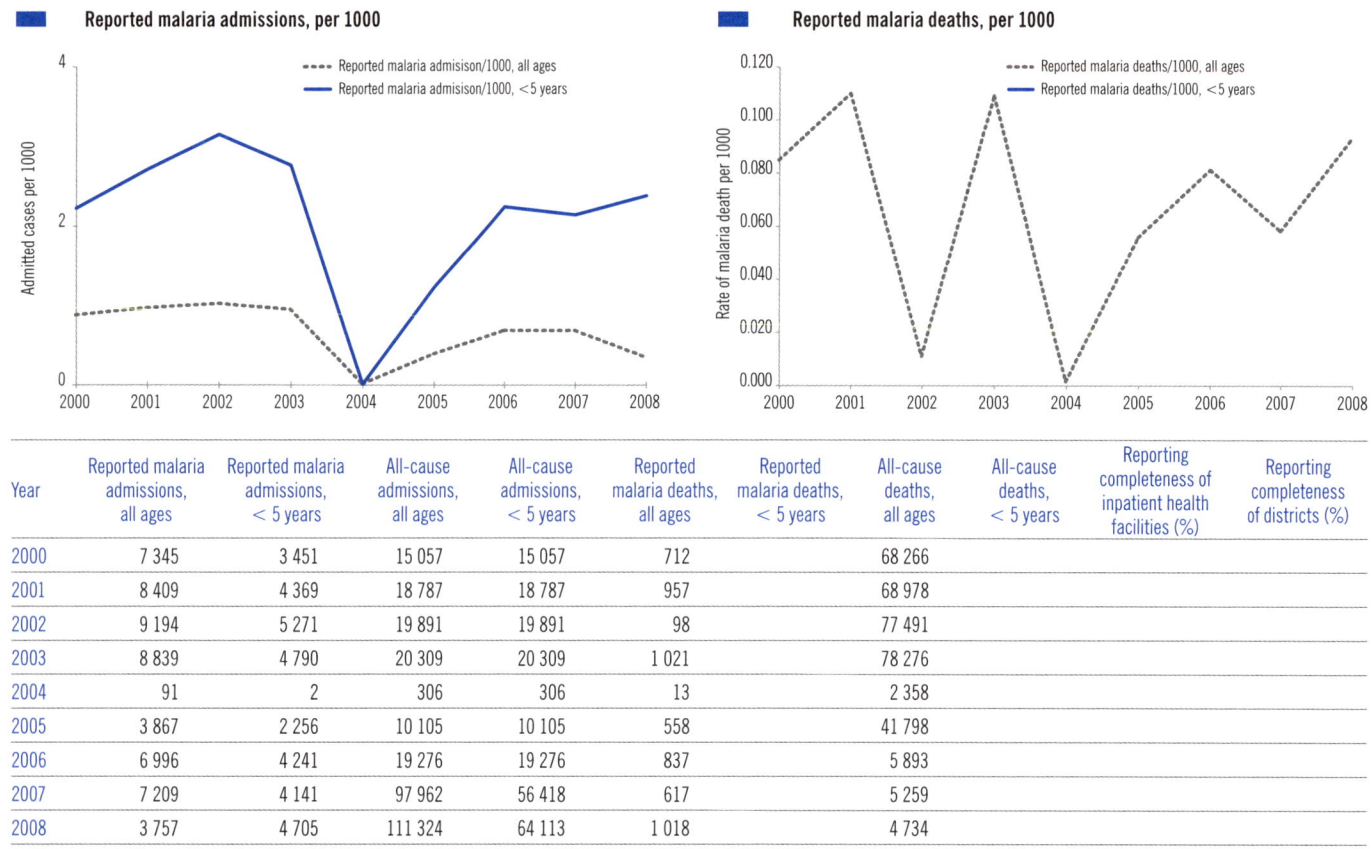

Reported malaria admissions, per 1000

- ---- Reported malaria admision/1000, all ages
- —— Reported malaria admision/1000, <5 years

Reported malaria deaths, per 1000

- ---- Reported malaria deaths/1000, all ages
- —— Reported malaria deaths/1000, <5 years

Year	Reported malaria admissions, all ages	Reported malaria admissions, < 5 years	All-cause admissions, all ages	All-cause admissions, < 5 years	Reported malaria deaths, all ages	Reported malaria deaths, < 5 years	All-cause deaths, all ages	All-cause deaths, < 5 years	Reporting completeness of inpatient health facilities (%)	Reporting completeness of districts (%)
2000	7 345	3 451	15 057	15 057	712		68 266			
2001	8 409	4 369	18 787	18 787	957		68 978			
2002	9 194	5 271	19 891	19 891	98		77 491			
2003	8 839	4 790	20 309	20 309	1 021		78 276			
2004	91	2	306	306	13		2 358			
2005	3 867	2 256	10 105	10 105	558		41 798			
2006	6 996	4 241	19 276	19 276	837		5 893			
2007	7 209	4 141	97 962	56 418	617		5 259			
2008	3 757	4 705	111 324	64 113	1 018		4 734			

II. INTERVENTION POLICIES AND STRATEGIES

Intervention	WHO-RECOMMENDED POLICIES / STRATEGIES	Yes or No	Year adopted	OPTIONAL POLICIES / STRATEGIES	Yes or No	Year adoped
Insecticide-treated nets (ITN)	Distribution of ITN/LLINs – Free	Yes	2003	Distribution – Antenatal care	Yes	2003
	Targeting all age groups	No	–	Distribution – EPI routine and campaign	Yes	2006
				Targeting children < 5 years and pregnant women	Yes	2003
				ITN distribution is subsidized	–	–
Indoor residual spraying (IRS)	IRS is a primary vector control intervention	No	–	Insecticide-resistance management implemented	Yes	2005
	DDT is used for IRS (public health) only	No	–	Where IRS is conducted, other options are also implemented, e.g. ITN	No	–
				IRS is used for prevention and control of epidemics	No	–
Intermittent preventive treatment (IPT)	IPT used to prevent malaria during pregnancy	Yes	2004			
Case management	Oral artemisinin monotherapies banned (prohibited from registration or removed from the system)	Yes	2007	Parasitological confirmation for patients ≥ 5 years only	–	–
	Parasitological confirmation for patients of all ages	Yes	–	Malaria diagnosis is free of charge in the public sector	Yes	–
	ACT is free of charge for < 5 years old in the public sector	Yes	–	ACT is free of charge for patients ≥ 5 years in the public sector	–	–
	Diagnosis of malaria of inpatients is based on parasitological confirmation	Yes	–	ACT is delivered at community level through community agents (beyond the health facilities)	Yes	–
	Pre-referral treatment with quinine or artemether IM or artesunate suppositories	No	–	Uncomplicated malaria cases are admitted	No	–
	Oversight regulation of case management in the private sectors	–	–			
	RDTs used at community level	Yes	–			

Antimalarial policy	Type of medicine	Year adopted	Results of therapeutic efficacy tests						
			Study year	No. of studies	Median	Minimum	Maximum	Percentiles: 25%	75%
First-line treatment of *P. falciparum* (unconfirmed)	AL, AS+AQ	–							
First-line treatment of *P. falciparum* (confirmed)	AL, AS+AQ	–							
Treatment failure of *P. falciparum*	QN(7d)	–							
Treatment of severe malaria	QN(7d)	–							
Treatment of *P. vivax*	–	–							

III. IMPLEMENTING MALARIA CONTROL

Coverage of ITN: survey data

- Households with at least one ITN (%)
- Children <5 years who slept under an ITN (%)
- Households with any net (%)

WHO 2010 Target

Percentage (y-axis: 0–100)
Years: 2000 2001 2002 2003 2004 2005 2006 2007 2008

Sources: MICS 2000, DHS 2004.

Coverage of IRS and ITN: programme data

No data

Access by febrile children to effective treatment: survey data

- Children <5 years with fever who took antimalarial drugs (%)
- Children <5 years with fever who took antimalarial drugs same or next day (%)
- Children <5 years years with fever who took ACT (%)

WHO 2010 Target

Percentage (y-axis: 0–100)
Years: 2000 2001 2002 2003 2004 2005 2006 2007 2008

Sources: MICS 2000.

Access to effective treatment: programme data

No data

Year	Pregnant women who slept under any net (%)	Pregnant women who slept under an ITN (%)	Children < 5 years with fever (%)	Febrile children < 5 years who sought treatment in HF (%)	Number of households protected by IRS	Number of people protected by IRS	Number of ITNs and/or LLINs	Number of 1st-line treatment courses received	Number of ACT treatment courses received
2000			–	–					
2001									
2002									
2003							104 118		
2004			–	–			10 000		
2005							128 293		
2006							267 000		
2007							83 000		
2008							126 000		

IV. FINANCING MALARIA CONTROL

Governmental and external financing

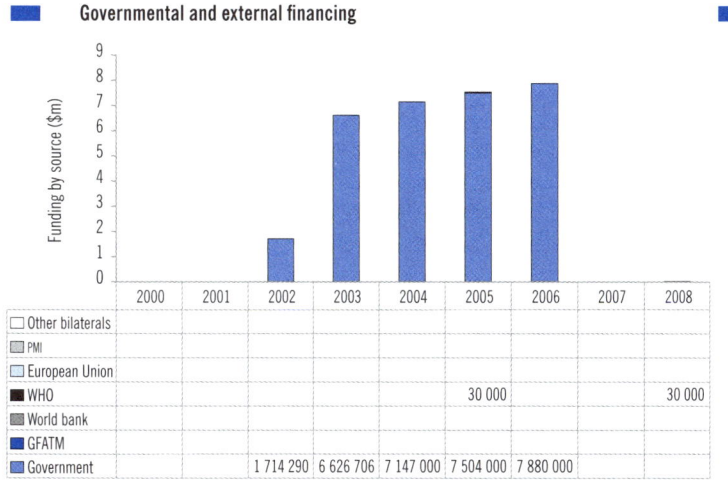

Funding by source ($m) (y-axis: 0–9)

	2000	2001	2002	2003	2004	2005	2006	2007	2008
Other bilaterals									
PMI									
European Union									
WHO						30 000			30 000
World bank									
GFATM									
Government			1 714 290	6 626 706	7 147 000	7 504 000	7 880 000		

Breakdown of expenditure by intervention in 2008

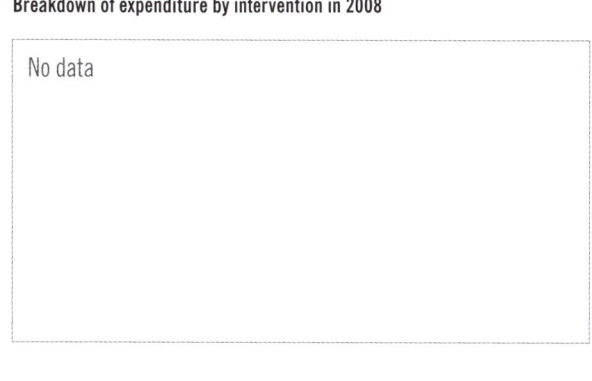

No data

V. SOURCE OF INFORMATION

PROGRAMME DATA		SURVEY AND OTHER DATA	
Reported cases	Surveillance data	Insecticide-treated nets (ITN)	MICS 2000, DHS 2004
Operational coverage of ITNs, IRS and access to medicines	Programme report	Treatment	MICS 2000
Financial data	Programme report	Use of health services	DHS 2004

COLOMBIA

About 18% of the population of Colombia is at risk for malaria. Transmission is highest in the upper Sinú River and lower Cauca River regions, in Urabá and on the Pacific coast. The number of reported malaria cases decreased from 231 233 in 2001 to 79 230 in 2008, and the number of reported malaria deaths fell from 58 in 2001 to 22 in 2008. About 28% of cases were due to *P. falciparum* in 2008. IRS is implemented selectively, protecting 69 000 households and 211 000 people in 2008. Over 280 000 LLINs were distributed in 2007 and 2008. The supply of first-line antimalarial drugs, including 46 350 courses of ACT, was sufficient to treat all reported cases. Funding for malaria control in 2008 reached US$ 18 million, of which US$ 17 million was financed by the Government, US$ 3 million by the Global Fund and US$ 200 000 by the United States Agency for International Development.

I. EPIDEMIOLOGICAL PROFILE

Population, endemicity and malaria burden

Population (in thousands)	2008	%
All age groups	45 012	
< 5 years	4 485	10
≥ 5 years	40 527	90

Population by malaria endemicity (in thousands)	2008	%
High transmission ≥ 1/1000	3 014	7
Low transmission (0–1/1000)	4 897	11
Malaria-free (0 cases)	37 101	82
Rural population	11 490	26

Vector and parasite profiles	
Major *Anopheles* species	*albimanus, darlingi, neivai, nunestovari, pseudopunctipenis*
Plasmodium species	*falciparum, vivax*

Stratification of burden (reported cases, per 1000)

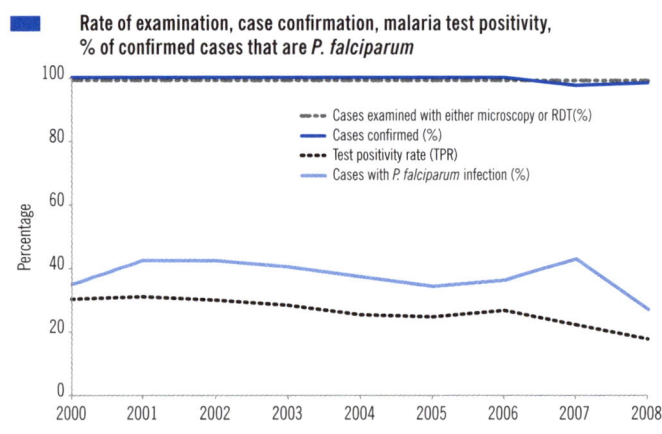

No data ⬚   0 ☐   0–1 ▨   1–100 ▨   > 100 ■

Trends in malaria morbidity and mortality

Reported malaria cases, per 1000

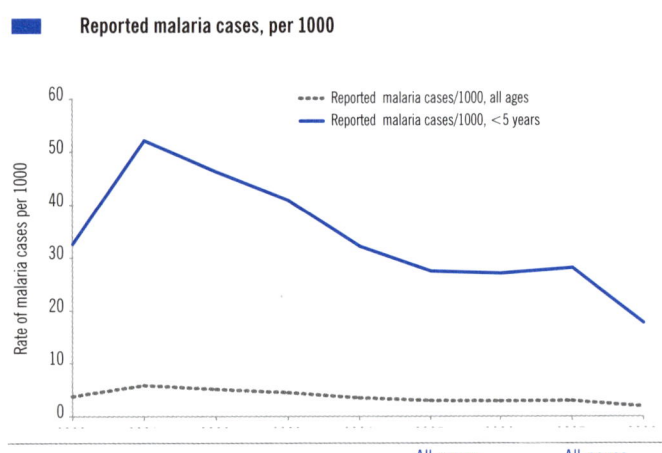

- - - Reported malaria cases/1000, all ages
— Reported malaria cases/1000, <5 years

Rate of examination, case confirmation, malaria test positivity, % of confirmed cases that are *P. falciparum*

- - - Cases examined with either microscopy or RDT(%)
— Cases confirmed (%)
····· Test positivity rate (TPR)
— Cases with *P. falciparum* infection (%)

Year	Reported malaria cases, all ages	Reported malaria cases, < 5 years	All-cause outpatient consultations, all ages	All-cause outpatient consultations, < 5 years	Examined	Positive	P. falciparum	Reporting completeness of outpatient health facilities (%)	Reporting completeness of districts (%)
2000	144 432	144 432			478 820	144 432	50 476		
2001	231 233	231 233			747 079	231 233	98 049		
2002	204 916	204 916			686 635	204 916	86 840		
2003	180 956	180 956			640 453	180 956	73 150		
2004	142 241	142 241			562 681	142 241	53 106		
2005	121 629	121 629			493 562	121 629	41 781		
2006	120 096	120 096			451 240	120 096	43 547		
2007	125 262	125 262			564 755	125 262	53 852		
2008	79 230	79 230			447 627	79 230	21 475		

Reported malaria admissions, per 1000

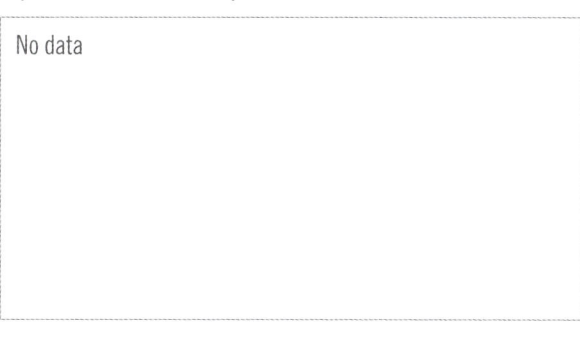

No data

Reported malaria deaths, per 1000

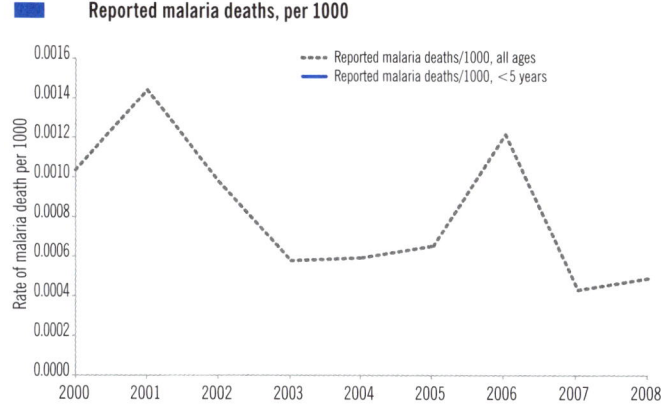

Year	Reported malaria admissions, all ages	Reported malaria admissions, < 5 years	All-cause admissions, all ages	All-cause admissions, < 5 years	Reported malaria deaths, all ages	Reported malaria deaths, < 5 years	All-cause deaths, all ages	All-cause deaths, < 5 years	Reporting completeness of inpatient health facilities (%)	Reporting completeness of districts (%)
2000					41					
2001					58					
2002					40					
2003					24					
2004					25					
2005					28					
2006					53					
2007					19					
2008	223	16			22	3				

II. INTERVENTION POLICIES AND STRATEGIES

Intervention	WHO-RECOMMENDED POLICIES / STRATEGIES	Yes or No	Year adopted	OPTIONAL POLICIES / STRATEGIES	Yes or No	Year adoped
Insecticide-treated nets (ITN)	Distribution of ITN/LLINs — Free	Yes	–	Distribution — Antenatal care	No	–
	Targeting all age groups	Yes	2005	Distribution — EPI routine and campaign	No	–
				Targeting children < 5 years and pregnant women	No	–
				ITN distribution is subsidized	No	–
Indoor residual spraying (IRS)	IRS is a primary vector control intervention	No	–	Insecticide-resistance management implemented	Yes	2005
	DDT is used for IRS (public health) only	No	–	Where IRS is conducted, other options are also implemented, e.g. ITN	Yes	2005
				IRS is used for prevention and control of epidemics	Yes	1950s
Intermittent preventive treatment (IPT)	IPT used to prevent malaria during pregnancy	No	–			
Case management	Oral artemisinin monotherapies banned (prohibited from registration or removed from the system)	–	–	Parasitological confirmation for patients ≥ 5 years only	No	–
	Parasitological confirmation for patients of all ages	Yes	1960s	Malaria diagnosis is free of charge in the public sector	Yes	–
	ACT is free of charge for < 5 years old in the public sector	Yes	2006	ACT is free of charge for patients ≥ 5 years in the public sector	Yes	2006
	Diagnosis of malaria of inpatients is based on parasitological confirmation	Yes	–	ACT is delivered at community level through community agents (beyond the health facilities)	No	–
	Pre-referral treatment with quinine or artemether IM or artesunate suppositories	No	–	Uncomplicated malaria cases are admitted	No	–
	Oversight regulation of case management in the private sectors	No	–			
	RDTs used at community level	Yes	2006			

Antimalarial policy	Type of medicine	Year adopted	Results of therapeutic efficacy tests						
			Study year	No. of studies	Median	Minimum	Maximum	Percentiles: 25%	75%
First-line treatment of *P. falciparum* (unconfirmed)	–	–							
First-line treatment of *P. falciparum* (confirmed)	AL	2006							
Treatment failure of *P. falciparum*	QN(3d) + CL(5d)	2004							
Treatment of severe malaria	QN(7d)	2004							
Treatment of *P. vivax*	CQ + PQ (7d)	1960s							

III. IMPLEMENTING MALARIA CONTROL

Coverage of ITN: survey data

No data

Coverage of IRS and ITN: programme data

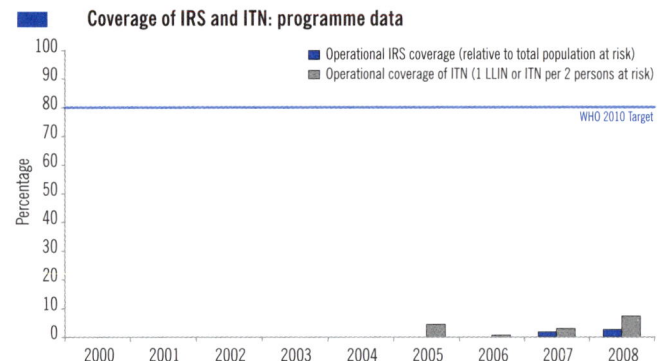

Access by febrile children to effective treatment: survey data

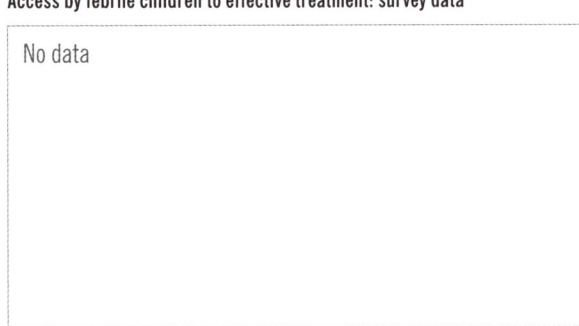

No data

Access to effective treatment: programme data

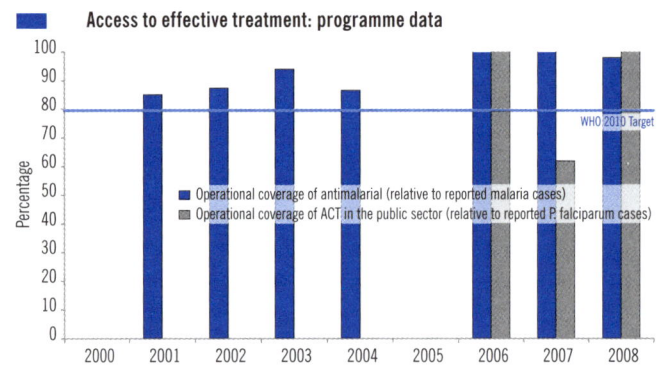

Year	Pregnant women who slept under any net (%)	Pregnant women who slept under an ITN (%)	Children < 5 years with fever (%)	Febrile children < 5 years who sought treatment in HF (%)	Number of households protected by IRS	Number of people protected by IRS	Number of ITNs and/or LLINs	Number of 1st-line treatment courses received	Number of ACT treatment courses received
2000			–	–					
2001								196 200	
2002								178 904	
2003								169 816	
2004								122 804	
2005							170 000		
2006							8 360	145 525	51 840
2007					28 728	143 640	87 394	155 132	33 240
2008					68 759	211 294	194 363	79 230	46 350

IV. FINANCING MALARIA CONTROL

Governmental and external financing

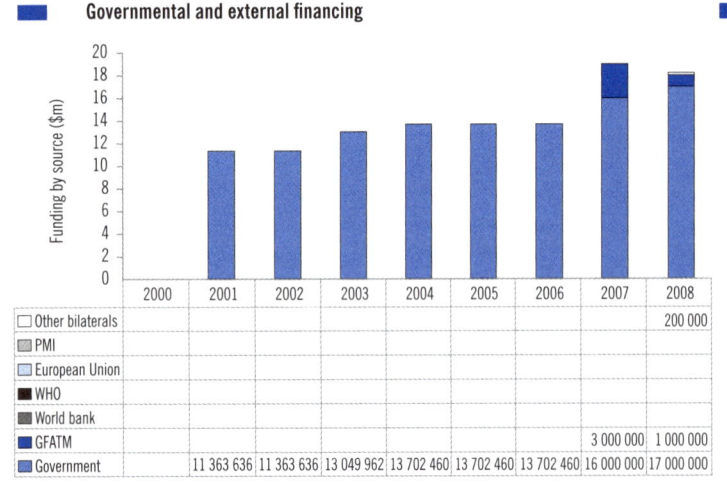

	2000	2001	2002	2003	2004	2005	2006	2007	2008
Other bilaterals									200 000
PMI									
European Union									
WHO									
World bank									
GFATM								3 000 000	1 000 000
Government		11 363 636	11 363 636	13 049 962	13 702 460	13 702 460	13 702 460	16 000 000	17 000 000

Breakdown of expenditure by intervention in 2008

No data

V. SOURCE OF INFORMATION

PROGRAMME DATA		SURVEY AND OTHER DATA	
Reported cases	Surveillance data	Insecticide-treated nets (ITN)	DHS 2000
Operational coverage of ITNs, IRS and access to medicines	Programme report	Treatment	No surveys
Financial data	Programme report	Use of health services	DHS 2004

CÔTE D'IVOIRE

Côte d'Ivoire had an estimated 8.0 million cases in 2006. Transmission occurs all year round throughout the country but is more seasonal in the north. None of the 1.25 million cases reported in 2006 was confirmed as malaria. There was no evidence of a systematic decrease in the number of malaria cases between 2001 and 2006. The number of malaria deaths increased, perhaps due to improved reporting. IRS is not carried out in Côte d'Ivoire. The national malaria control programme distributed only 1.6 million ITNs between 2006 and 2008. The 2006 multiple indicator cluster survey showed that only 27% of households owned a mosquito net, and just 6% had an ITN. Despite the adoption of ACT as treatment policy in 2003, the programme delivered only 476 000 ACT treatment courses in 2007, which represents 37% of the reported malaria cases in need of treatment. The multiple indicator cluster survey showed that only 3% of febrile children were given ACT. Funding for malaria control increased from less than US$ 2 million in 2002 to over US$ 27 million in 2008 funded by the Global Fund, government and UN agencies.

I.   EPIDEMIOLOGICAL PROFILE

Population, endemicity and malaria burden

Population (in thousands)	2008	%
All age groups	20 591	
< 5 years	3 139	15
≥ 5 years	17 452	85

Population by malaria endemicity (in thousands)	2008	%
High transmission ≥ 1/1000	20 591	100
Low transmission (0–1/1000)	0	0
Malaria-free (0 cases)	0	0
Rural population	10 537	51

Vector and parasite profiles

Major *Anopheles* species	*gambiae, arabiensis, funestus, brochieri, coustani, Hancocki, hargreavesi, melas, moucheti, moucheti, nili, paludis, pharoensis*
Plasmodium species	*falciparum, vivax*

Stratification of burden (reported cases, per 1000)

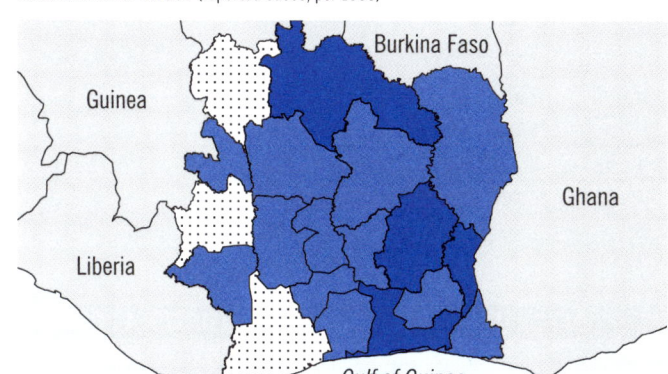

Trends in malaria morbidity and mortality

Reported malaria cases, per 1000

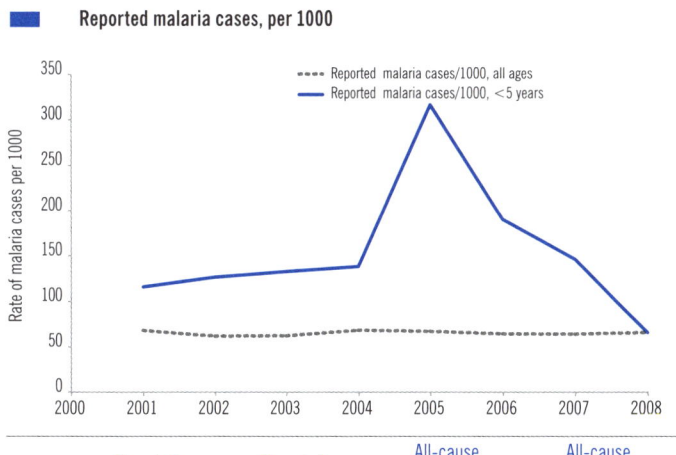

- - - Reported malaria cases/1000, all ages
— Reported malaria cases/1000, <5 years

Rate of examination, case confirmation, malaria test positivity, % of confirmed cases that are *P. falciparum*

No data

Year	Reported malaria cases, all ages	Reported malaria cases, < 5 years	All-cause outpatient consultations, all ages	All-cause outpatient consultations, < 5 years	Examined	Positive	*P. falciparum*	Reporting completeness of outpatient health facilities (%)	Reporting completeness of districts (%)
2000									
2001	1 193 288	321 361	1 969 077	397 679				80	61
2002	1 109 751	359 073	2 318 879	519 240				82	63
2003	1 136 810	384 982	2 368 584	450 098				86	54
2004	1 275 138	409 063	2 349 636	452 086				82	56
2005	1 280 914	952 056	2 664 516					84	58
2006	1 253 408	582 242	3 632 014					58	65
2007	1 277 670	454 725	2 449 332	563 363					
2008	1 343 654	208 459	3 001 009	394 090					

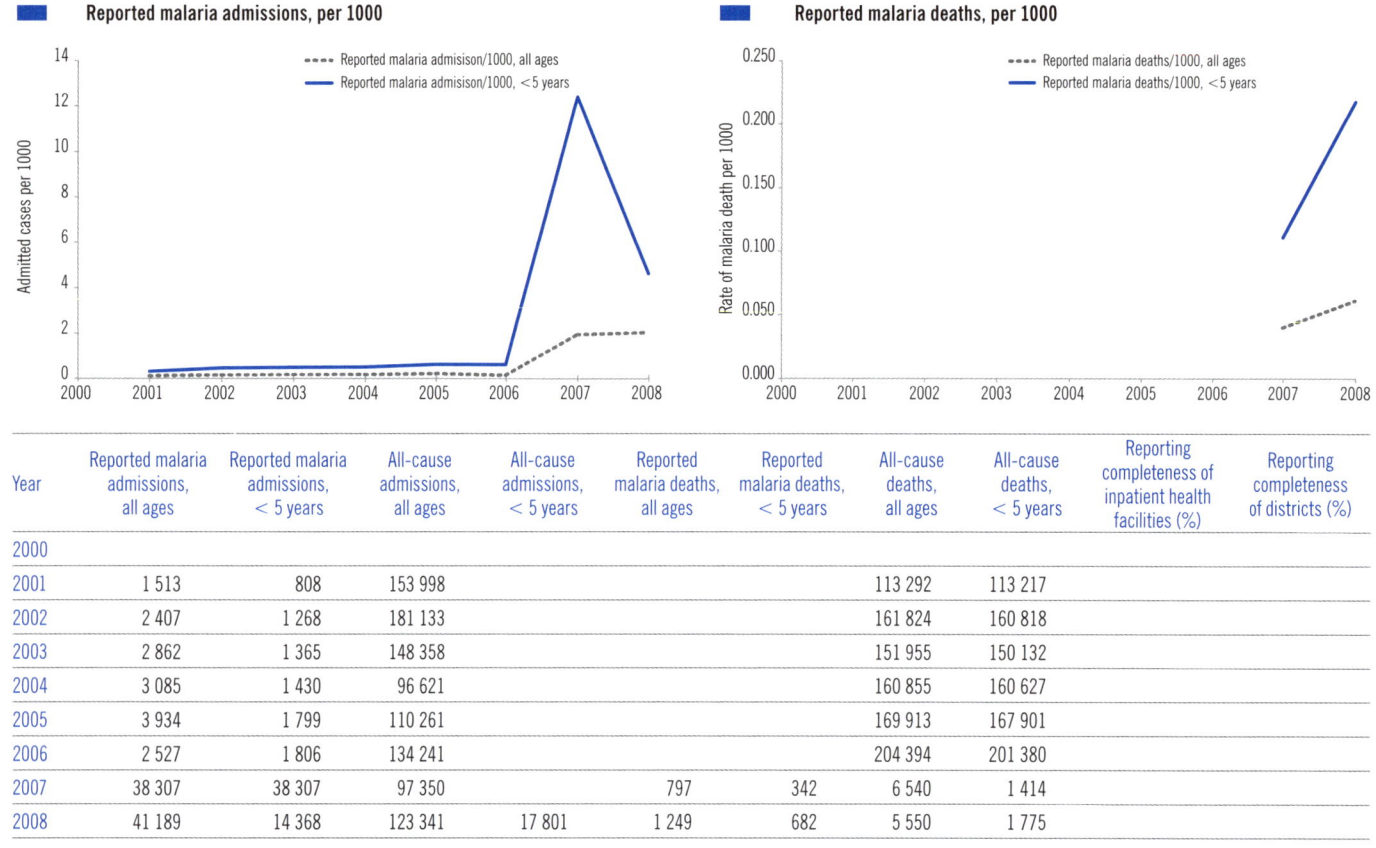

Reported malaria admissions, per 1000
- ---- Reported malaria admisison/1000, all ages
- —— Reported malaria admisison/1000, <5 years

Reported malaria deaths, per 1000
- ---- Reported malaria deaths/1000, all ages
- —— Reported malaria deaths/1000, <5 years

Year	Reported malaria admissions, all ages	Reported malaria admissions, < 5 years	All-cause admissions, all ages	All-cause admissions, < 5 years	Reported malaria deaths, all ages	Reported malaria deaths, < 5 years	All-cause deaths, all ages	All-cause deaths, < 5 years	Reporting completeness of inpatient health facilities (%)	Reporting completeness of districts (%)
2000										
2001	1 513	808	153 998				113 292	113 217		
2002	2 407	1 268	181 133				161 824	160 818		
2003	2 862	1 365	148 358				151 955	150 132		
2004	3 085	1 430	96 621				160 855	160 627		
2005	3 934	1 799	110 261				169 913	167 901		
2006	2 527	1 806	134 241				204 394	201 380		
2007	38 307	38 307	97 350		797	342	6 540	1 414		
2008	41 189	14 368	123 341	17 801	1 249	682	5 550	1 775		

II. INTERVENTION POLICIES AND STRATEGIES

Intervention	WHO-RECOMMENDED POLICIES / STRATEGIES	Yes or No	Year adopted	OPTIONAL POLICIES / STRATEGIES	Yes or No	Year adoped
Insecticide-treated nets (ITN)	Distribution of ITN/LLINs – Free	Yes	2006	Distribution – Antenatal care	Yes	2006
	Targeting all age groups	Yes	2005	Distribution – EPI routine and campaign	Yes	2006
				Targeting children < 5 years and pregnant women	Yes	2005
				ITN distribution is subsidized	No	–
Indoor residual spraying (IRS)	IRS is a primary vector control intervention	No	–	Insecticide-resistance management implemented	Yes	1998
	DDT is used for IRS (public health) only	No	–	Where IRS is conducted, other options are also implemented, e.g. ITN	No	–
				IRS is used for prevention and control of epidemics	No	–
Intermittent preventive treatment (IPT)	IPT used to prevent malaria during pregnancy	Yes	2005			
Case management	Oral artemisinin monotherapies banned (prohibited from registration or removed from the system)	Yes	2005	Parasitological confirmation for patients ≥ 5 years only	Yes	2005
	Parasitological confirmation for patients of all ages	No	–	Malaria diagnosis is free of charge in the public sector	No	–
	ACT is free of charge for < 5 years old in the public sector	No	–	ACT is free of charge for patients ≥ 5 years in the public sector	No	–
	Diagnosis of malaria of inpatients is based on parasitological confirmation	Yes	1997	ACT is delivered at community level through community agents (beyond the health facilities)	No	–
	Pre-referral treatment with quinine or artemether IM or artesunate suppositories	No	–	Uncomplicated malaria cases are admitted	No	–
	Oversight regulation of case management in the private sectors	No	–			
	RDTs used at community level	No	–			

				Results of therapeutic efficacy tests						
Antimalarial policy	Type of medicine	Year adopted	Study year	No. of studies	Median	Minimum	Maximum	Percentiles:	25%	75%
First-line treatment of *P. falciparum* (unconfirmed)	AS+AQ	2003	20008–2009	2	0	0	0		0	0
First-line treatment of *P. falciparum* (confirmed)	AS+AQ	2003								
Treatment failure of *P. falciparum*	AL	2003	2005–2009	4	2.0999	0	7.4		0.8	5
Treatment of severe malaria	QN(7d)	2003								
Treatment of *P. vivax*	–	–								

III. IMPLEMENTING MALARIA CONTROL

Coverage of ITN: survey data

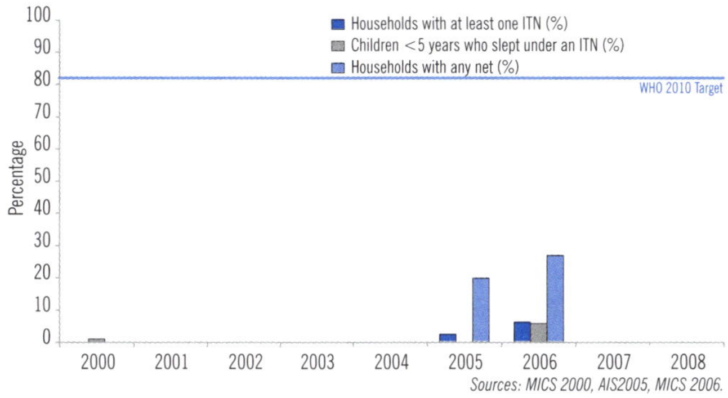

- ■ Households with at least one ITN (%)
- ■ Children <5 years who slept under an ITN (%)
- ■ Households with any net (%)

WHO 2010 Target

Percentage — years 2000–2008

Sources: MICS 2000, AIS2005, MICS 2006.

Coverage of IRS and ITN: programme data

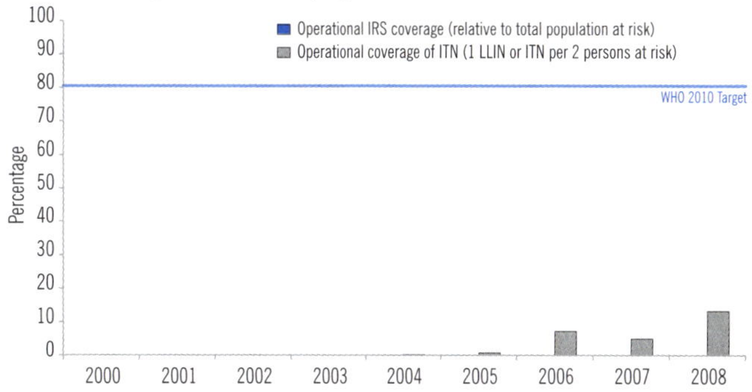

- ■ Operational IRS coverage (relative to total population at risk)
- ■ Operational coverage of ITN (1 LLIN or ITN per 2 persons at risk)

WHO 2010 Target

Percentage — years 2000–2008

Access by febrile children to effective treatment: survey data

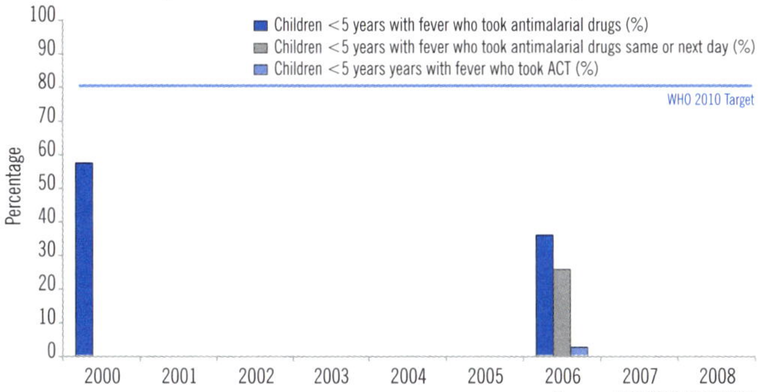

- ■ Children <5 years with fever who took antimalarial drugs (%)
- ■ Children <5 years with fever who took antimalarial drugs same or next day (%)
- ■ Children <5 years years with fever who took ACT (%)

WHO 2010 Target

Percentage — years 2000–2008

Sources: MICS 2000, MICS 2006

Access to effective treatment: programme data

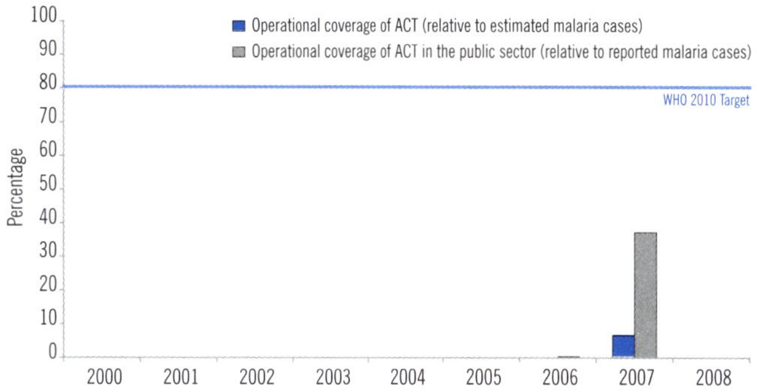

- ■ Operational coverage of ACT (relative to estimated malaria cases)
- ■ Operational coverage of ACT in the public sector (relative to reported malaria cases)

WHO 2010 Target

Percentage — years 2000–2008

Year	Pregnant women who slept under any net (%)	Pregnant women who slept under an ITN (%)	Children < 5 years with fever (%)	Febrile children < 5 years who sought treatment in HF (%)	Number of households protected by IRS	Number of people protected by IRS	Number of ITNs and/or LLINs	Number of 1st-line treatment courses received	Number of ACT treatment courses received
2000			–	–					
2001									
2002									
2003								5 000	
2004								12 000	
2005			–	–				53 696	971 683	
2006			–	–				371 816	1 102 879	4 875
2007								169 832	721 314	476 203
2008								1 034 486		

IV. FINANCING MALARIA CONTROL

Governmental and external financing

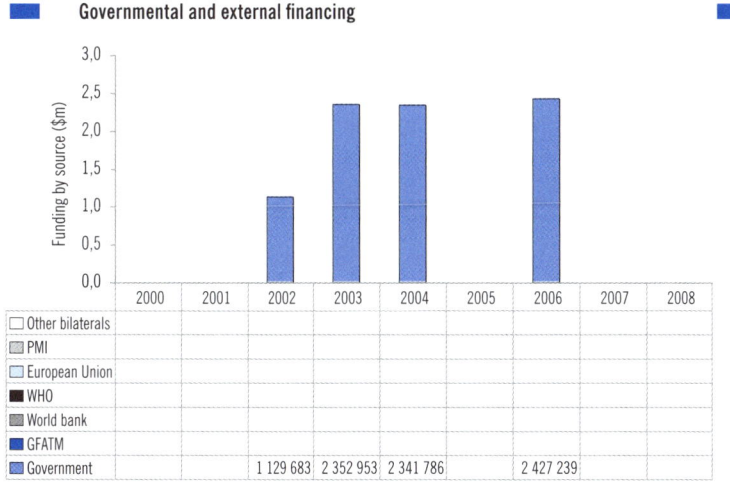

	2000	2001	2002	2003	2004	2005	2006	2007	2008
☐ Other bilaterals									
▨ PMI									
☐ European Union									
■ WHO									
▨ World bank									
■ GFATM									
■ Government			1 129 683	2 352 953	2 341 786		2 427 239		

Breakdown of expenditure by intervention in 2008

No data

V. SOURCE OF INFORMATION

PROGRAMME DATA		SURVEY AND OTHER DATA	
Reported cases	Surveillance data	Insecticide-treated nets (ITN)	MICS 2000, AIS 2005, MICS 2006
Operational coverage of ITNs, IRS and access to medicines	Programme report	Treatment	MICS 2000, MICS 2006
Financial data	Programme report	Use of health services	MICS 2006

DEMOCRATIC REPUBLIC OF THE CONGO

The Democratic Republic of the Congo, with 61 million people, accounted for an estimated 11% of all estimated malaria cases in the WHO African Region in 2006. Transmission occurs all year round, but with seasonal variation. Almost none of the 5 million reported suspected malaria cases in 2008, largely due to *P. falciparum*, are confirmed. The number of malaria deaths reported by the programme was 18 928 in 2008 alone. The programme delivered a total of about 11.2 million LLINs during 2006–2008, adequate to protect about 37% of the population. IRS was begun in 2008 in selected districts, covering only 83 000 people at risk. The programme delivered a total of 1.7 million ACT treatment courses in public facilities in 2008, covering only 32% of the treatment needs in those facilities. Funding for malaria increased from US$ 20 million in 2005 to over US$ 50 million in 2008, mainly from the World Bank and the Global Fund, with about US$ 2 million annually from the Government.

I. EPIDEMIOLOGICAL PROFILE

Population, endemicity and malaria burden

Population (in thousands)	2008	%
All age groups	64 704	
< 5 years	21 944	34
≥ 5 years	42 760	66

Population by malaria endemicity (in thousands)	2008	%
High transmission ≥ 1/1000	62 763	97
Low transmission (0–1/1000)	1 941	3
Malaria-free (0 cases)	0	0
Rural population	64 704	100

Vector and parasite profiles

Major *Anopheles* species	gambiae, arabiensis, funestus, brochieri, coustani, hancocki, hargreavesi, melas, moucheti, moucheti, paludis, pharoensis
Plasmodium species	falciparum, vivax

Stratification of burden (reported cases, per 1000)

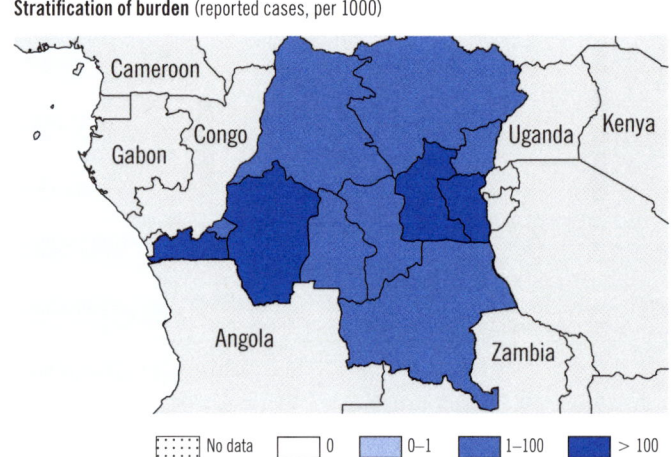

No data | 0 | 0–1 | 1–100 | > 100

Trends in malaria morbidity and mortality

Reported malaria cases, per 1000

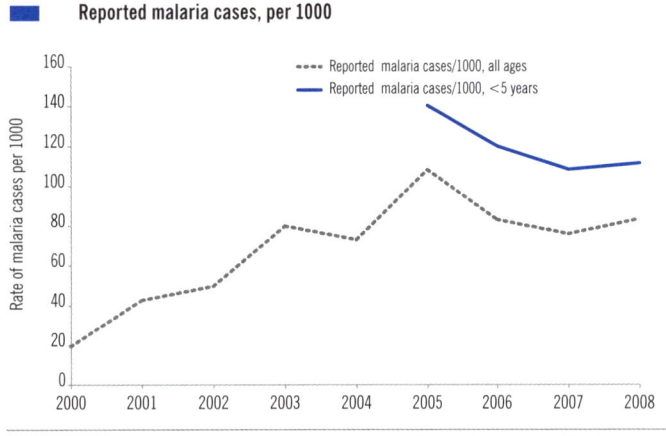

- - - Reported malaria cases/1000, all ages
—— Reported malaria cases/1000, <5 years

Rate of examination, case confirmation, malaria test positivity, % of confirmed cases that are *P. falciparum*

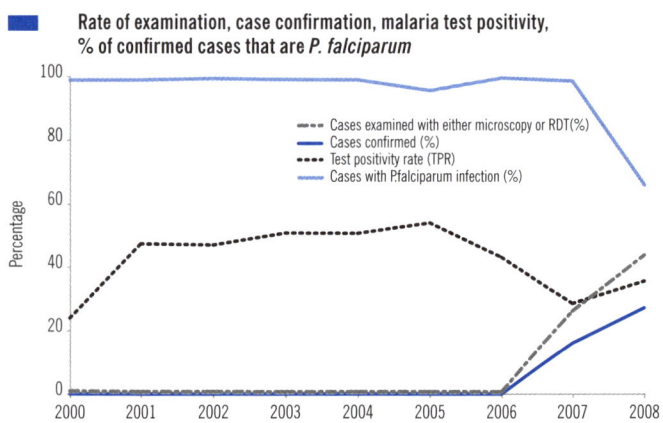

- - - Cases examined with either microscopy or RDT(%)
—— Cases confirmed (%)
····· Test positivity rate (TPR)
—— Cases with P.falciparum infection (%)

Year	Reported malaria cases, all ages	Reported malaria cases, < 5 years	All-cause outpatient consultations, all ages	All-cause outpatient consultations, < 5 years	Examined	Positive	P. falciparum	Reporting completeness of outpatient health facilities (%)	Reporting completeness of districts (%)
2000	964 623		1 045 630		3 758	897	889		
2001	2 199 247		2 259 025		3 244	1 531	1 517		
2002	2 640 168		2 771 867		3 704	1 735	1 727		
2003	4 386 638		4 548 049		4 820	2 438	2 418		
2004	4 133 514				5 320	2 684	2 659		
2005	6 334 608	2 650 284	6 994 007		5 531	2 971	2 844		
2006	5 008 959	2 380 353	6 291 164	2 735 273	4 779	2 050	2 043		
2007	4 730 484	2 260 081	9 301 888	4 109 716	1 207 850	759 059	1 642	48	
2008	5 371 196	2 450 304	10 314 473	4 455 022	2 314 880	1 462 300	1 196	53	

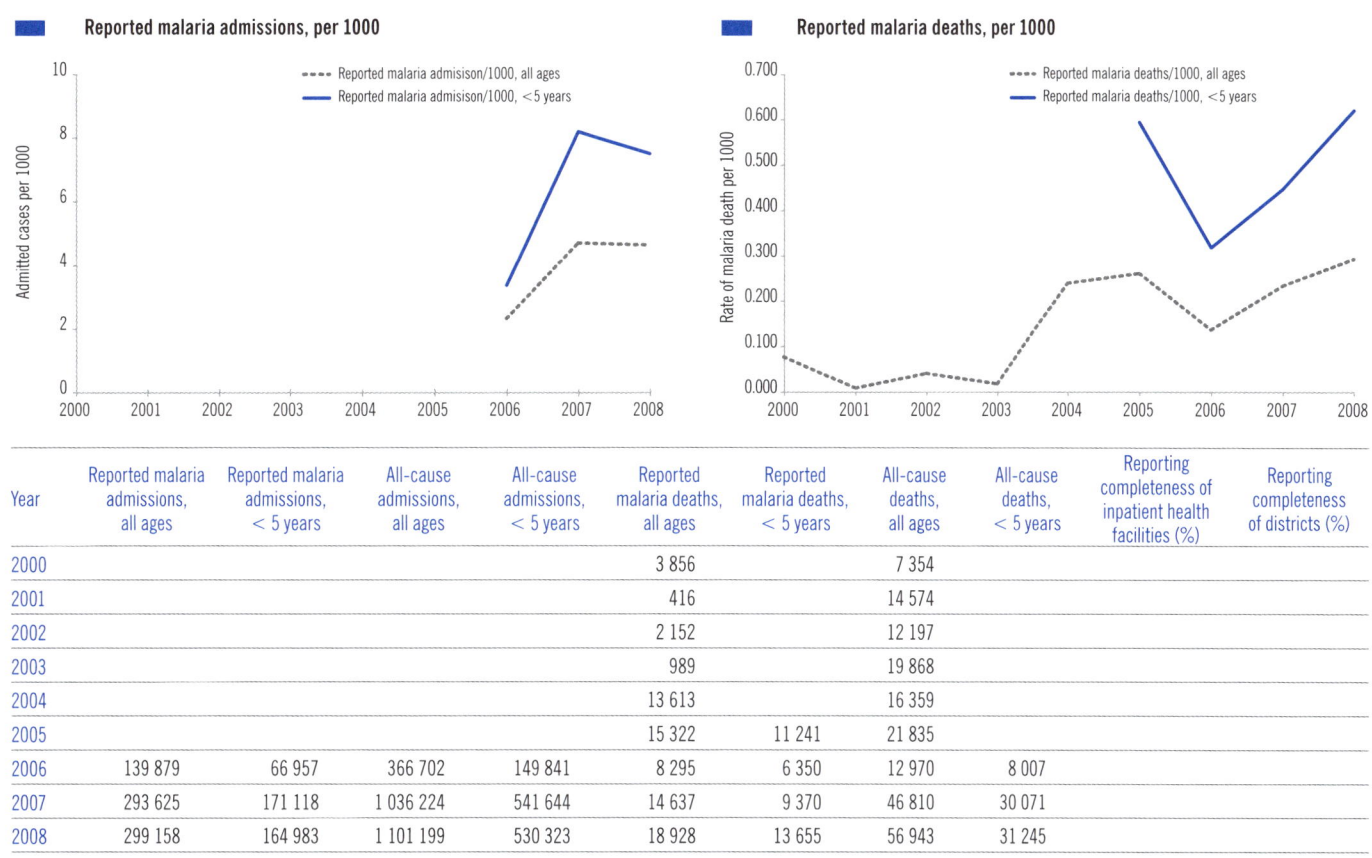

Reported malaria admissions, per 1000

- ···· Reported malaria admisison/1000, all ages
- —— Reported malaria admisison/1000, <5 years

Reported malaria deaths, per 1000

- ···· Reported malaria deaths/1000, all ages
- —— Reported malaria deaths/1000, <5 years

Year	Reported malaria admissions, all ages	Reported malaria admissions, < 5 years	All-cause admissions, all ages	All-cause admissions, < 5 years	Reported malaria deaths, all ages	Reported malaria deaths, < 5 years	All-cause deaths, all ages	All-cause deaths, < 5 years	Reporting completeness of inpatient health facilities (%)	Reporting completeness of districts (%)
2000					3 856		7 354			
2001					416		14 574			
2002					2 152		12 197			
2003					989		19 868			
2004					13 613		16 359			
2005					15 322	11 241	21 835			
2006	139 879	66 957	366 702	149 841	8 295	6 350	12 970	8 007		
2007	293 625	171 118	1 036 224	541 644	14 637	9 370	46 810	30 071		
2008	299 158	164 983	1 101 199	530 323	18 928	13 655	56 943	31 245		

II. INTERVENTION POLICIES AND STRATEGIES

Intervention	WHO-RECOMMENDED POLICIES / STRATEGIES	Yes or No	Year adopted	OPTIONAL POLICIES / STRATEGIES	Yes or No	Year adoped
Insecticide-treated nets (ITN)	Distribution of ITN/LLINs – Free	Yes	2006	Distribution – Antenatal care	Yes	2003
	Targeting all age groups	Yes	2008	Distribution – EPI routine and campaign	Yes	2003
				Targeting children < 5 years and pregnant women	Yes	2006
				ITN distribution is subsidized	Yes	2003
Indoor residual spraying (IRS)	IRS is a primary vector control intervention	Yes	2008	Insecticide-resistance management implemented	Yes	2008
	DDT is used for IRS (public health) only	Yes	2008	Where IRS is conducted, other options are also implemented, e.g. ITN	Yes	2008
				IRS is used for prevention and control of epidemics	Yes	2008
Intermittent preventive treatment (IPT)	IPT used to prevent malaria during pregnancy	Yes	2004			
Case management	Oral artemisinin monotherapies banned (prohibited from registration or removed from the system)	Yes	2007	Parasitological confirmation for patients ≥ 5 years only	Yes	–
	Parasitological confirmation for patients of all ages	Yes	–	Malaria diagnosis is free of charge in the public sector	No	–
	ACT is free of charge for < 5 years old in the public sector	No	–	ACT is free of charge for patients ≥ 5 years in the public sector	No	–
	Diagnosis of malaria of inpatients is based on parasitological confirmation	Yes	2009	ACT is delivered at community level through community agents (beyond the health facilities)	Yes	2007
	Pre-referral treatment with quinine or artemether IM or artesunate suppositories	No	–	Uncomplicated malaria cases are admitted	No	–
	Oversight regulation of case management in the private sectors	Yes	2005			
	RDTs used at community level	No	–			

				Results of therapeutic efficacy tests						
Antimalarial policy	Type of medicine	Year adopted	Study year	No. of studies	Median	Minimum	Maximum	Percentiles:	25%	75%
First-line treatment of *P. falciparum* (unconfirmed)	AS+AQ	2005	2003–2005	8	6.2	0	19		2.5	6.8
First-line treatment of *P. falciparum* (confirmed)	AS+AQ	2005								
Treatment failure of *P. falciparum*	QN(7d)	2005								
Treatment of severe malaria	QN(7d)	2005								
Treatment of *P. vivax*	–	–								

III. IMPLEMENTING MALARIA CONTROL

Coverage of ITN: survey data

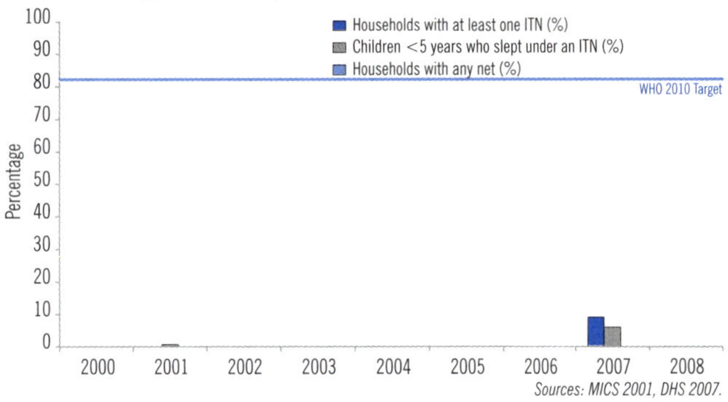

- Households with at least one ITN (%)
- Children <5 years who slept under an ITN (%)
- Households with any net (%)

WHO 2010 Target

Percentage — years 2000–2008

Sources: MICS 2001, DHS 2007.

Coverage of IRS and ITN: programme data

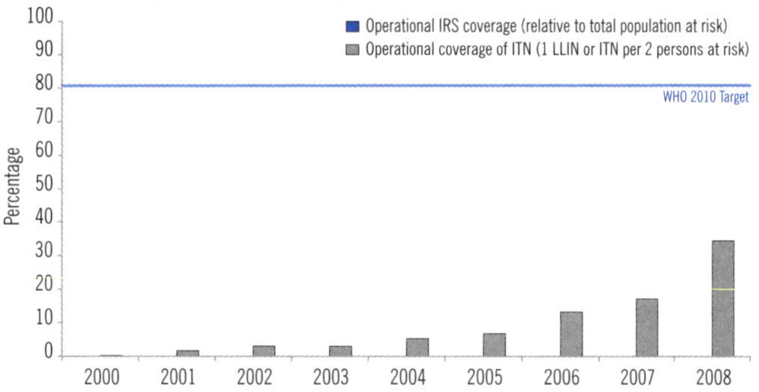

- Operational IRS coverage (relative to total population at risk)
- Operational coverage of ITN (1 LLIN or ITN per 2 persons at risk)

WHO 2010 Target

Percentage — years 2000–2008

Access by febrile children to effective treatment: survey data

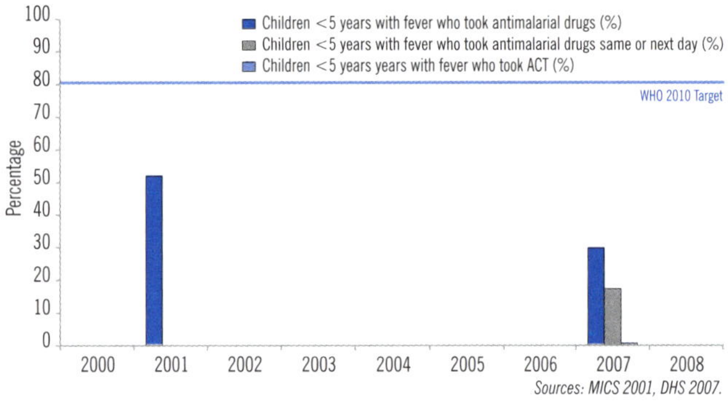

- Children <5 years with fever who took antimalarial drugs (%)
- Children <5 years with fever who took antimalarial drugs same or next day (%)
- Children <5 years years with fever who took ACT (%)

WHO 2010 Target

Percentage — years 2000–2008

Sources: MICS 2001, DHS 2007.

Access to effective treatment: programme data

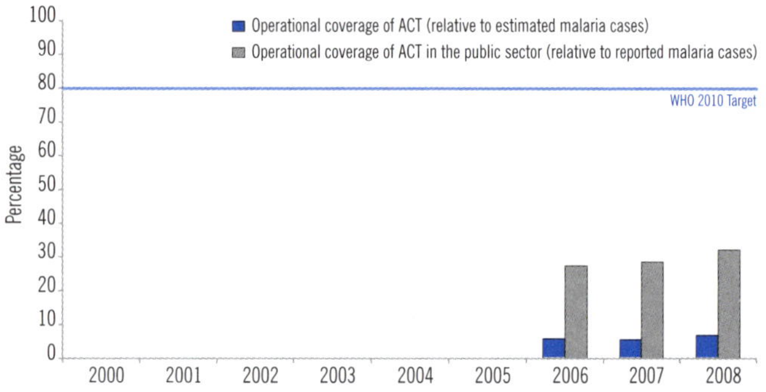

- Operational coverage of ACT (relative to estimated malaria cases)
- Operational coverage of ACT in the public sector (relative to reported malaria cases)

WHO 2010 Target

Percentage — years 2000–2008

Year	Pregnant women who slept under any net (%)	Pregnant women who slept under an ITN (%)	Children < 5 years with fever (%)	Febrile children < 5 years who sought treatment in HF (%)	Number of households protected by IRS	Number of people protected by IRS	Number of ITNs and/or LLINs	Number of 1st-line treatment courses received	Number of ACT treatment courses received
2000							70 000		
2001			–	–			400 000		
2002							583 650		
2003							338 856		
2004							877 131		
2005							791 135		
2006							3 153 026	1 373 318	1 373 318
2007			–	–			2 385 684	1 348 304	1 348 304
2008					22 000	82 975	5 788 513	1 723 655	1 723 655

IV. FINANCING MALARIA CONTROL

Governmental and external financing

Funding by source ($m) — years 2000–2008

Breakdown of expenditure by intervention in 2008

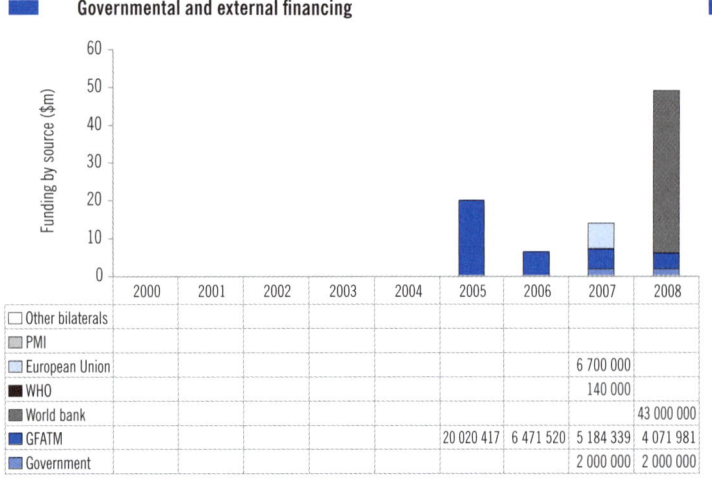

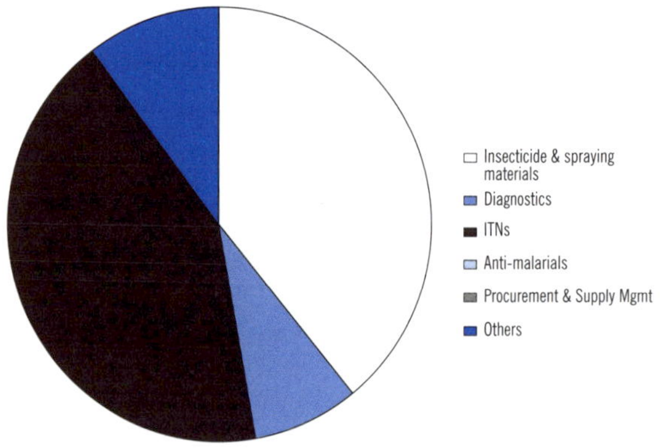

- □ Insecticide & spraying materials
- ■ Diagnostics
- ■ ITNs
- ■ Anti-malarials
- ■ Procurement & Supply Mgmt
- ■ Others

	2000	2001	2002	2003	2004	2005	2006	2007	2008
□ Other bilaterals									
■ PMI									
□ European Union								6 700 000	
■ WHO								140 000	
■ World bank									43 000 000
■ GFATM						20 020 417	6 471 520	5 184 339	4 071 981
■ Government								2 000 000	2 000 000

V. SOURCE OF INFORMATION

PROGRAMME DATA		SURVEY AND OTHER DATA	
Reported cases	Surveillance data	Insecticide-treated nets (ITN)	MICS 2001, DHS 2007
Operational coverage of ITNs, IRS and access to medicines	Programme report	Treatment	MICS 2001, DHS 2007
Financial data	Programme report	Use of health services	MICS 2001

ETHIOPIA

Ethiopia had approximately 4% of all cases in the African Region in 2006. Malaria is present everywhere except in the central highlands. Epidemics are frequent, the last having occurred in 2003–2004. Over half the cases are caused by *P. falciparum*. The number of reported malaria cases decreased from an average of 3.2 million (excluding the epidemic year, 2004) to 2 532 645 in 2008, of which over 986 000 were tested (39%) by either microscopy or a RDT, and 460 000 cases were confirmed. The reported number of malaria deaths in children under 5 years fell from an average of 1866 during 2001–2006 to only 1169 in 2008 (a decrease of over 37%). The programme distributed 19.6 million LLINs between 2006 and 2008, targeting 40 million people at risk. The percentage of households with one ITN increased from 3% nationwide in 2005 to 66% in 2007. IRS was expanded to cover 5.6 million households, protecting 28 million people at risk. Nearly 4 million treatment courses of ACT were delivered in 2007 and 8 million in 2008, which was adequate to cover all reported cases in the public sector. The recent decrease in the number of cases and deaths coincides with rapid expansion of control efforts. Funding increased from US$ 2.7 million in 2001 to over US$ 200 million between 2004 and 2007, mainly from the Global Fund and the United States President's Malaria Initiative. The Government provides about US$ 5 million annually. With the round 8 Global Fund grant, the programme has secured over US$ 150 million for the next five years.

I. EPIDEMIOLOGICAL PROFILE

Population, endemicity and malaria burden

Population (in thousands)	2008	%
All age groups	80 713	
< 5 years	13 323	17
≥ 5 years	67 390	83

Population by malaria endemicity (in thousands)	2008	%
High transmission ≥ 1/1000	1 022	1
Low transmission (0–1/1000)	53 128	66
Malaria-free (0 cases)	26 564	33
Rural population	67 057	83

Vector and parasite profiles

Major *Anopheles* species	*arabiensis, funestus, coustani, nili, paludis, pharoensis, quadriannulatus*
Plasmodium species	*falciparum, vivax*

Stratification of burden (reported cases, per 1000)

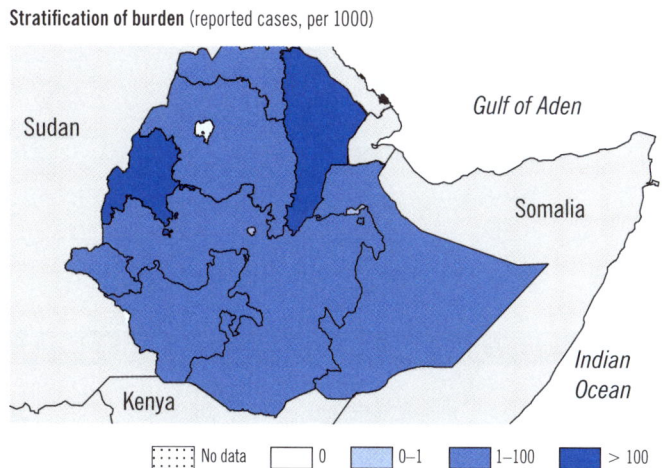

No data | 0 | 0–1 | 1–100 | > 100

Trends in malaria morbidity and mortality

Reported malaria cases, per 1000

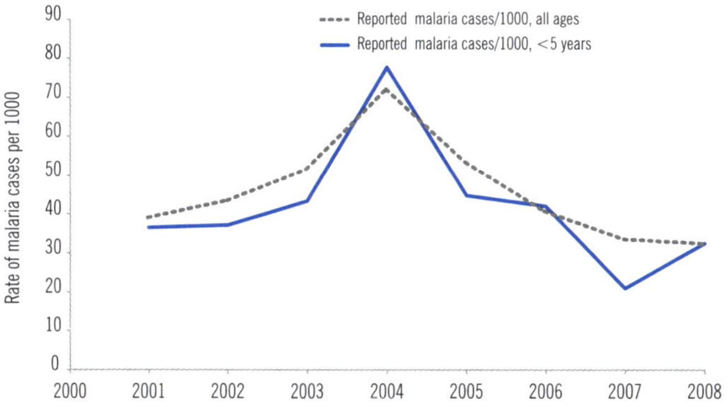

- ····· Reported malaria cases/1000, all ages
- —— Reported malaria cases/1000, <5 years

Rate of examination, case confirmation, malaria test positivity, % of confirmed cases that are *P. falciparum*

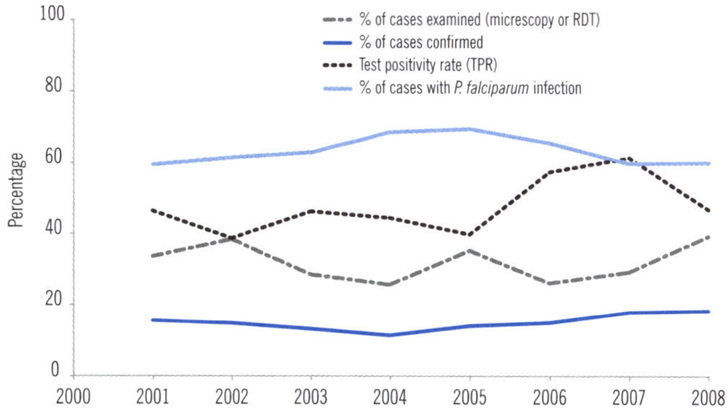

- ----- % of cases examined (microscopy or RDT)
- —— % of cases confirmed
- ······ Test positivity rate (TPR)
- —— % of cases with *P. falciparum* infection

Year	Reported malaria cases, all ages	Reported malaria cases, < 5 years	All-cause outpatient consultations, all ages	All-cause outpatient consultations, < 5 years	Examined	Positive	*P. falciparum*	Reporting completeness of outpatient health facilities (%)	Reporting completeness of districts (%)
2000									
2001	2 555 314	428 089	11 097 537		851 942	392 377	233 218		
2002	2 929 685	441 811	10 916 435		1 115 167	427 795	262 623		
2003	3 582 097	522 491	11 660 924		1 010 925	463 797	291 403		
2004	5 170 614	948 587	12 264 096		1 312 422	578 904	396 621		
2005	3 901 957	554 262	14 353 595		1 364 194	538 942	374 335		
2006	3 038 565	528 603	24 620 248		785 209	447 780	293 326		
2007	2 557 152	268 854	24 737 524		739 627	451 816	269 514		
2008	2 532 645	422 248	18 835 927	519 099	986 323	458 561	274 657		

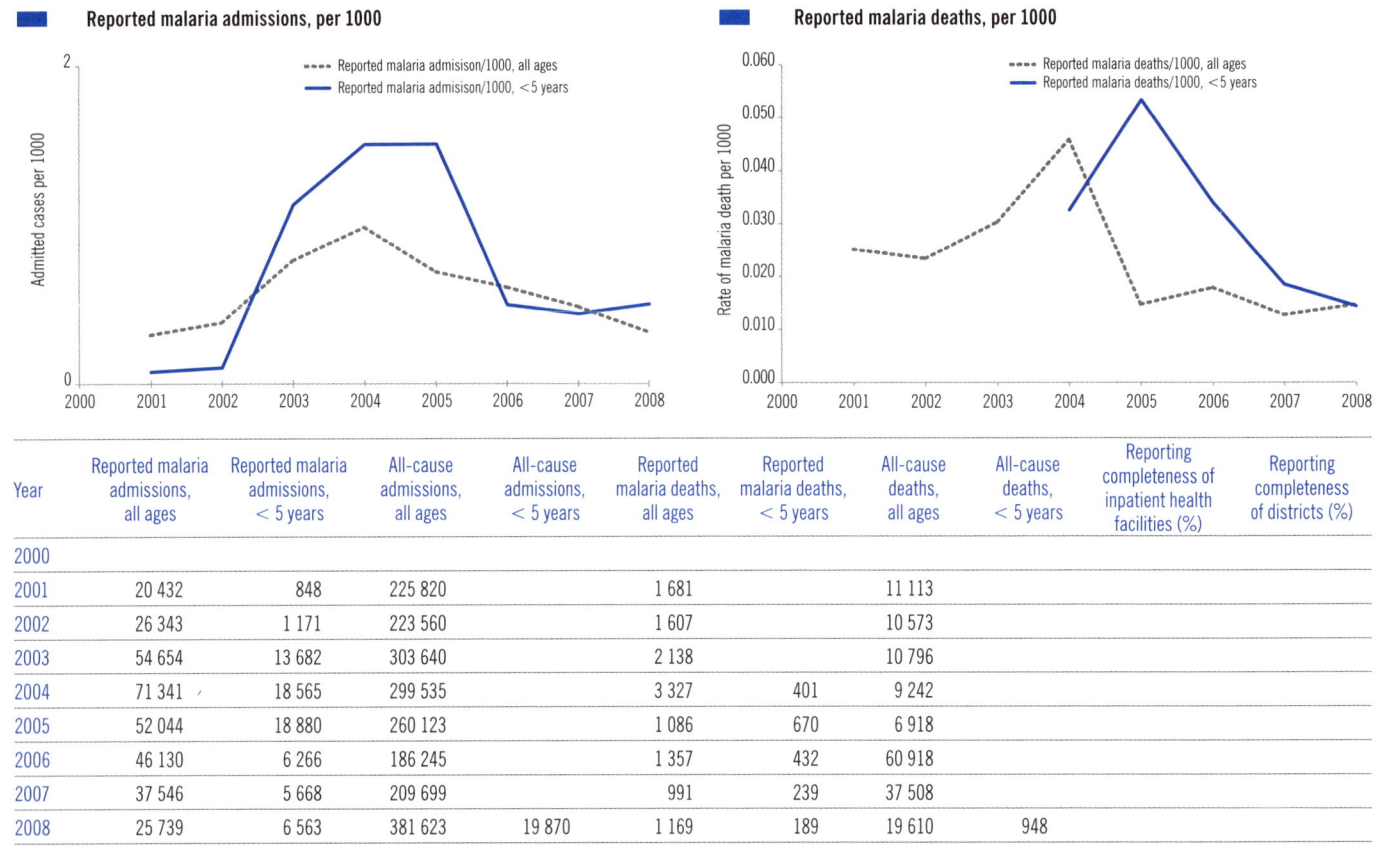

Reported malaria admissions, per 1000

- ---- Reported malaria admission/1000, all ages
- —— Reported malaria admission/1000, <5 years

Admitted cases per 1000

Reported malaria deaths, per 1000

- ---- Reported malaria deaths/1000, all ages
- —— Reported malaria deaths/1000, <5 years

Rate of malaria death per 1000

Year	Reported malaria admissions, all ages	Reported malaria admissions, < 5 years	All-cause admissions, all ages	All-cause admissions, < 5 years	Reported malaria deaths, all ages	Reported malaria deaths, < 5 years	All-cause deaths, all ages	All-cause deaths, < 5 years	Reporting completeness of inpatient health facilities (%)	Reporting completeness of districts (%)
2000										
2001	20 432	848	225 820		1 681		11 113			
2002	26 343	1 171	223 560		1 607		10 573			
2003	54 654	13 682	303 640		2 138		10 796			
2004	71 341	18 565	299 535		3 327	401	9 242			
2005	52 044	18 880	260 123		1 086	670	6 918			
2006	46 130	6 266	186 245		1 357	432	60 918			
2007	37 546	5 668	209 699		991	239	37 508			
2008	25 739	6 563	381 623	19 870	1 169	189	19 610	948		

II. INTERVENTION POLICIES AND STRATEGIES

Intervention	WHO-RECOMMENDED POLICIES / STRATEGIES	Yes or No	Year adopted	OPTIONAL POLICIES / STRATEGIES	Yes or No	Year adoped
Insecticide-treated nets (ITN)	Distribution of ITN/LLINs – Free	Yes	2004	Distribution – Antenatal care	No	–
	Targeting all age groups	Yes	2004	Distribution – EPI routine and campaign	Yes	2006
				Targeting children < 5 years and pregnant women	Yes	2001
				ITN distribution is subsidized	Yes	2004
Indoor residual spraying (IRS)	IRS is a primary vector control intervention	Yes	1997	Insecticide-resistance management implemented	Yes	1997
	DDT is used for IRS (public health) only	Yes	1998	Where IRS is conducted, other options are also implemented, e.g. ITN	Yes	1997
				IRS is used for prevention and control of epidemics	Yes	1998
Intermittent preventive treatment (IPT)	IPT used to prevent malaria during pregnancy	No	–			
Case management	Oral artemisinin monotherapies banned (prohibited from registration or removed from the system)	Yes	1997	Parasitological confirmation for patients ≥ 5 years only	No	–
	Parasitological confirmation for patients of all ages	Yes	1997	Malaria diagnosis is free of charge in the public sector	Yes	2004
	ACT is free of charge for < 5 years old in the public sector	Yes	2004	ACT is free of charge for patients ≥ 5 years in the public sector	Yes	2004
	Diagnosis of malaria of inpatients is based on parasitological confirmation	Yes	1997	ACT is delivered at community level through community agents (beyond the health facilities)	Yes	2004
	Pre-referral treatment with quinine or artemether IM or artesunate suppositories	Yes	1997	Uncomplicated malaria cases are admitted	No	–
	Oversight regulation of case management in the private sectors	No	–			
	RDTs used at community level	Yes	2004			

					Results of therapeutic efficacy tests					
Antimalarial policy	Type of medicine	Year adopted	Study year	No. of studies	Median	Minimum	Maximum	Percentiles:	25%	75%
First-line treatment of *P. falciparum* (unconfirmed)	AL	2004	2003–2008	8	0	0	3.4		0	2.9
First-line treatment of *P. falciparum* (confirmed)	AL	2004								
Treatment failure of *P. falciparum*	QN(7d)	2004								
Treatment of severe malaria	QN(7d)	2004								
Treatment of *P. vivax*	CQ	2004								

III. IMPLEMENTING MALARIA CONTROL

Coverage of ITN: survey data

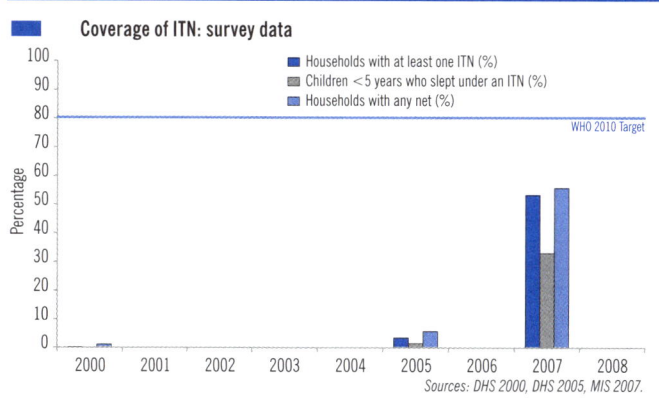

Sources: DHS 2000, DHS 2005, MIS 2007.

Coverage of IRS and ITN: programme data

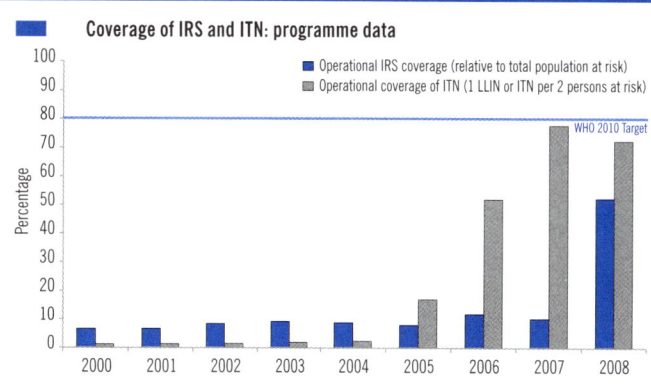

Access by febrile children to effective treatment: survey data

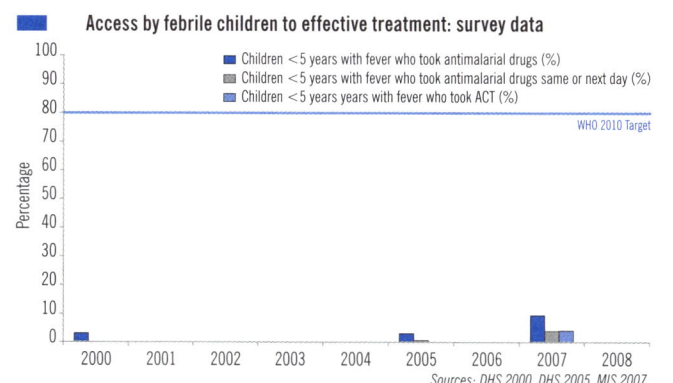

Sources: DHS 2000, DHS 2005, MIS 2007.

Access to effective treatment: programme data

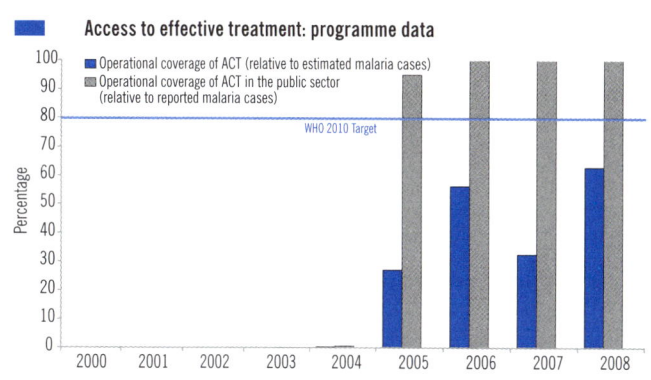

Year	Pregnant women who slept under any net (%)	Pregnant women who slept under an ITN (%)	Children < 5 years with fever (%)	Febrile children < 5 years who sought treatment in HF (%)	Number of households protected by IRS	Number of people protected by IRS	Number of ITNs and/or LLINs	Number of 1st-line treatment courses received	Number of ACT treatment courses received
2000			–	–	568 780	2 843 898	250 000		
2001					711 376	2 960 986	280 000		
2002					768 430	3 826 898	320 000		
2003					517 925	4 298 183	430 000		
2004					521 010	4 228 465	550 000	9 725 000	25 000
2005	2	1	–	–	594 521	3 912 903	4 243 157	3 500 000	3 193 993
2006					702 959	5 984 485	9 070 718	6 950 000	6 806 744
2007	37	35	–	–	2 523 902	5 303 213	7 178 443	5 450 400	4 032 640
2008					5 641 275	28 206 375	3 316 696		8 000 000

IV. FINANCING MALARIA CONTROL

Governmental and external financing

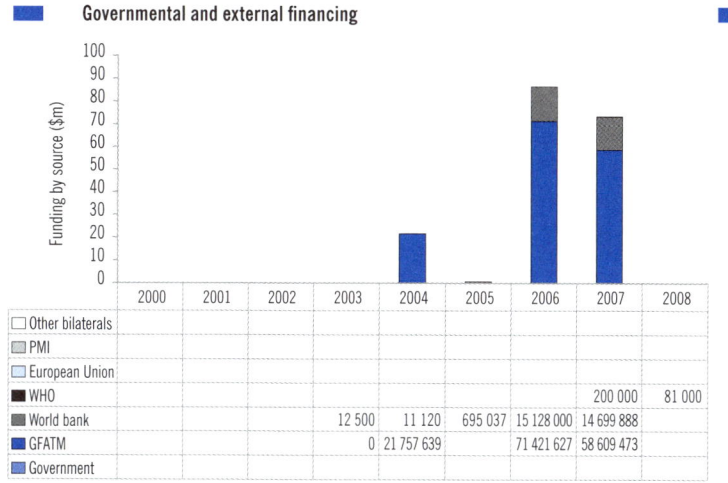

Breakdown of expenditure by intervention in 2008

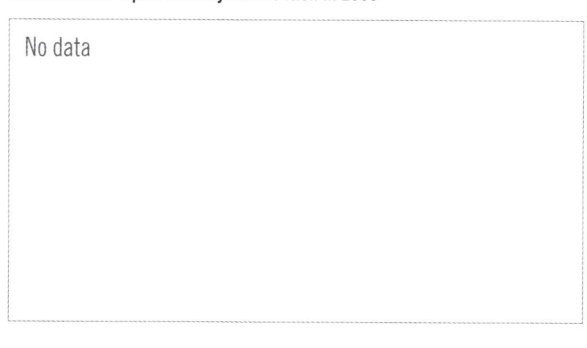

No data

V. SOURCE OF INFORMATION

PROGRAMME DATA		SURVEY AND OTHER DATA	
Reported cases	Surveillance data	Insecticide-treated nets (ITN)	DHS 2000, DHS 2005, MIS 2007
Operational coverage of ITNs, IRS and access to medicines	Programme report	Treatment	DHS 2000, DHS 2005, MIS 2007
Financial data	Programme report	Use of health services	DHS 1997

GHANA

Ghana had an estimated 8.3 million malaria cases in 2006 and 3.2 million in 2008. Most cases are caused by *P. falciparum*; 26% of the reported cases were confirmed in 2008. There was no evidence of a reduction in the number of cases between 2001 and 2007, and the numbers of reported inpatient cases and deaths have increased. It is not known if the rise is due to better reporting or a change in the incidence of malaria. The programme delivered about 4.7 million LLINs during 2006–2008, adequate to cover 40% of the population at risk. The programme implemented IRS covering 68 000 households, protecting about 600 000 people at risk in selected areas in 2008. In the 2008 demographic and health survey, 33% of households owned an ITN, and only 19% of children under 5 had slept under an ITN the previous night. While 24% of febrile children received an antimalarial drug, only 12% were given ACT. Funding for malaria control increased from almost nothing in 2005 to about US$ 90 million during 2006–2008, with annual expenditure of US$ 30 million. Major funding is provided by the Government, the Global Fund, the World Bank and the United States President's Malaria Initiative.

I. EPIDEMIOLOGICAL PROFILE

Population, endemicity and malaria burden

Population (in thousands)	2008	%
All age groups	23 351	
< 5 years	3 319	14
≥ 5 years	20 032	86

Population by malaria endemicity (in thousands)	2008	%
High transmission ≥ 1/1000	23 351	100
Low transmission (0–1/1000)	0	0
Malaria-free (0 cases)	0	0
Rural population	11 675	50

Vector and parasite profiles

Major *Anopheles* species	*gambiae, funestus, brochieri, coustani, flavicosta, hancocki, hargreavesi, melas, nili, paludis, pharoensis*
Plasmodium species	*falciparum, vivax*

Stratification of burden (reported cases, per 1000)

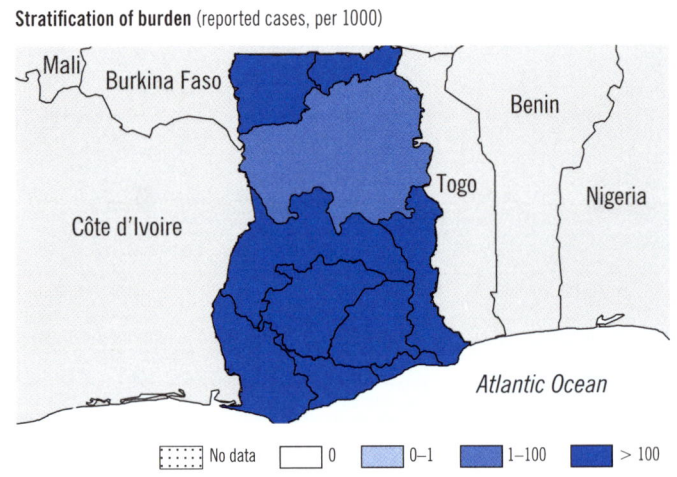

No data   0   0–1   1–100   > 100

Trends in malaria morbidity and mortality

Reported malaria cases, per 1000

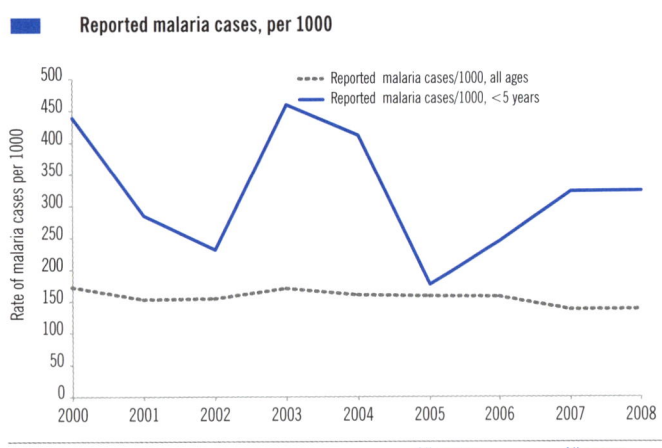

Rate of examination, case confirmation, malaria test positivity, % of confirmed cases that are *P. falciparum*

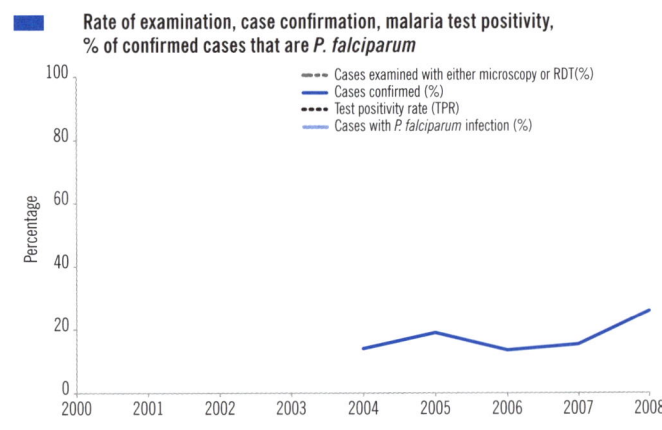

Year	Reported malaria cases, all ages	Reported malaria cases, < 5 years	All-cause outpatient consultations, all ages	All-cause outpatient consultations, < 5 years	Examined	Positive	*P. falciparum*	Reporting completeness of outpatient health facilities (%)	Reporting completeness of districts (%)
2000	3 349 528	1 303 685	7 000 000	2 591 570				32	52
2001	3 044 844	856 872	6 904 408	1 518 970				32	52
2002	3 140 893	705 288	7 253 794	1 679 257				32	52
2003	3 552 896	1 421 148	8 129 510	1 900 809				30	57
2004	3 416 033	1 289 874	7 540 470	1 318 900		475 441		30	56
2005	3 452 969	562 941	7 753 845	1 757 833		655 093		31	81
2006	3 511 452	789 952	9 114 401	1 712 728		472 255		31	65
2007	3 123 147	1 056 331	9 259 343	3 417 098		476 484		32	70
2008	3 200 147	1 074 267	10 323 853	2 191 381	827 436	827 438		25	81

Reported malaria admissions, per 1000

Legend:
- Reported malaria admision/1000, all ages
- Reported malaria admision/1000, <5 years

Reported malaria deaths, per 1000

Legend:
- Reported malaria deaths/1000, all ages
- Reported malaria deaths/1000, <5 years

Year	Reported malaria admissions, all ages	Reported malaria admissions, < 5 years	All-cause admissions, all ages	All-cause admissions, < 5 years	Reported malaria deaths, all ages	Reported malaria deaths, < 5 years	All-cause deaths, all ages	All-cause deaths, < 5 years	Reporting completeness of inpatient health facilities (%)	Reporting completeness of districts (%)
2000	84 091	27 478	263 269	98 507	6 108	3 952	18 323	8 872		
2001	87 236	38 911	268 598	102 397	1 717	1 717	7 805	6 265		
2002	116 600	38 340	310 793	100 895	2 376	2 376	8 714	5 913		
2003	115 401	45 648	517 566	120 126	2 103	2 103	7 636	5 983		
2004	132 566	46 886	844 091	123 384	1 575	1 575	5 727	5 887		
2005	118 449	31 644	483 038	174 522	2 037	2 037	6 610	4 532		
2006	122 928	51 407	356 000	97 860	3 125	3 125	15 102	4 988		
2007	157 628	22 019	556 036	113 952	4 622	4 622	18 395	5 263		
2008	272 802	99 217	900 242	181 427	3 889	1 697	21 246	4 907		

II.   INTERVENTION POLICIES AND STRATEGIES

Intervention	WHO-RECOMMENDED POLICIES / STRATEGIES	Yes or No	Year adopted	OPTIONAL POLICIES / STRATEGIES	Yes or No	Year adoped
Insecticide-treated nets (ITN)	Distribution of ITN/LLINs – Free	Yes	2006	Distribution – Antenatal care	Yes	1999
	Targeting all age groups	No	–	Distribution – EPI routine and campaign	Yes	2000
				Targeting children < 5 years and pregnant women	Yes	1999
				ITN distribution is subsidized	Yes	1997
Indoor residual spraying (IRS)	IRS is a primary vector control intervention	Yes	2005	Insecticide-resistance management implemented	Yes	2004
	DDT is used for IRS (public health) only	No	–	Where IRS is conducted, other options are also implemented, e.g. ITN	Yes	2005
				IRS is used for prevention and control of epidemics	Yes	2004
Intermittent preventive treatment (IPT)	IPT used to prevent malaria during pregnancy	Yes	2003			
Case management	Oral artemisinin monotherapies banned (prohibited from registration or removed from the system)	Yes	2006	Parasitological confirmation for patients ≥ 5 years only	Yes	1997
	Parasitological confirmation for patients of all ages	No	–	Malaria diagnosis is free of charge in the public sector	No	–
	ACT is free of charge for < 5 years old in the public sector	No	–	ACT is free of charge for patients ≥ 5 years in the public sector	No	–
	Diagnosis of malaria of inpatients is based on parasitological confirmation	No	–	ACT is delivered at community level through community agents (beyond the health facilities)	Yes	2008
	Pre-referral treatment with quinine or artemether IM or artesunate suppositories	Yes	1998	Uncomplicated malaria cases are admitted	No	–
	Oversight regulation of case management in the private sectors	Yes	1997			
	RDTs used at community level	No	–			

Antimalarial policy	Type of medicine	Year adopted	Results of therapeutic efficacy tests					
			Study year	No. of studies	Median	Minimum	Maximum	Percentiles: 25% 75%
First-line treatment of *P. falciparum* (unconfirmed)	AL, AS+AQ	2004						
First-line treatment of *P. falciparum* (confirmed)	AL, AS+AQ	2004						
Treatment failure of *P. falciparum*	QN(7d)	2004						
Treatment of severe malaria	QN(7d)	2004						
Treatment of *P. vivax*	–	–						

III. IMPLEMENTING MALARIA CONTROL

Coverage of ITN: survey data

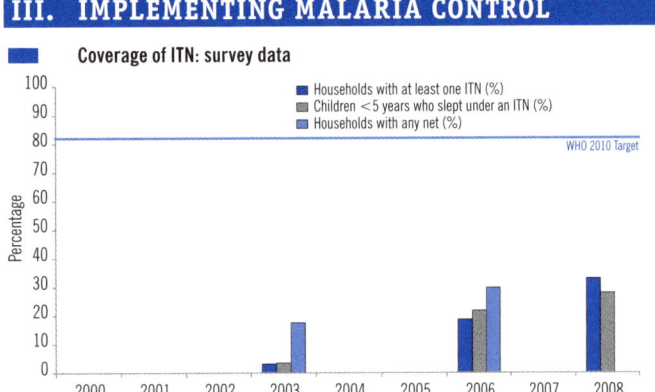

Sources: DHS 2003, MISC 2006, DHS 2008.

Coverage of IRS and ITN: programme data

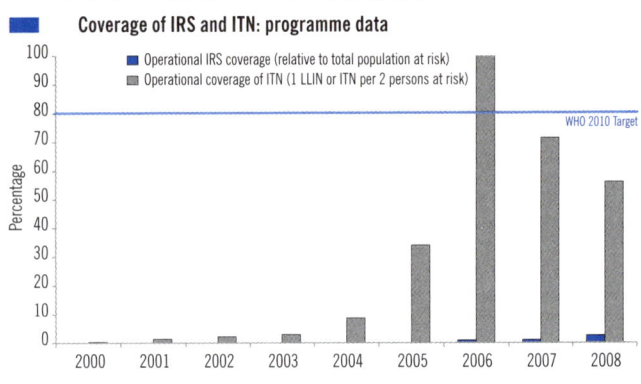

Access by febrile children to effective treatment: survey data

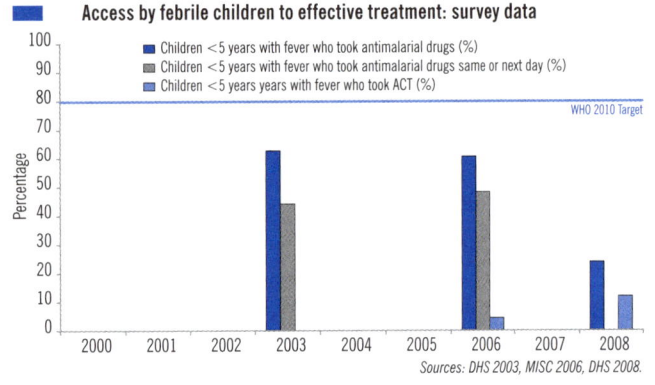

Sources: DHS 2003, MISC 2006, DHS 2008.

Access to effective treatment: programme data

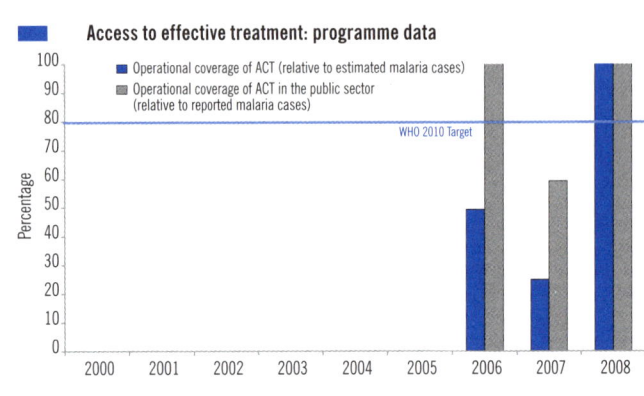

Year	Pregnant women who slept under any net (%)	Pregnant women who slept under an ITN (%)	Children < 5 years with fever (%)	Febrile children < 5 years who sought treatment in HF (%)	Number of households protected by IRS	Number of people protected by IRS	Number of ITNs and/or LLINs	Number of 1st-line treatment courses received	Number of ACT treatment courses received
2000							15 000		
2001							60 000		
2002							742 000		
2003		3	–	–			85 000		
2004							375 000		
2005							618 855		
2006			–	–	134 000	200 000	2 100 000	3 600 000	3 600 000
2007					154 000	240 000	1 477 538	2 018 967	1 852 967
2008			–	–	68 252	601 973	2 100 000	9 616 195	9 783 983

IV. FINANCING MALARIA CONTROL

Governmental and external financing

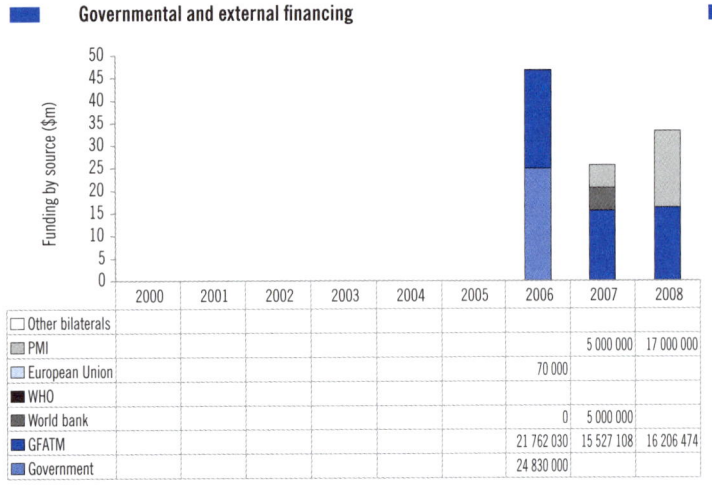

	2000	2001	2002	2003	2004	2005	2006	2007	2008
Other bilaterals									
PMI								5 000 000	17 000 000
European Union							70 000		
WHO									
World bank							0	5 000 000	
GFATM							21 762 030	15 527 108	16 206 474
Government							24 830 000		

Breakdown of expenditure by intervention in 2008

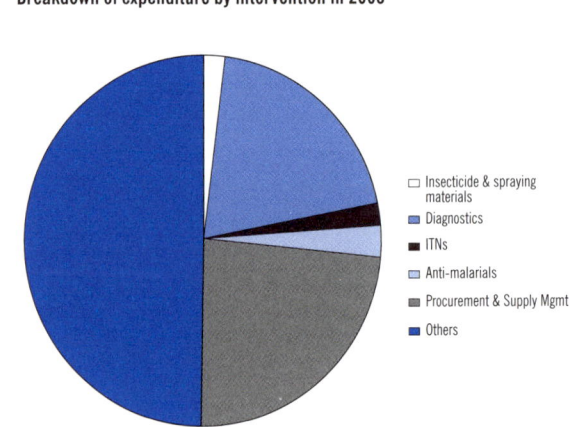

V. SOURCE OF INFORMATION

PROGRAMME DATA		SURVEY AND OTHER DATA	
Reported cases	Surveillance data	Insecticide-treated nets (ITN)	DHS 2003, MICS 2006, DHS 2008
Operational coverage of ITNs, IRS and access to medicines	Programme report	Treatment	DHS 2003, MICS 2006, DHS 2008
Financial data	Programme report	Use of health services	DHS 2003

INDIA

India accounts for approximately two thirds of the confirmed cases reported in the South-East Asia Region. In 2008, 96 million slides were examined, from which 1.5 million cases were confirmed. The number of cases has fallen from more than 2 million confirmed in 2000 to 1.5 million cases in 2008. About half the cases confirmed are due to *P. falciparum*. Five states account for 60% of cases: Orissa, Chhattisgarh, Madhya Pradesh, Jharkhand and West Bengal. Other highly endemic states include Arunachal Pradesh, Assam, Meghalaya and Tripura. A demographic and household survey carried out in 2005–2006 found that 36% of households owned a mosquito net. IRS has been the main method of mosquito control, covering about 54 million people at risk. The programme delivered 7.2 million ITNs, more than 1.5 million first-line treatments and 600 000 courses of ACT during 2008, enough to treat over two thirds of *P. falciparum* malaria cases. Funding for malaria programmes from domestic and external sources increased from US$ 54 million in 2001 to US$ 110 million in 2008, of which 65% was from the Government.

I. EPIDEMIOLOGICAL PROFILE

Population, endemicity and malaria burden

Population (in thousands)	2008	%
All age groups	1 181 412	
< 5 years	126 642	11
≥ 5 years	1 054 770	89

Population by malaria endemicity (in thousands)	2008	%
High transmission ≥ 1/1000	307 189	26
Low transmission (0–1/1000)	755 223	64
Malaria-free (0 cases)	118 999	10
Rural population	833 321	71

Vector and parasite profiles

Major *Anopheles* species	stephensi, culicifacies, dirus, fluviatilis, minimus, philippinensis
Plasmodium species	falciparum, vivax

Stratification of burden (reported cases, per 1000)

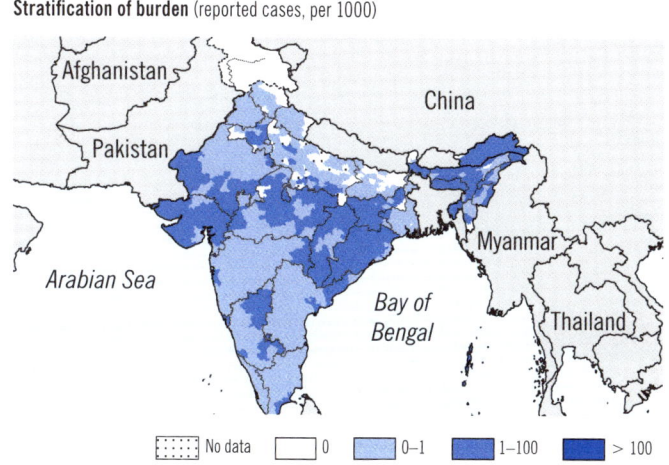

No data | 0 | 0–1 | 1–100 | > 100

Trends in malaria morbidity and mortality

Reported malaria cases, per 1000

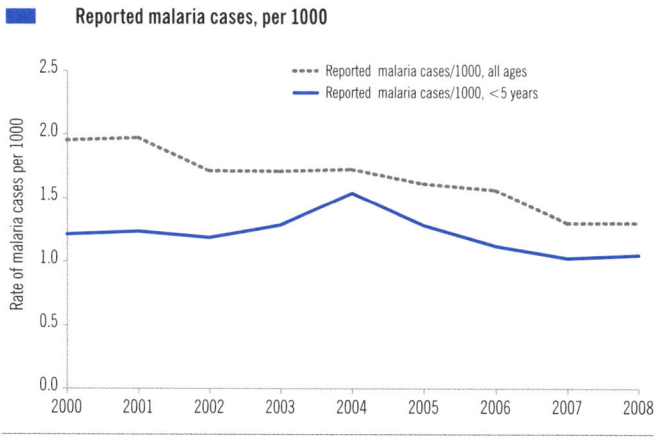

- - - - Reported malaria cases/1000, all ages
—— Reported malaria cases/1000, <5 years

Rate of examination, case confirmation, malaria test positivity, % of confirmed cases that are *P. falciparum*

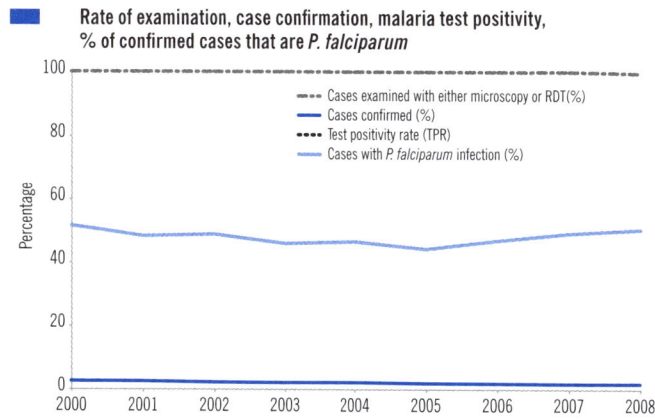

- - - Cases examined with either microscopy or RDT(%)
—— Cases confirmed (%)
···· Test positivity rate (TPR)
—— Cases with *P. falciparum* infection (%)

Year	Reported malaria cases, all ages	Reported malaria cases, < 5 years	All-cause outpatient consultations, all ages	All-cause outpatient consultations, < 5 years	Examined	Positive	P. falciparum	Reporting completeness of outpatient health facilities (%)	Reporting completeness of districts (%)
2000	2 031 790	153 500			86 790 375	2 031 790	1 045 170	100	100
2001	2 085 484	156 700			90 389 019	2 085 484	1 005 236	100	100
2002	1 841 227	150 605			91 617 725	1 841 227	897 446	100	100
2003	1 869 403	163 573			99 136 143	1 869 403	857 101	100	100
2004	1 915 363	196 064			97 111 526	1 915 363	890 152	100	100
2005	1 816 569	163 471			104 120 792	1 816 569	805 077	100	100
2006	1 785 109	142 463			106 606 703	1 785 109	838 555	100	100
2007	1 508 927	129 937			94 925 988	1 508 927	725 502	100	100
2008	1 532 467	132 431			95 368 303	1 532 467	771 670	100	100

Reported malaria admissions, per 1000

No data

Reported malaria deaths, per 1000

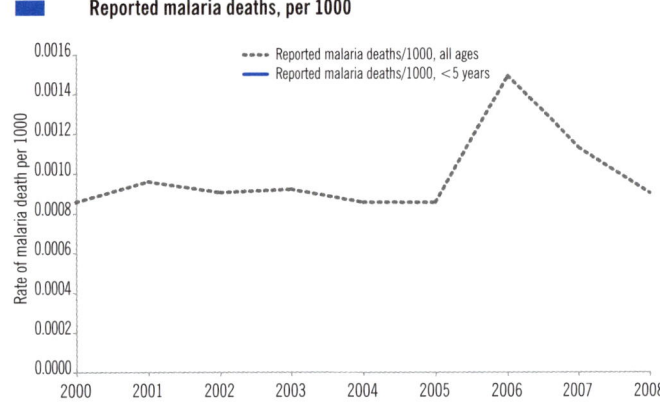

Year	Reported malaria admissions, all ages	Reported malaria admissions, < 5 years	All-cause admissions, all ages	All-cause admissions, < 5 years	Reported malaria deaths, all ages	Reported malaria deaths, < 5 years	All-cause deaths, all ages	All-cause deaths, < 5 years	Reporting completeness of inpatient health facilities (%)	Reporting completeness of districts (%)
2000					892				100	100
2001					1 015				100	100
2002					973				100	100
2003					1 006				100	100
2004					949				100	100
2005					963				100	100
2006					1 708				100	100
2007					1 311				100	100
2008					1 061				100	100

II.   INTERVENTION POLICIES AND STRATEGIES

Intervention	WHO-RECOMMENDED POLICIES / STRATEGIES	Yes or No	Year adopted	OPTIONAL POLICIES / STRATEGIES	Yes or No	Year adoped
Insecticide-treated nets (ITN)	Distribution of ITN/LLINs – Free	Yes	2001	Distribution – Antenatal care	Yes	2003
	Targeting all age groups	Yes	2001	Distribution – EPI routine and campaign	No	–
				Targeting children < 5 years and pregnant women	No	–
				ITN distribution is subsidized	No	–
Indoor residual spraying (IRS)	IRS is a primary vector control intervention	Yes	2000	Insecticide-resistance management implemented	Yes	2000
	DDT is used for IRS (public health) only	Yes	2000	Where IRS is conducted, other options are also implemented, e.g. ITN	Yes	2001
				IRS is used for prevention and control of epidemics	Yes	2000
Intermittent preventive treatment (IPT)	IPT used to prevent malaria during pregnancy	No	–			
Case management	Oral artemisinin monotherapies banned (prohibited from registration or removed from the system)	Yes	2009	Parasitological confirmation for patients ≥ 5 years only	No	–
	Parasitological confirmation for patients of all ages	Yes	2000	Malaria diagnosis is free of charge in the public sector	Yes	2000
	ACT is free of charge for < 5 years old in the public sector	Yes	2006	ACT is free of charge for patients ≥ 5 years in the public sector	Yes	2006
	Diagnosis of malaria of inpatients is based on parasitological confirmation	Yes	2000	ACT is delivered at community level through community agents (beyond the health facilities)	Yes	2007
	Pre-referral treatment with quinine or artemether IM or artesunate suppositories	Yes	2000	Uncomplicated malaria cases are admitted	No	–
	Oversight regulation of case management in the private sectors	Yes	2000			
	RDTs used at community level	Yes	2006			

Antimalarial policy	Type of medicine	Year adopted	Results of therapeutic efficacy tests						
			Study year	No. of studies	Median	Minimum	Maximum	Percentiles: 25%	75%
First-line treatment of *P. falciparum* (unconfirmed)	CQ+PQ	2007							
First-line treatment of *P. falciparum* (confirmed)	AS+SP	2007							
Treatment failure of *P. falciparum*	–	–							
Treatment of severe malaria	AM, QN	2007							
Treatment of *P. vivax*	CQ+PQ(14d)	2007							

III. IMPLEMENTING MALARIA CONTROL

Coverage of ITN: survey data

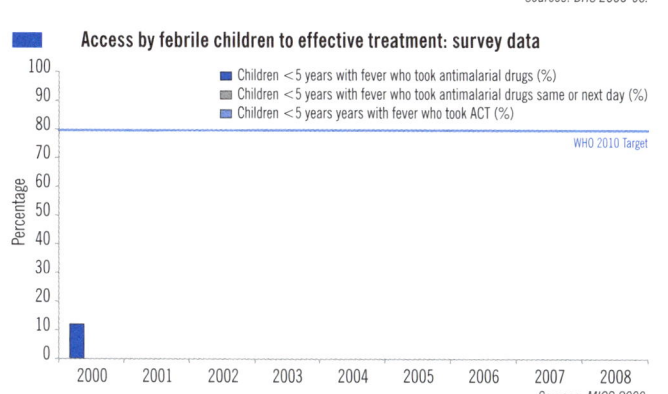

Sources: DHS 2005-06.

Coverage of IRS and ITN: programme data

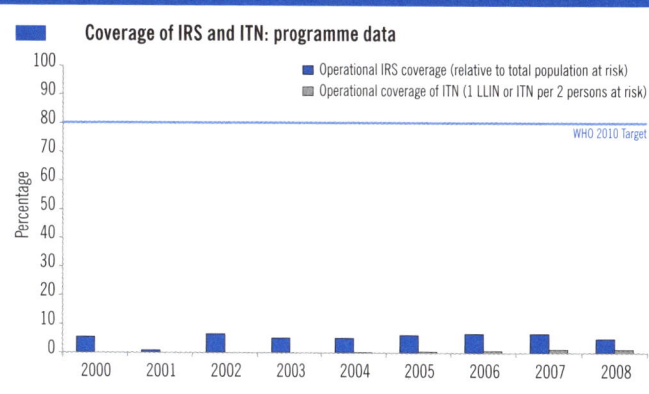

Access by febrile children to effective treatment: survey data

Sources: MICS 2000.

Access to effective treatment: programme data

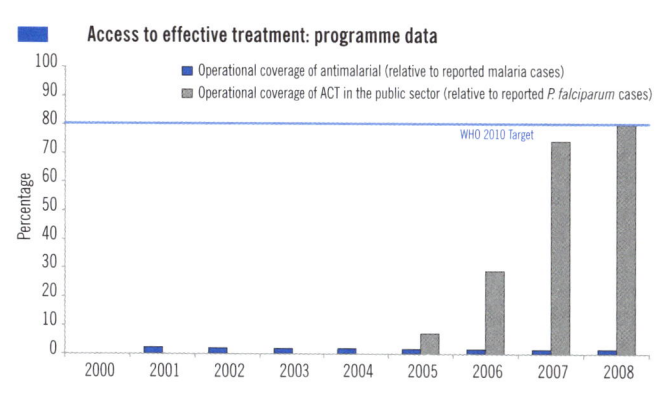

Year	Pregnant women who slept under any net (%)	Pregnant women who slept under an ITN (%)	Children < 5 years with fever (%)	Febrile children < 5 years who sought treatment in HF (%)	Number of households protected by IRS	Number of people protected by IRS	Number of ITNs and/or LLINs	Number of 1st-line treatment courses received	Number of ACT treatment courses received
2000			–	–		51 650 476			
2001						7 787 823	175 000	2 085 484	
2002						63 575 991	90 000	1 842 019	
2003						50 754 459	230 000	1 869 403	
2004						52 118 040	1 200 000	1 915 363	
2005			–	–		62 935 123	2 720 000	1 816 342	57 700
2006						69 457 913	3 950 000	1 780 777	242 300
2007						70 853 795	7 000 000	1 508 927	550 000
2008						53 773 347	7 240 000	1 532 497	622 000

IV. FINANCING MALARIA CONTROL

Governmental and external financing

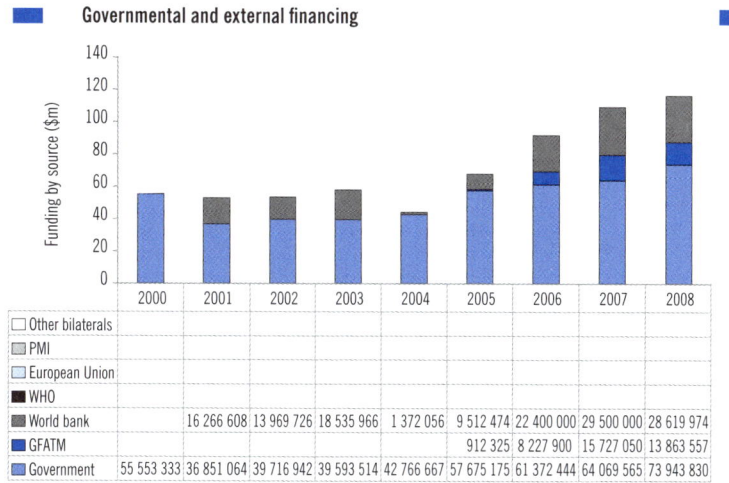

	2000	2001	2002	2003	2004	2005	2006	2007	2008
Other bilaterals									
PMI									
European Union									
WHO									
World bank		16 266 608	13 969 726	18 535 966	1 372 056	9 512 474	22 400 000	29 500 000	28 619 974
GFATM						912 325	8 227 900	15 727 050	13 863 557
Government	55 553 333	36 851 064	39 716 942	39 593 514	42 766 667	57 675 175	61 372 444	64 069 565	73 943 830

Breakdown of expenditure by intervention in 2008

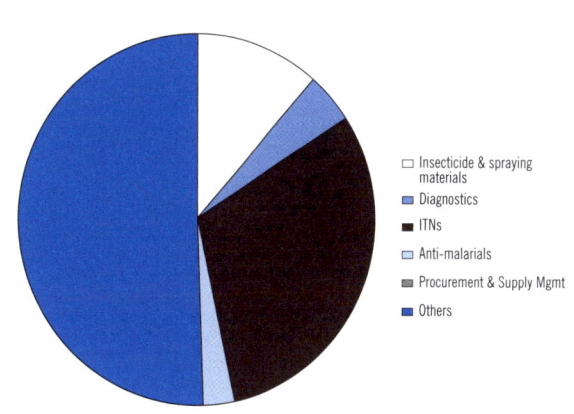

- ☐ Insecticide & spraying materials
- ◼ Diagnostics
- ◼ ITNs
- ☐ Anti-malarials
- ◼ Procurement & Supply Mgmt
- ◼ Others

V. SOURCE OF INFORMATION

PROGRAMME DATA

Reported cases	Surveillance data
Operational coverage of ITNs, IRS and access to medicines	Programme report
Financial data	Programme report

SURVEY AND OTHER DATA

Insecticide-treated nets (ITN)	DHS 2005-06
Treatment	MICS 2000
Use of health services	DHS 2005

INDONESIA

Malaria transmission is higher in the forest areas, particularly in the eastern part of the country, where about 113 million people of the 227 million total population live. The number of reported cases decreased from 2.8 million in 2001 to 1.2 million in 2008. Only 20% of the reported cases were confirmed, of which nearly 50% were due to *P. falciparum*. Inpatient data are incomplete, so that trends in admissions or deaths cannot be assessed. Widescale vector control against malaria was not reported, other than the delivery of 2 million LLINs in 2006 and 250 000 conventional ITNs in 2007. IRS implementation is not recorded consistently, although it remains a national policy. The programme delivered 327 000 ACT courses in 2008, sufficient to treat all confirmed *P. falciparum* cases in the public sector. In the 2008 demographic and heath survey, 65% of households had at least one ITN and 68% of children under 5 had slept under an ITN the previous night. External funding for malaria control appears to have increased, from less than US$ 2 million in 2000 to more than US$ 15 million in 2008, mainly from the Global Fund, United Nations agencies and the Government.

I. EPIDEMIOLOGICAL PROFILE

Population, endemicity and malaria burden

Population (in thousands)	2008	%
All age groups	227 345	
< 5 years	20 891	9
≥ 5 years	206 454	91

Population by malaria endemicity (in thousands)	2008	%
High transmission ≥ 1/1000	83 536	37
Low transmission (0–1/1000)	30 760	14
Malaria-free (0 cases)	113 049	50
Rural population	110 149	48

Vector and parasite profiles

Major *Anopheles* species	*acoitnus, balabacensis, bancrofti, , barbirostris, farauti, ftuviatilis, karwari, koliensis, letifer, maculatus, minimus, nigerrimus, punctulatus, subpictus, sundaicus, umbrosus*
Plasmodium species	*falciparum, vivax*

Stratification of burden (reported cases, per 1000)

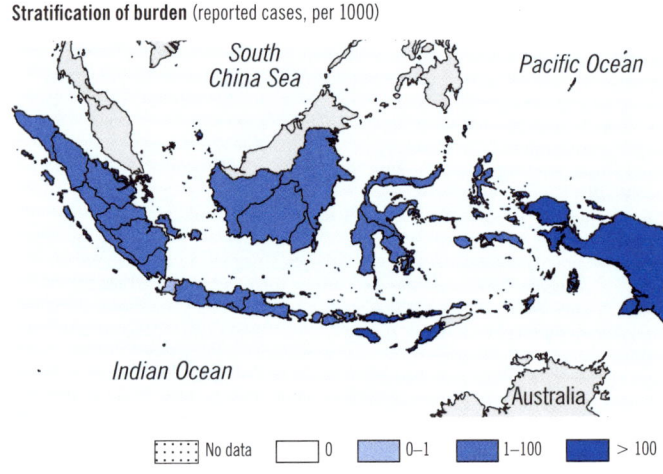

No data / 0 / 0–1 / 1–100 / > 100

Trends in malaria morbidity and mortality

Reported malaria cases, per 1000

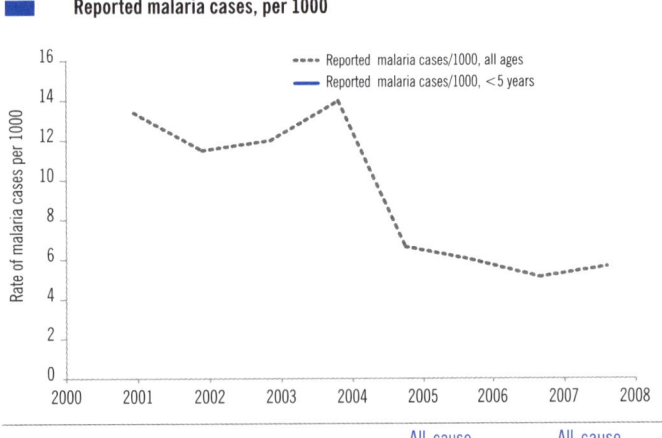

Rate of examination, case confirmation, malaria test positivity, % of confirmed cases that are *P. falciparum*

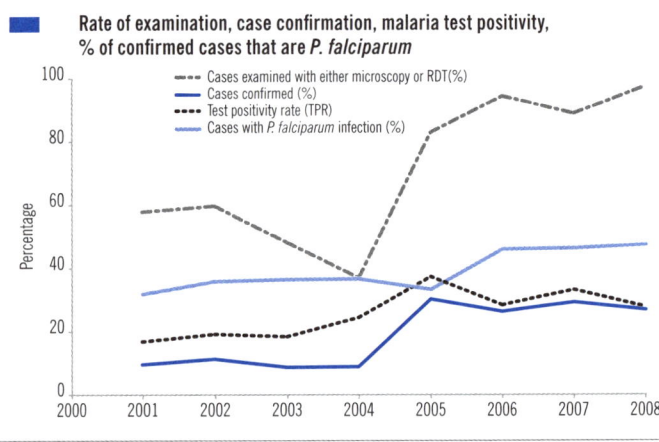

Year	Reported malaria cases, all ages	Reported malaria cases, < 5 years	All-cause outpatient consultations, all ages	All-cause outpatient consultations, < 5 years	Examined	Positive	P. falciparum	Reporting completeness of outpatient health facilities (%)	Reporting completeness of districts (%)
2000									
2001	2 776 477				1 604 573	267 592	85 596		
2002	2 416 039				1 440 320	273 793	98 430		
2003	2 554 223				1 224 232	223 074	81 591		
2004	3 016 262				1 109 801	268 852	98 729		
2005	1 445 831				1 197 621	437 323	146 209		
2006	1 320 581				1 246 324	347 597	160 147		
2007	1 140 424				1 012 681	333 793	155 050		
2008	1 275 192				1 243 744	343 048	163 222		

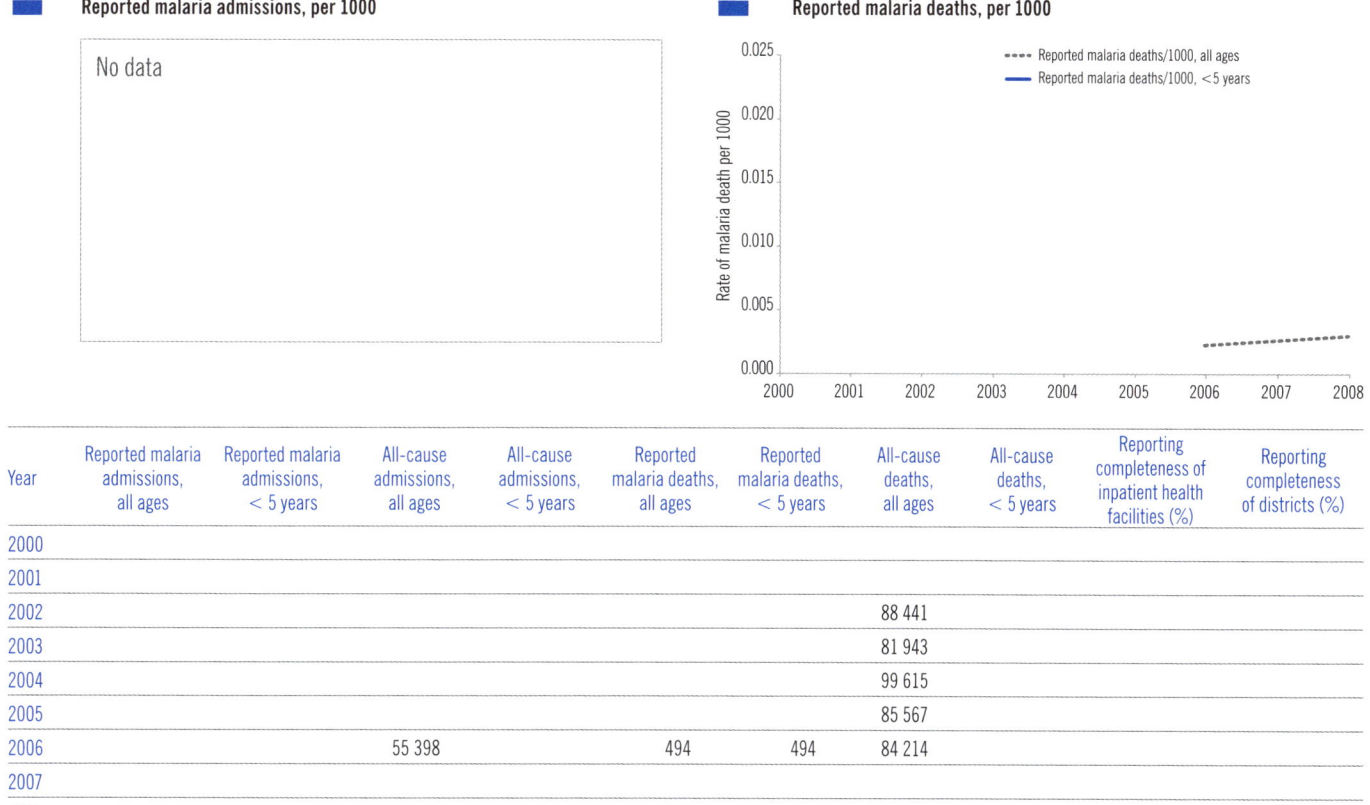

Reported malaria admissions, per 1000

No data

Reported malaria deaths, per 1000

---- Reported malaria deaths/1000, all ages
— Reported malaria deaths/1000, <5 years

Year	Reported malaria admissions, all ages	Reported malaria admissions, < 5 years	All-cause admissions, all ages	All-cause admissions, < 5 years	Reported malaria deaths, all ages	Reported malaria deaths, < 5 years	All-cause deaths, all ages	All-cause deaths, < 5 years	Reporting completeness of inpatient health facilities (%)	Reporting completeness of districts (%)
2000										
2001										
2002							88 441			
2003							81 943			
2004							99 615			
2005							85 567			
2006		55 398			494	494	84 214			
2007										
2008					669		92 917			

II.   INTERVENTION POLICIES AND STRATEGIES

Intervention	WHO-RECOMMENDED POLICIES / STRATEGIES	Yes or No	Year adopted	OPTIONAL POLICIES / STRATEGIES	Yes or No	Year adoped
Insecticide-treated nets (ITN)	Distribution of ITN/LLINs – Free	Yes	2003	Distribution – Antenatal care	Yes	2005
	Targeting all age groups	Yes	2003	Distribution – EPI routine and campaign	Yes	2005
				Targeting children < 5 years and pregnant women	Yes	2005
				ITN distribution is subsidized	–	–
Indoor residual spraying (IRS)	IRS is a primary vector control intervention	No	–	Insecticide-resistance management implemented	Yes	2000
	DDT is used for IRS (public health) only	No	–	Where IRS is conducted, other options are also implemented, e.g. ITN	Yes	2000
				IRS is used for prevention and control of epidemics	Yes	2000
Intermittent preventive treatment (IPT)	IPT used to prevent malaria during pregnancy	No	–			
Case management	Oral artemisinin monotherapies banned (prohibited from registration or removed from the system)	Yes	2003	Parasitological confirmation for patients ≥ 5 years only	–	–
	Parasitological confirmation for patients of all ages	Yes	2000	Malaria diagnosis is free of charge in the public sector	Yes	–
	ACT is free of charge for < 5 years old in the public sector	Yes	2003	ACT is free of charge for patients ≥ 5 years in the public sector	Yes	–
	Diagnosis of malaria of inpatients is based on parasitological confirmation	No	–	ACT is delivered at community level through community agents (beyond the health facilities)	No	–
	Pre-referral treatment with quinine or artemether IM or artesunate suppositories	Yes	2004	Uncomplicated malaria cases are admitted	Yes	2000
	Oversight regulation of case management in the private sectors	–	–			
	RDTs used at community level	No	–			

Antimalarial policy	Type of medicine	Year adopted	Results of therapeutic efficacy tests						
			Study year	No. of studies	Median	Minimum	Maximum	Percentiles: 25%	75%
First-line treatment of *P. falciparum* (unconfirmed)	CQ+PQ	2004							
First-line treatment of *P. falciparum* (confirmed)	DHA-PPQ, AS+AQ+PQ	2009							
Treatment failure of *P. falciparum*	QN+D+PQ	2004							
Treatment of severe malaria	AM, QN	2004							
Treatment of *P. vivax*	CQ+PQ(14d)	2004							

III. IMPLEMENTING MALARIA CONTROL

Coverage of ITN: survey data

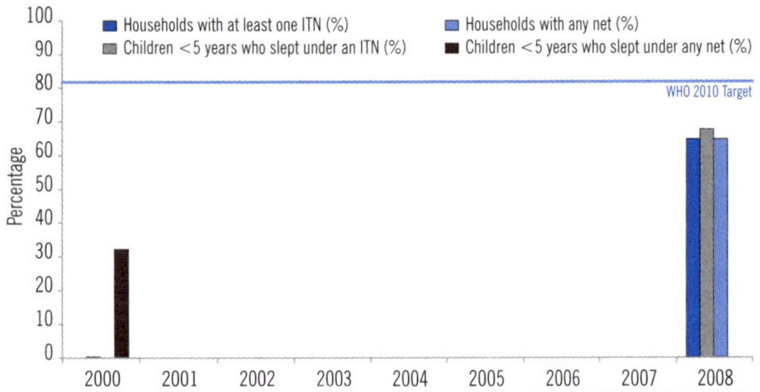

- Households with at least one ITN (%)
- Households with any net (%)
- Children <5 years who slept under an ITN (%)
- Children <5 years who slept under any net (%)

Sources: MICS 2000, National 2008.

Coverage of IRS and ITN: programme data

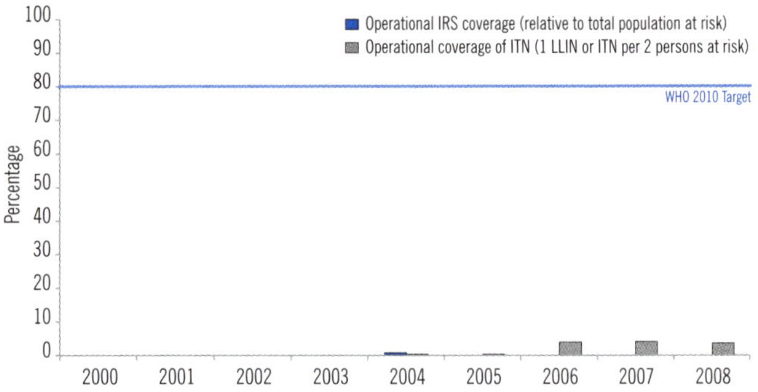

- Operational IRS coverage (relative to total population at risk)
- Operational coverage of ITN (1 LLIN or ITN per 2 persons at risk)

Access by febrile children to effective treatment: survey data

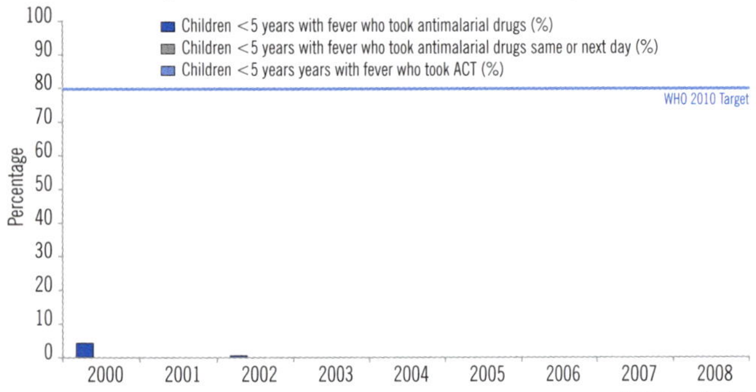

- Children <5 years with fever who took antimalarial drugs (%)
- Children <5 years with fever who took antimalarial drugs same or next day (%)
- Children <5 years years with fever who took ACT (%)

Sources: MICS 2000.

Access to effective treatment: programme data

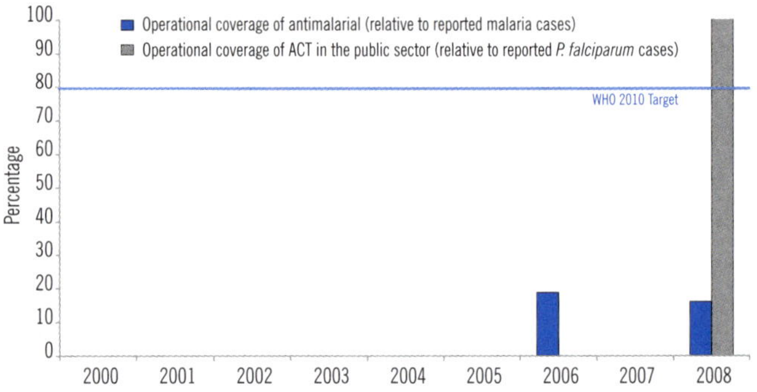

- Operational coverage of antimalarial (relative to reported malaria cases)
- Operational coverage of ACT in the public sector (relative to reported *P. falciparum* cases)

Year	Pregnant women who slept under any net (%)	Pregnant women who slept under an ITN (%)	Children < 5 years with fever (%)	Febrile children < 5 years who sought treatment in HF (%)	Number of households protected by IRS	Number of people protected by IRS	Number of ITNs and/or LLINs	Number of 1st-line treatment courses received	Number of ACT treatment courses received
2000			–	–					
2001									
2002			–	–					
2003									
2004						749 500	155 000		
2005									
2006							2 000 000	250 000	
2007					40 000		250 000		
2008					1 383			338 629	327 440

IV. FINANCING MALARIA CONTROL

Governmental and external financing

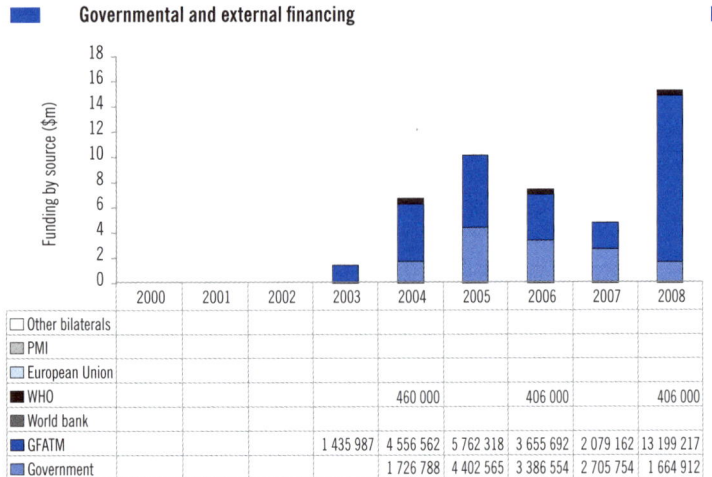

	2000	2001	2002	2003	2004	2005	2006	2007	2008
Other bilaterals									
PMI									
European Union									
WHO					460 000		406 000		406 000
World bank									
GFATM				1 435 987	4 556 562	5 762 318	3 655 692	2 079 162	13 199 217
Government					1 726 788	4 402 565	3 386 554	2 705 754	1 664 912

Breakdown of expenditure by intervention in 2008

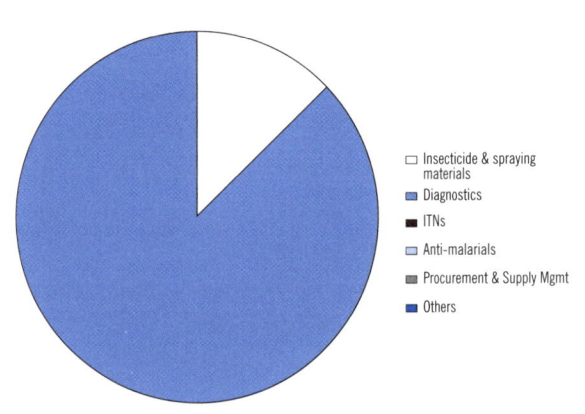

- Insecticide & spraying materials
- Diagnostics
- ITNs
- Anti-malarials
- Procurement & Supply Mgmt
- Others

V. SOURCE OF INFORMATION

PROGRAMME DATA		SURVEY AND OTHER DATA	
Reported cases	Surveillance data	Insecticide-treated nets (ITN)	MICS 2000
Operational coverage of ITNs, IRS and access to medicines	Programme report	Treatment	MICS 2000, DHS 2002-03
Financial data	Programme report	Use of health services	DHS 2002

KENYA

Kenya had an estimated 15 million malaria cases in 2006. The majority are due to *P. falciparum*. Almost all the reported 9 million suspected malaria cases in 2007 were unconfirmed. The number of reported cases increased between 2001 and 2007; it is not known whether this represents improved reporting or an increase in incidence. No reports of malaria deaths were provided for 2008, although about 40 000 deaths were reported in 2006. The national malaria control programme distributed 10.4 million LLINs during 2006–2008, adequate to cover 31% of the population at risk. IRS is implemented in selected districts, covering 307 207 households in 2008 and protecting about 3 million people at risk. About 5 million ACT treatment courses were delivered in 2006, fewer than would be needed to treat all reported malaria cases in the public sector. There were no data on ACTs delivered in 2007 and 2008. In the 2008 demographic and health survey, 48% of households owned an ITN, 39% of children under 5 had slept under an ITN the previous night and 8% of febrile children received ACT treatment. Funding for malaria control increased from less than US$ 1 million in 2003 to about US$ 62 million in 2008, mainly from the Global Fund, the United States President's Malaria Initiative, the United Kingdom Department for International Development and nongovernmental organizations.

I. EPIDEMIOLOGICAL PROFILE

Population, endemicity and malaria burden

Population (in thousands)	2008	%
All age groups	38 765	
< 5 years	6 540	17
≥ 5 years	32 226	83

Population by malaria endemicity (in thousands)	2008	%
High transmission ≥ 1/1000	13 991	36
Low transmission (0–1/1000)	15 417	40
Malaria-free (0 cases)	9 357	24
Rural population	30 411	78

Vector and parasite profiles

Major *Anopheles* species	*gambiae, arabiensis, funestus, melas, nili, paludis, pharoensis*
Plasmodium species	*falciparum, vivax*

Stratification of burden (reported cases, per 1000)

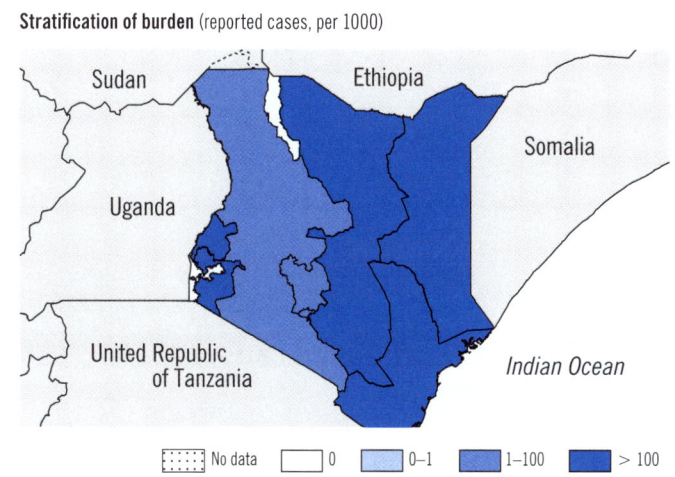

No data | 0 | 0–1 | 1–100 | > 100

Trends in malaria morbidity and mortality

Reported malaria cases, per 1000

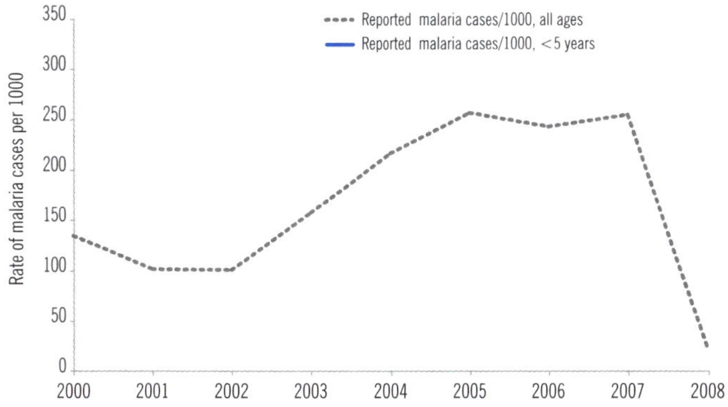

- Reported malaria cases/1000, all ages
- Reported malaria cases/1000, <5 years

Rate of examination, case confirmation, malaria test positivity, % of confirmed cases that are *P. falciparum*

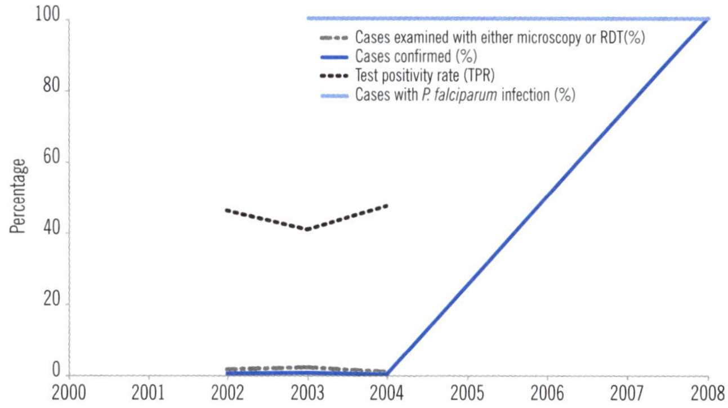

- Cases examined with either microscopy or RDT(%)
- Cases confirmed (%)
- Test positivity rate (TPR)
- Cases with *P. falciparum* infection (%)

Year	Reported malaria cases, all ages	Reported malaria cases, < 5 years	All-cause outpatient consultations, all ages	All-cause outpatient consultations, < 5 years	Examined	Positive	*P. falciparum*	Reporting completeness of outpatient health facilities (%)	Reporting completeness of districts (%)
2000	4 216 531								
2001	3 262 931		10 443 984						
2002	3 319 399		9 944 058		43 643	20 049			
2003	5 338 008		15 067 165		96 893	39 383	39 383		
2004	7 545 541		22 691 025		59 995	28 328	28 328		
2005	9 181 224		33 256 138						
2006	8 926 058		28 955 219						
2007	9 610 691		31 168 878						
2008									

Reported malaria admissions, per 1000

No data

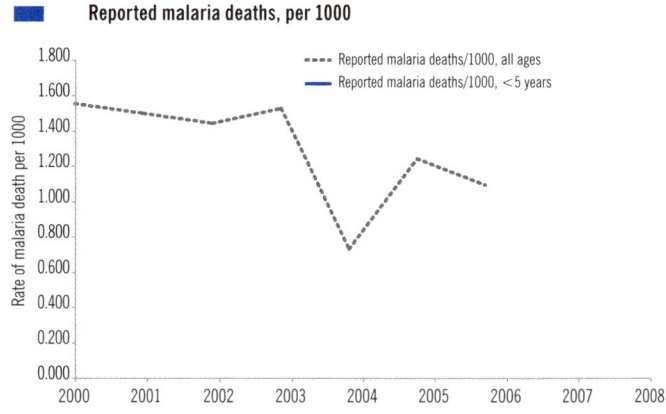

Reported malaria deaths, per 1000

---- Reported malaria deaths/1000, all ages
—— Reported malaria deaths/1000, < 5 years

Year	Reported malaria admissions, all ages	Reported malaria admissions, < 5 years	All-cause admissions, all ages	All-cause admissions, < 5 years	Reported malaria deaths, all ages	Reported malaria deaths, < 5 years	All-cause deaths, all ages	All-cause deaths, < 5 years	Reporting completeness of inpatient health facilities (%)	Reporting completeness of districts (%)
2000					48 767		214 864			
2001					48 286		199 358			
2002		116 276			47 697		200 549			
2003		126 678			51 842		213 164			
2004		530 640			25 403		123 674			
2005					44 328		194 885			
2006		1 288 423			40 079		216 158			
2007										
2008		234 576								

II. INTERVENTION POLICIES AND STRATEGIES

Intervention	WHO-RECOMMENDED POLICIES / STRATEGIES	Yes or No	Year adopted	OPTIONAL POLICIES / STRATEGIES	Yes or No	Year adoped
Insecticide-treated nets (ITN)	Distribution of ITN/LLINs — Free	Yes	2006	Distribution — Antenatal care	Yes	2005
	Targeting all age groups	No	–	Distribution — EPI routine and campaign	Yes	2006
				Targeting children < 5 years and pregnant women	Yes	2001
				ITN distribution is subsidized	Yes	2002
Indoor residual spraying (IRS)	IRS is a primary vector control intervention	No	–	Insecticide-resistance management implemented	No	–
	DDT is used for IRS (public health) only	No	–	Where IRS is conducted, other options are also implemented, e.g. ITN	Yes	2003
				IRS is used for prevention and control of epidemics	Yes	2003
Intermittent preventive treatment (IPT)	IPT used to prevent malaria during pregnancy	Yes	2001			
Case management	Oral artemisinin monotherapies banned (prohibited from registration or removed from the system)	Yes	2006	Parasitological confirmation for patients ≥ 5 years only	No	–
	Parasitological confirmation for patients of all ages	No	–	Malaria diagnosis is free of charge in the public sector	Yes	2006
	ACT is free of charge for < 5 years old in the public sector	Yes	2006	ACT is free of charge for patients ≥ 5 years in the public sector	Yes	2006
	Diagnosis of malaria of inpatients is based on parasitological confirmation	Yes	1997	ACT is delivered at community level through community agents (beyond the health facilities)	No	–
	Pre-referral treatment with quinine or artemether IM or artesunate suppositories	Yes	2006	Uncomplicated malaria cases are admitted	No	–
	Oversight regulation of case management in the private sectors	No	–			
	RDTs used at community level	No	–			

				Results of therapeutic efficacy tests					
Antimalarial policy	Type of medicine	Year adopted	Study year	No. of studies	Median	Minimum	Maximum	Percentiles: 25%	75%
First-line treatment of *P. falciparum* (unconfirmed)	AL	2004							
First-line treatment of *P. falciparum* (confirmed)	AL	2004							
Treatment failure of *P. falciparum*	QN(7d)	2004							
Treatment of severe malaria	QN(7d)	2004							
Treatment of *P. vivax*	–	–							

III. IMPLEMENTING MALARIA CONTROL

Coverage of ITN: survey data

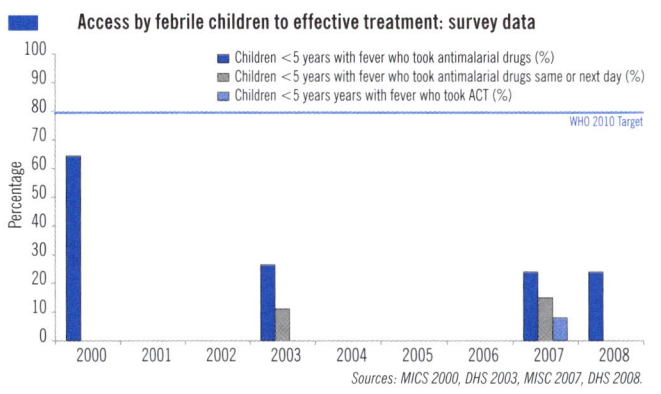

Sources: MICS 2000, DHS 2003, MISC 2007, DHS 2008.

Coverage of IRS and ITN: programme data

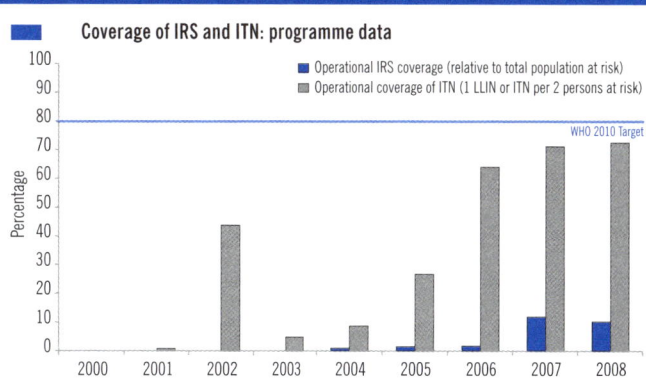

Access by febrile children to effective treatment: survey data

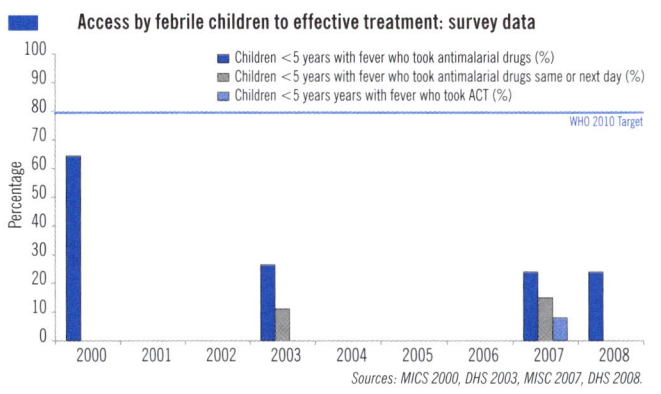

Sources: MICS 2000, DHS 2003, MISC 2007, DHS 2008.

Access to effective treatment: programme data

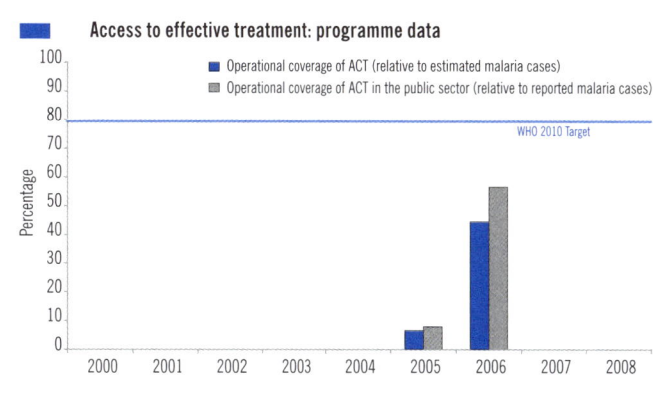

Year	Pregnant women who slept under any net (%)	Pregnant women who slept under an ITN (%)	Children < 5 years with fever (%)	Febrile children < 5 years who sought treatment in HF (%)	Number of households protected by IRS	Number of people protected by IRS	Number of ITNs and/or LLINs	Number of 1st-line treatment courses received	Number of ACT treatment courses received
2000			–	–					
2001							120 010		
2002							5 550 563		
2003	13	5	–	–			643 218		
2004					300 000	300 000	1 169 600		
2005					350 000	465 000	3 655 576	723 333	723 333
2006					380 000	550 000	7 102 752	5 049 000	5 049 000
2007			–	–	390 058	3 459 207	1 996 875		
2008			–	–	307 207	3 061 966	2 786 742		

IV. FINANCING MALARIA CONTROL

Governmental and external financing

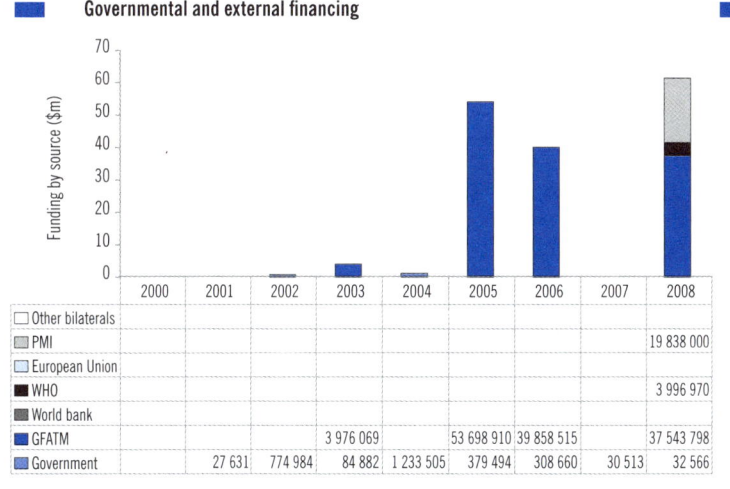

	2000	2001	2002	2003	2004	2005	2006	2007	2008
☐ Other bilaterals									
▨ PMI									19 838 000
☐ European Union									
■ WHO									3 996 970
■ World bank									
■ GFATM				3 976 069		53 698 910	39 858 515		37 543 798
■ Government		27 631	774 984	84 882	1 233 505	379 494	308 660	30 513	32 566

Breakdown of expenditure by intervention in 2008

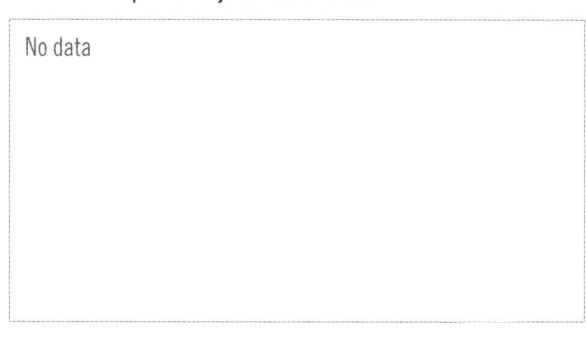

No data

V. SOURCE OF INFORMATION

PROGRAMME DATA		SURVEY AND OTHER DATA	
Reported cases	Surveillance data	Insecticide-treated nets (ITN)	MICS 2000, DHS 2003, MIS 2007, DHS 2008
Operational coverage of ITNs, IRS and access to medicines	Programme report	Treatment	MICS 2000, DHS 2003, MIS 2007, DHS 2008
Financial data	Programme report	Use of health services	DHS 2003

MADAGASCAR

Transmission occurs all year round in the north, with seasonal peaks between September and June elsewhere. About 70% of the population live in low-transmission areas, prone to epidemics, whereas the remainder inhabit high-transmission areas. The reported number of malaria cases dropped from an average of 1.4 million in 2001–2006 to only 352 000 cases in 2008 (76% decrease); only 89 000 cases were confirmed. The percentage of suspected cases tested increased from 2% in 2003 to 85% in 2008 as a result of the introduction of RDTs in 2007. The number of inpatient malaria cases also decreased, from an average of 10 283 during 2001–2006 to 5367 in 2008 (a decrease of 47%). Similarly, the number of malaria deaths during this period decreased from an average of 665 to 276 (decrease of 58%). In spite of limitations due to under reporting, the marked decreases in numbers of cases and deaths perhaps reflect the growing use of ITN, IRS and ACTs. The national malaria control programme distributed nearly 3.6 million LLINs during the period 2006–2008, covering half the target population. IRS has also increased since 2003, covering 1.3 million households and protecting 6.5 million people at risk (34%) in 2008. The national malaria control programme reported that 1 167 480 malaria cases received ACT. In a national household survey in 2008, 59% of households had an ITN and 60% of children under 5 had slept under an ITN the previous night. Funding for malaria control has increased every year, from about US$ 2 million in 2004 to over US$ 23 million in 2008, mainly from the Global Fund, United Nations agencies, the United States President's Malaria Initiative and other bilateral agencies.

I. EPIDEMIOLOGICAL PROFILE

Population, endemicity and malaria burden

Population (in thousands)	2008	%
All age groups	19 111	
< 5 years	3 060	16
≥ 5 years	16 051	84

Population by malaria endemicity (in thousands)	2008	%
High transmission ≥ 1/1000	5 758	30
Low transmission (0–1/1000)	13 352	70
Malaria-free (0 cases)	0	0
Rural population	13 480	71

Vector and parasite profiles	
Major *Anopheles* species	*gambiae, arabiensis, funestus, coustani, flavicosta, merus, pharoensis*
Plasmodium species	*falciparum, vivax*

Stratification of burden (reported cases, per 1000)

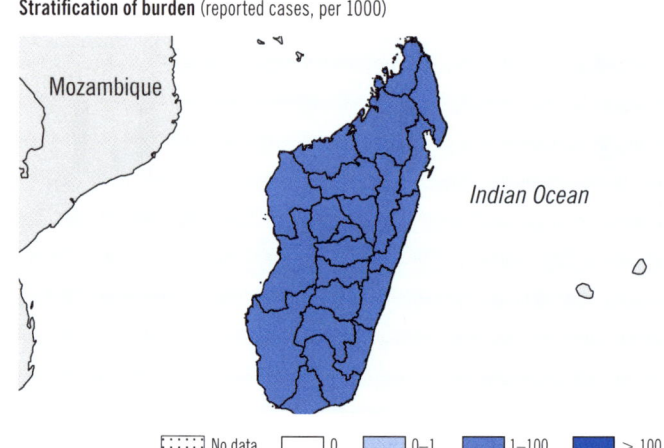

No data | 0 | 0–1 | 1–100 | > 100

Trends in malaria morbidity and mortality

Reported malaria cases, per 1000

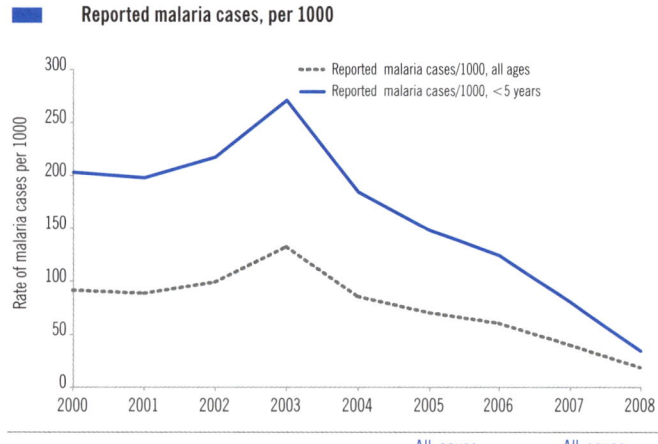

- Reported malaria cases/1000, all ages
- Reported malaria cases/1000, <5 years

Rate of examination, case confirmation, malaria test positivity, % of confirmed cases that are *P. falciparum*

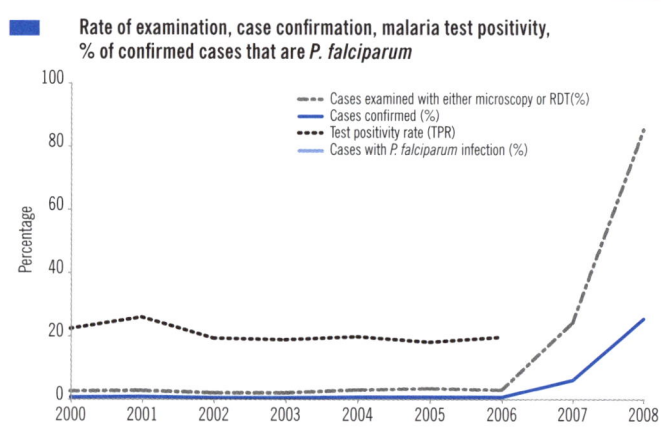

- Cases examined with either microscopy or RDT(%)
- Cases confirmed (%)
- Test positivity rate (TPR)
- Cases with *P. falciparum* infection (%)

Year	Reported malaria cases, all ages	Reported malaria cases, < 5 years	All-cause outpatient consultations, all ages	All-cause outpatient consultations, < 5 years	Examined	Positive	*P. falciparum*	Reporting completeness of outpatient health facilities (%)	Reporting completeness of districts (%)
2000	1 392 483	553 350	7 425 845	2 435 584	31 575	6 946		100	85
2001	1 386 291	549 457	7 163 740	2 307 873	33 354	8 538		99	81
2002	1 598 919	612 724	8 189 035	3 641 821	27 752	5 272		98	75
2003	2 198 297	774 142	11 693 122	3 588 525	37 333	6 909		96	85
2004	1 458 408	534 201	8 091 929	2 451 234	39 174	7 638		93	87
2005	1 229 385	434 849	7 296 934	2 118 281	37 943	6 753		92	84
2006	1 087 563	370 356	6 991 184	1 957 387	29 318	5 689		85	85
2007	736 194	243 638	6 900 024	1 859 232	175 595	43 674		86	90
2008	352 520	106 090	6 809 115	1 793 241	299 000	89 138		73	73

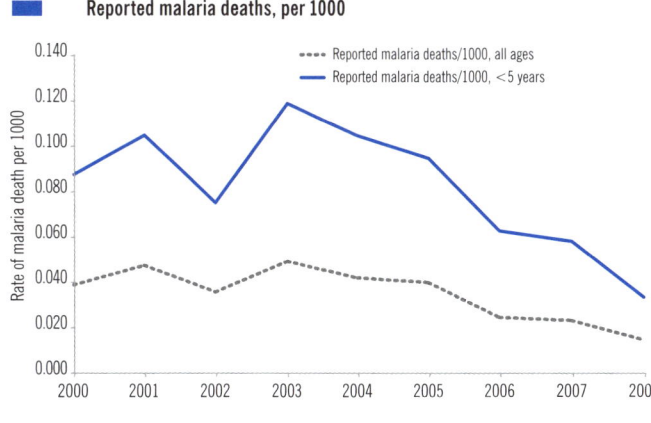

Reported malaria admissions, per 1000

- - - - Reported malaria admisison/1000, all ages
—— Reported malaria admisison/1000, <5 years

Reported malaria deaths, per 1000

- - - - Reported malaria deaths/1000, all ages
—— Reported malaria deaths/1000, <5 years

Year	Reported malaria admissions, all ages	Reported malaria admissions, < 5 years	All-cause admissions, all ages	All-cause admissions, < 5 years	Reported malaria deaths, all ages	Reported malaria deaths, < 5 years	All-cause deaths, all ages	All-cause deaths, < 5 years	Reporting completeness of inpatient health facilities (%)	Reporting completeness of districts (%)
2000	8 514	2 883	84 020	12 528	591	238	4 023	1 107		
2001	9 826	3 298	88 853	12 177	742	290	4 300	1 078		
2002	8 730	2 758	80 604	11 376	575	211	3 897	1 975		
2003	11 795	3 790	106 283	15 176	817	339	4 849	1 308		
2004	9 753	3 192	93 960	12 085	715	302	4 148	1 058		
2005	12 346	3 819	108 313	13 570	699	277	4 229	1 021		
2006	9 246	2 479	88 303	10 387	441	186	3 357	717		
2007	8 190	2 537	102 157	12 794	428	175	3 721	793		
2008	5 367	1 521	118 882	9 094	276	102	2 830	566		

II. INTERVENTION POLICIES AND STRATEGIES

Intervention	WHO-RECOMMENDED POLICIES / STRATEGIES	Yes or No	Year adopted	OPTIONAL POLICIES / STRATEGIES	Yes or No	Year adoped
Insecticide-treated nets (ITN)	Distribution of ITN/LLINs – Free	Yes	2004	Distribution – Antenatal care	Yes	2005
	Targeting all age groups	Yes	2009	Distribution – EPI routine and campaign	Yes	2007
				Targeting children < 5 years and pregnant women	Yes	2000
				ITN distribution is subsidized	Yes	2000
Indoor residual spraying (IRS)	IRS is a primary vector control intervention	Yes	1998	Insecticide-resistance management implemented	Yes	1998
	DDT is used for IRS (public health) only	No	–	Where IRS is conducted, other options are also implemented, e.g. ITN	Yes	1998
				IRS is used for prevention and control of epidemics	Yes	1998
Intermittent preventive treatment (IPT)	IPT used to prevent malaria during pregnancy	Yes	2006			
Case management	Oral artemisinin monotherapies banned (prohibited from registration or removed from the system)	Yes	2005	Parasitological confirmation for patients ≥ 5 years only	No	–
	Parasitological confirmation for patients of all ages	Yes	2006	Malaria diagnosis is free of charge in the public sector	Yes	2006
	ACT is free of charge for < 5 years old in the public sector	Yes	2006	ACT is free of charge for patients ≥ 5 years in the public sector	Yes	2006
	Diagnosis of malaria of inpatients is based on parasitological confirmation	No	–	ACT is delivered at community level through community agents (beyond the health facilities)	Yes	2008
	Pre-referral treatment with quinine or artemether IM or artesunate suppositories	No	–	Uncomplicated malaria cases are admitted	No	–
	Oversight regulation of case management in the private sectors	–	–			
	RDTs used at community level	No	–			

				Results of therapeutic efficacy tests					
Antimalarial policy	Type of medicine	Year adopted	Study year	No. of studies	Median	Minimum	Maximum	Percentiles: 25%	75%
First-line treatment of *P. falciparum* (unconfirmed)	AS + AQ	2006	2006–2007	10	0	0	8.7	0	6.9
First-line treatment of *P. falciparum* (confirmed)	AS + AQ	2006							
Treatment failure of *P. falciparum*	QN(7d)	2006							
Treatment of severe malaria	QN(7d)	2006							
Treatment of *P. vivax*	–	–							

III. IMPLEMENTING MALARIA CONTROL

Coverage of ITN: survey data

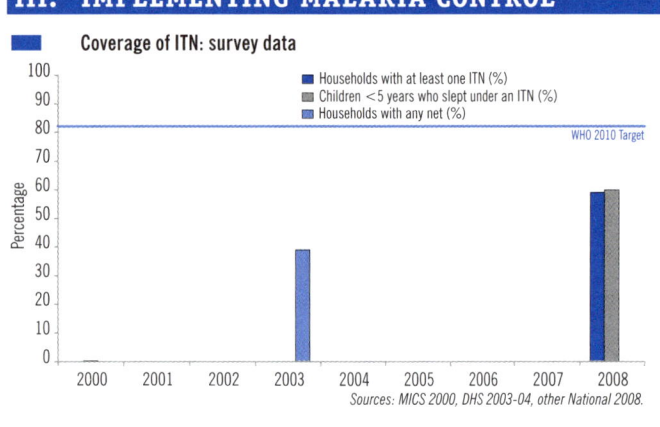

Legend:
- Households with at least one ITN (%)
- Children <5 years who slept under an ITN (%)
- Households with any net (%)

WHO 2010 Target

Sources: MICS 2000, DHS 2003-04, other National 2008.

Coverage of IRS and ITN: programme data

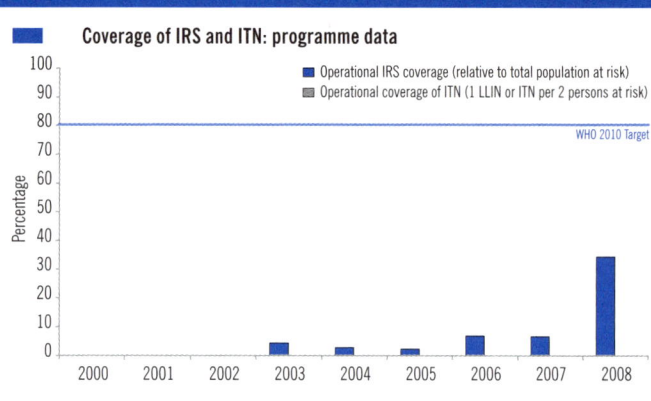

Legend:
- Operational IRS coverage (relative to total population at risk)
- Operational coverage of ITN (1 LLIN or ITN per 2 persons at risk)

WHO 2010 Target

Access by febrile children to effective treatment: survey data

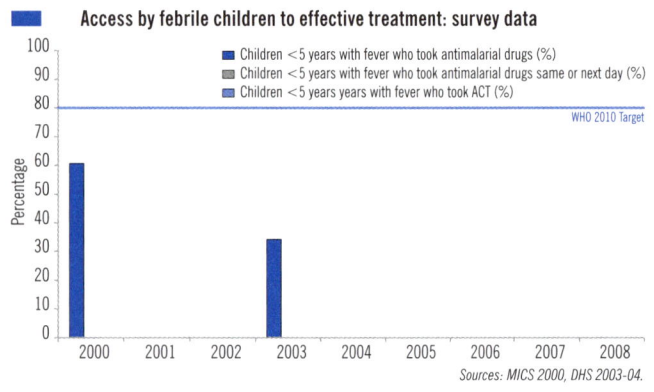

Legend:
- Children <5 years with fever who took antimalarial drugs (%)
- Children <5 years with fever who took antimalarial drugs same or next day (%)
- Children <5 years years with fever who took ACT (%)

WHO 2010 Target

Sources: MICS 2000, DHS 2003-04.

Access to effective treatment: programme data

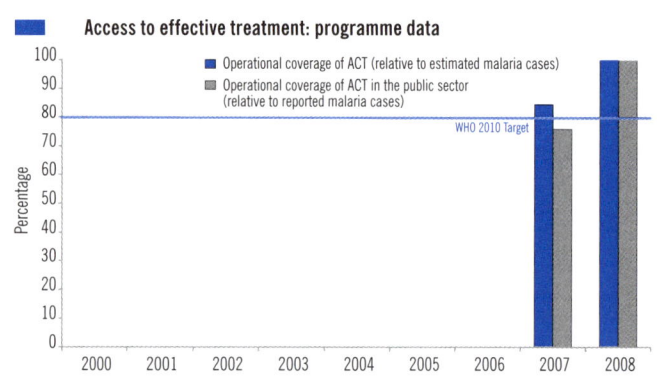

Legend:
- Operational coverage of ACT (relative to estimated malaria cases)
- Operational coverage of ACT in the public sector (relative to reported malaria cases)

WHO 2010 Target

Year	Pregnant women who slept under any net (%)	Pregnant women who slept under an ITN (%)	Children < 5 years with fever (%)	Febrile children < 5 years who sought treatment in HF (%)	Number of households protected by IRS	Number of people protected by IRS	Number of ITNs and/or LLINs	Number of 1st-line treatment courses received	Number of ACT treatment courses received
2000				–					
2001							41 060		
2002							77 139		
2003			–	–	143 617	736 145	115 051		
2004					100 907	485 395	488 700		
2005					84 030	409 155	869 450		
2006					251 100	1 250 000	1 614 187		
2007					248 269	1 241 344	3 359 244		558 000
2008			–	–	1 312 811	6 564 056	907 739		1 167 480

IV. FINANCING MALARIA CONTROL

Governmental and external financing

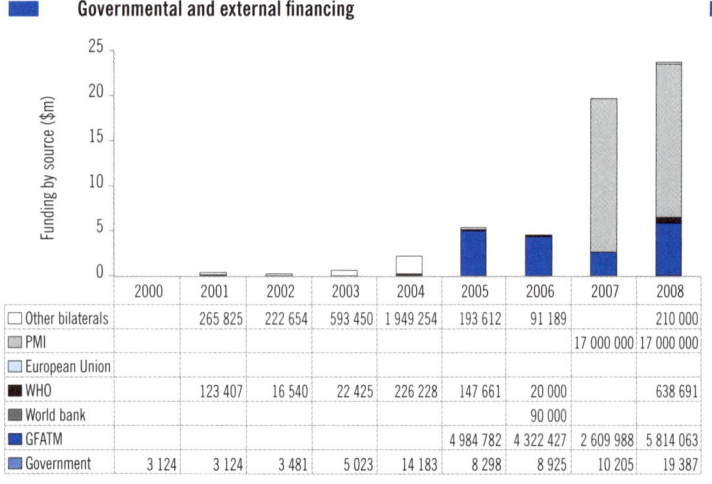

	2000	2001	2002	2003	2004	2005	2006	2007	2008
Other bilaterals		265 825	222 654	593 450	1 949 254	193 612	91 189		210 000
PMI								17 000 000	17 000 000
European Union									
WHO		123 407	16 540	22 425	226 228	147 661	20 000		638 691
World bank							90 000		
GFATM						4 984 782	4 322 427	2 609 988	5 814 063
Government	3 124	3 124	3 481	5 023	14 183	8 298	8 925	10 205	19 387

Breakdown of expenditure by intervention in 2008

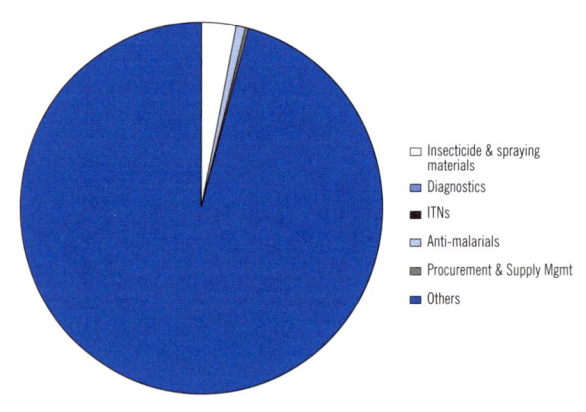

Legend:
- Insecticide & spraying materials
- Diagnostics
- ITNs
- Anti-malarials
- Procurement & Supply Mgmt
- Others

V. SOURCE OF INFORMATION

PROGRAMME DATA		SURVEY AND OTHER DATA	
Reported cases	Surveillance data	Insecticide-treated nets (ITN)	MICS 2000, DHS 2003-04, Other Nat.
Operational coverage of ITNs, IRS and access to medicines	Programme report	Treatment	MICS 2000, DHS 2003-04
Financial data	Programme report	Use of health services	DHS 2003

MALAWI

Malaria is endemic in all parts of the country, with seasonal peaks between December and June. The majority of cases are caused by *P. falciparum*, but most suspected cases are not parasitologically tested. The numbers of malaria cases and deaths reported through the surveillance system were either stable or showed an increasing trend. It is not known whether this is due to improved reporting or an increased incidence. The national malaria control programme distributed over 4.5 million ITNs between 2006 and 2008, of which about 1.2 million were LLINs. In the 2006 multiple indicator cluster survey, 38% of households had at least an ITN, and 25% of children under 5 had slept under an ITN the previous night. Only 25% of febrile children under 5 years were treated with any antimalarial medicine. Although ACT was adopted as the recommended method of treatment in 2007, the national malaria control programme did not report delivery of ACT in recent years. Funding for malaria has increased significantly over the past 3 years, reaching a total of US$ 49 million in 2007 and US$ 41 million in 2008. Most of the funding was provided by the Global Fund, the United States President's Malaria Initiative and United Nations agencies.

I.   EPIDEMIOLOGICAL PROFILE

Population, endemicity and malaria burden

Population (in thousands)	2008	%
All age groups	14 846	
< 5 years	2 591	17
≥ 5 years	12 255	83

Population by malaria endemicity (in thousands)	2008	%
High transmission ≥ 1/1000	14 846	100
Low transmission (0–1/1000)	0	0
Malaria-free (0 cases)	0	0
Rural population	12 061	81

Vector and parasite profiles

Major *Anopheles* species	*gambiae, funestus, coustani, paludis, pharoensis*
Plasmodium species	*falciparum, vivax*

Stratification of burden (reported cases, per 1000)

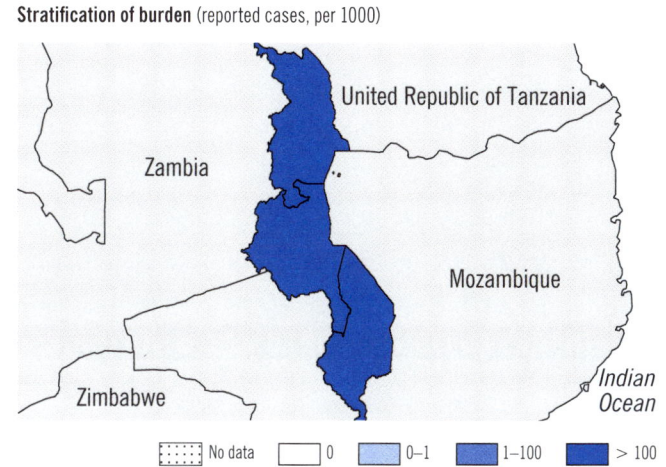

Trends in malaria morbidity and mortality

■ **Reported malaria cases, per 1000**

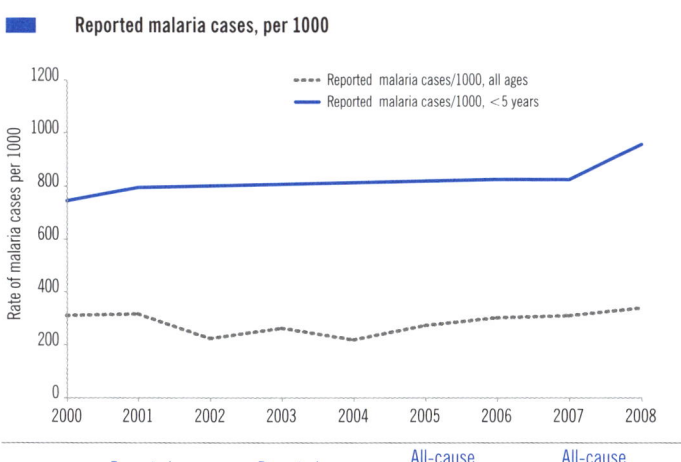

- - - Reported malaria cases/1000, all ages
— Reported malaria cases/1000, <5 years

■ **Rate of examination, case confirmation, malaria test positivity, % of confirmed cases that are *P. falciparum***

No data

Year	Reported malaria cases, all ages	Reported malaria cases, < 5 years	All-cause outpatient consultations, all ages	All-cause outpatient consultations, < 5 years	Examined	Positive	*P. falciparum*	Reporting completeness of outpatient health facilities (%)	Reporting completeness of districts (%)
2000	3 646 212	1 658 012							
2001	3 823 796	1 815 628							
2002	2 784 001								
2003	3 358 960								
2004	2 871 098								
2005	3 688 389		15 753 331						
2006	4 204 468	2 065 004	14 014 893						
2007	4 442 197	2 096 425	6 172 195						
2008	4 986 779	2 473 208	10 183 764						

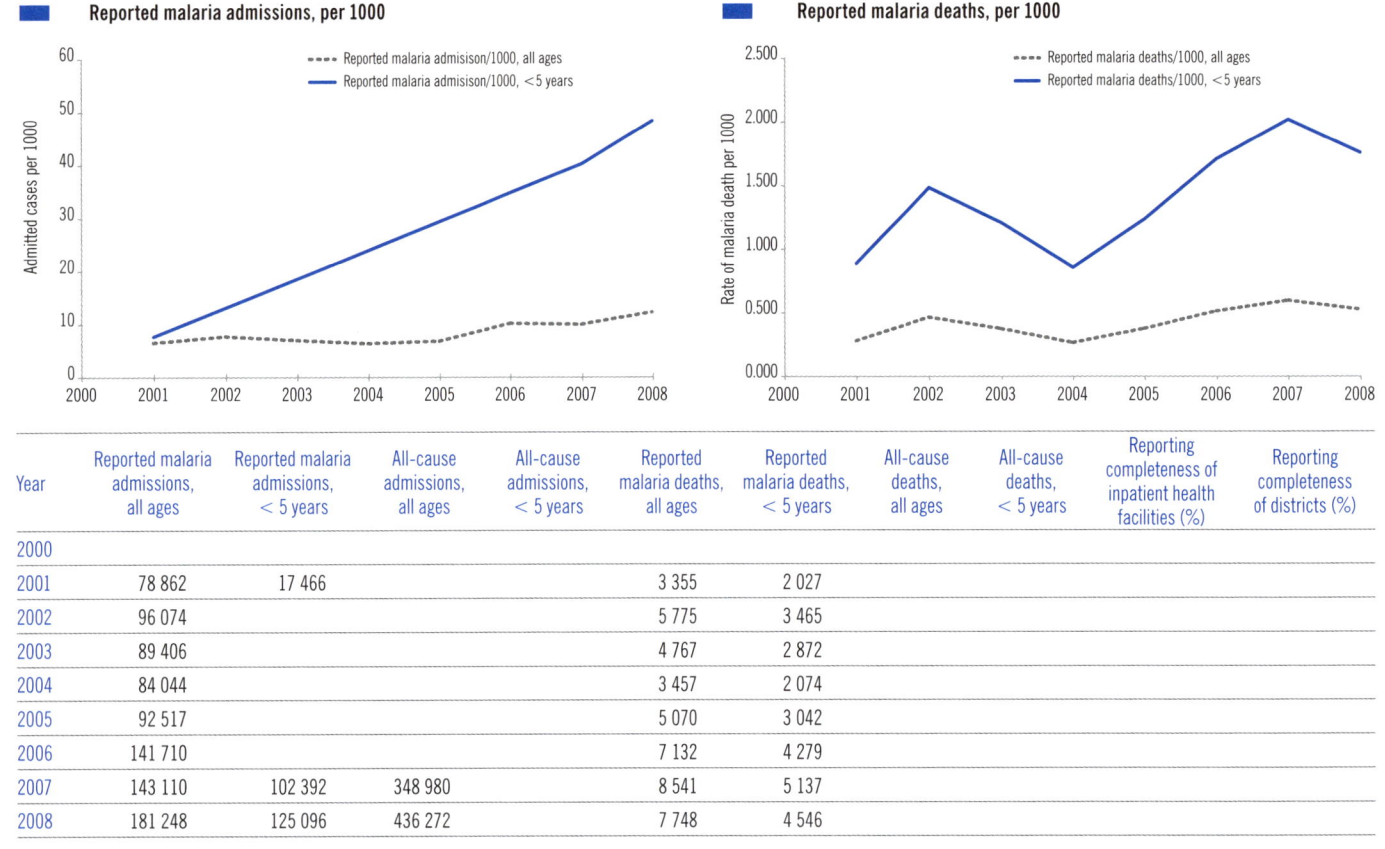

Reported malaria admissions, per 1000

- - - - Reported malaria admission/1000, all ages
———— Reported malaria admission/1000, <5 years

Reported malaria deaths, per 1000

- - - - Reported malaria deaths/1000, all ages
———— Reported malaria deaths/1000, <5 years

Year	Reported malaria admissions, all ages	Reported malaria admissions, < 5 years	All-cause admissions, all ages	All-cause admissions, < 5 years	Reported malaria deaths, all ages	Reported malaria deaths, < 5 years	All-cause deaths, all ages	All-cause deaths, < 5 years	Reporting completeness of inpatient health facilities (%)	Reporting completeness of districts (%)
2000										
2001	78 862	17 466			3 355	2 027				
2002	96 074				5 775	3 465				
2003	89 406				4 767	2 872				
2004	84 044				3 457	2 074				
2005	92 517				5 070	3 042				
2006	141 710				7 132	4 279				
2007	143 110	102 392	348 980		8 541	5 137				
2008	181 248	125 096	436 272		7 748	4 546				

II. INTERVENTION POLICIES AND STRATEGIES

Intervention	WHO-RECOMMENDED POLICIES / STRATEGIES	Yes or No	Year adopted	OPTIONAL POLICIES / STRATEGIES	Yes or No	Year adoped
Insecticide-treated nets (ITN)	Distribution of ITN/LLINs – Free	Yes	2006	Distribution – Antenatal care	Yes	2002
	Targeting all age groups	Yes	2008	Distribution – EPI routine and campaign	No	–
				Targeting children < 5 years and pregnant women	Yes	2002
				ITN distribution is subsidized	–	–
Indoor residual spraying (IRS)	IRS is a primary vector control intervention	No	–	Insecticide-resistance management implemented	No	–
	DDT is used for IRS (public health) only	No	–	Where IRS is conducted, other options are also implemented, e.g. ITN	Yes	2005
				IRS is used for prevention and control of epidemics	No	–
Intermittent preventive treatment (IPT)	IPT used to prevent malaria during pregnancy	Yes	–			
Case management	Oral artemisinin monotherapies banned (prohibited from registration or removed from the system)	Yes	2006	Parasitological confirmation for patients ≥ 5 years only	–	–
	Parasitological confirmation for patients of all ages	No	–	Malaria diagnosis is free of charge in the public sector	–	–
	ACT is free of charge for < 5 years old in the public sector	Yes	2007	ACT is free of charge for patients ≥ 5 years in the public sector	–	–
	Diagnosis of malaria of inpatients is based on parasitological confirmation	–	–	ACT is delivered at community level through community agents (beyond the health facilities)	–	–
	Pre-referral treatment with quinine or artemether IM or artesunate suppositories	Yes	–	Uncomplicated malaria cases are admitted	–	–
	Oversight regulation of case management in the private sectors	–	–			
	RDTs used at community level	–	–			

Antimalarial policy	Type of medicine	Year adopted	Study year	No. of studies	Results of therapeutic efficacy tests Median	Minimum	Maximum	Percentiles: 25%	75%
First-line treatment of *P. falciparum* (unconfirmed)	AL	2007	2005	1	7.1	7.1	7.1	7.1	7.1
First-line treatment of *P. falciparum* (confirmed)	AL	2007							
Treatment failure of *P. falciparum*	AS+AQ	2007	2005	2	1.8	0	3.599	0	3.599
Treatment of severe malaria	QN(7d)	2007							
Treatment of *P. vivax*	–	–							

III. IMPLEMENTING MALARIA CONTROL

Coverage of ITN: survey data

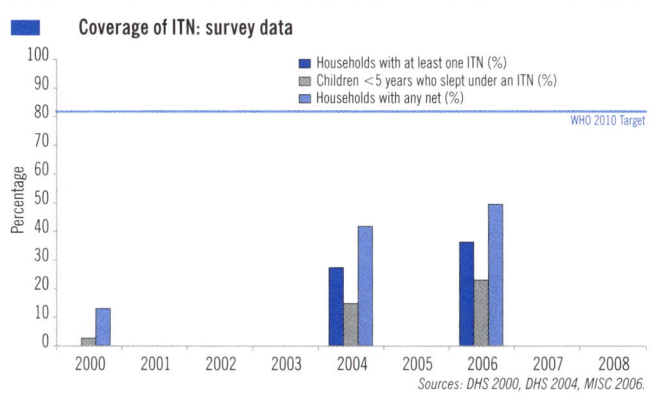

Sources: DHS 2000, DHS 2004, MISC 2006.

Coverage of IRS and ITN: programme data

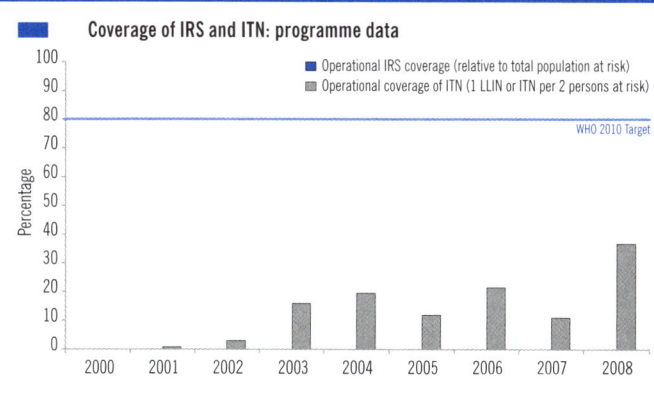

Access by febrile children to effective treatment: survey data

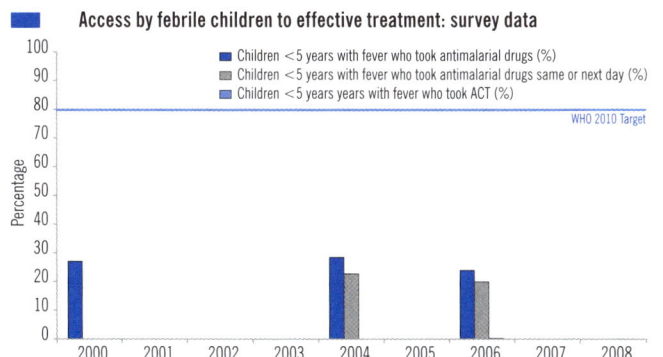

Sources: DHS 2000, DHS 2004, MISC 2006.

Access to effective treatment: programme data

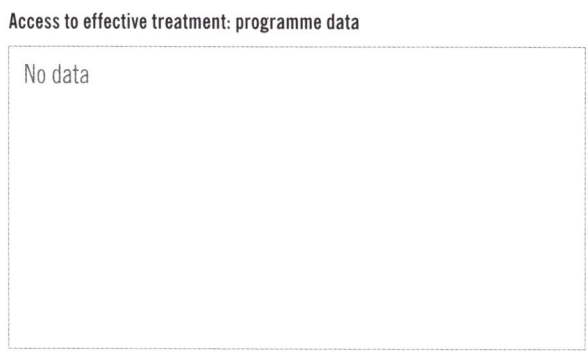

No data

Year	Pregnant women who slept under any net (%)	Pregnant women who slept under an ITN (%)	Children < 5 years with fever (%)	Febrile children < 5 years who sought treatment in HF (%)	Number of households protected by IRS	Number of people protected by IRS	Number of ITNs and/or LLINs	Number of 1st-line treatment courses received	Number of ACT treatment courses received
2000			–						
2001							46 062		
2002							185 968		
2003							1 029 884		
2004	19	15	–	–			1 295 498		
2005							815 620	27 903 000	
2006			–	–			1 508 735	27 903 000	
2007							673 238		
2008							2 354 094		

IV. FINANCING MALARIA CONTROL

Governmental and external financing

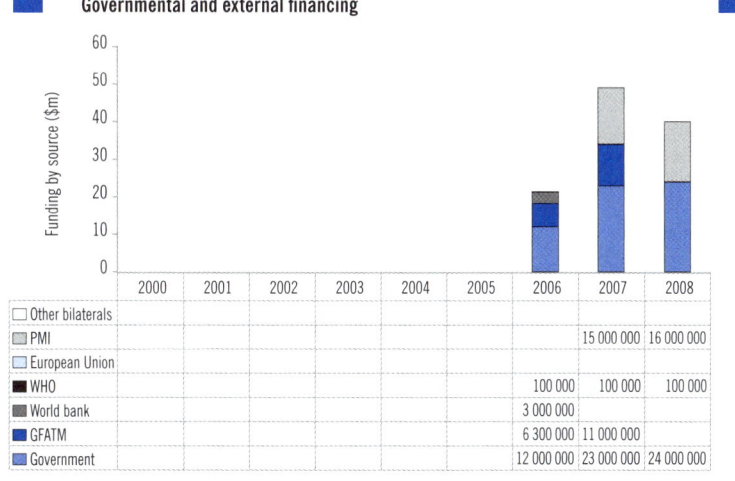

	2000	2001	2002	2003	2004	2005	2006	2007	2008
☐ Other bilaterals									
☐ PMI								15 000 000	16 000 000
☐ European Union									
■ WHO							100 000	100 000	100 000
■ World bank							3 000 000		
■ GFATM							6 300 000	11 000 000	
■ Government							12 000 000	23 000 000	24 000 000

Breakdown of expenditure by intervention in 2008

No data

V. SOURCE OF INFORMATION

PROGRAMME DATA		SURVEY AND OTHER DATA	
Reported cases	Surveillance data	Insecticide-treated nets (ITN)	DHS 2000, DHS 2004, MICS 2006
Operational coverage of ITNs, IRS and access to medicines	Programme report	Treatment	DHS 2000, DHS 2004, MICS 2006
Financial data	Programme report	Use of health services	DHS 2004

MALI

While the entire population is at risk, over 90% of the population live in high-transmission areas. Malaria transmission is more intensive in the southern part of the country, with seasonal peaks between May and November. Almost all cases are caused by *P. falciparum*, but most suspected cases are not parasitologically tested, despite recent improvements in diagnostic services. The number of reported suspected malaria cases has increased in recent years, and the number of reported deaths increased more than twofold between 2001 and 2008. It is not known whether the increase was due to improved reporting or to an increase in incidence. During 2006–2008, the national malaria control programme distributed nearly 3.7 million LLINs, of which 3 million were delivered in the 2007 mass campaign. The programme conducted IRS in 2007, covering 87 000 households and protecting over 405 000 people at risk. Over 2.8 million ACT treatment courses were delivered in 2008, adequate to treat all the malaria cases reported from the public sector. In the 2006 demographic and health survey, 50% of households owned an ITN and 41% of children under 5 had slept under an ITN the previous night. In the 2006 demographic and health survey, 32% of febrile children received any antimalarial medicine, but only 2% received ACT. Although Government expenditure on malaria control is unknown, funding for malaria increased to US$ 27 million in 2008, mainly from the Global Fund, the World Bank, the United States President's Malaria Initiative, United Nations agencies and other bilateral agencies and nongovernmental organizations.

I. EPIDEMIOLOGICAL PROFILE

Population, endemicity and malaria burden

Population (in thousands)	2008	%
All age groups	12 706	
< 5 years	2 207	17
≥ 5 years	10 499	83

Population by malaria endemicity (in thousands)	2008	%
High transmission ≥ 1/1000	11 435	90
Low transmission (0–1/1000)	1 271	10
Malaria-free (0 cases)	0	0
Rural population	8 620	68

Vector and parasite profiles

Major *Anopheles* species	gambiae, arabiensis, funestus, brochieri, coustani, flavicosta, hancocki, nili, paludis, pharoensis
Plasmodium species	falciparum, vivax

Stratification of burden (reported cases, per 1000)

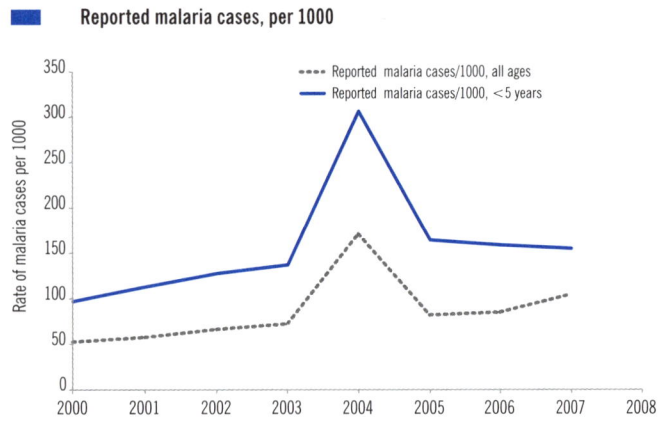

No data | 0 | 0–1 | 1–100 | > 100

Trends in malaria morbidity and mortality

Reported malaria cases, per 1000

- - - - Reported malaria cases/1000, all ages
——— Reported malaria cases/1000, < 5 years

Rate of examination, case confirmation, malaria test positivity, % of confirmed cases that are *P. falciparum*

No data

Year	Reported malaria cases, all ages	Reported malaria cases, < 5 years	All-cause outpatient consultations, all ages	All-cause outpatient consultations, < 5 years	Examined	Positive	P. falciparum	Reporting completeness of outpatient health facilities (%)	Reporting completeness of districts (%)
2000	546 634	177 969	1 685 072	548 814					
2001	612 896	211 018	2 065 677	665 692					
2002	723 077	243 390	2 289 524	736 139					
2003	809 428	267 133	2 533 291	794 023					
2004	1 969 214	611 680	2 626 206	815 931					
2005	962 706	335 701	2 652 526	870 359					
2006	1 022 592	332 495	3 126 181	902 043					
2007	1 291 853	332 262	3 442 514	980 295				33	100
2008									

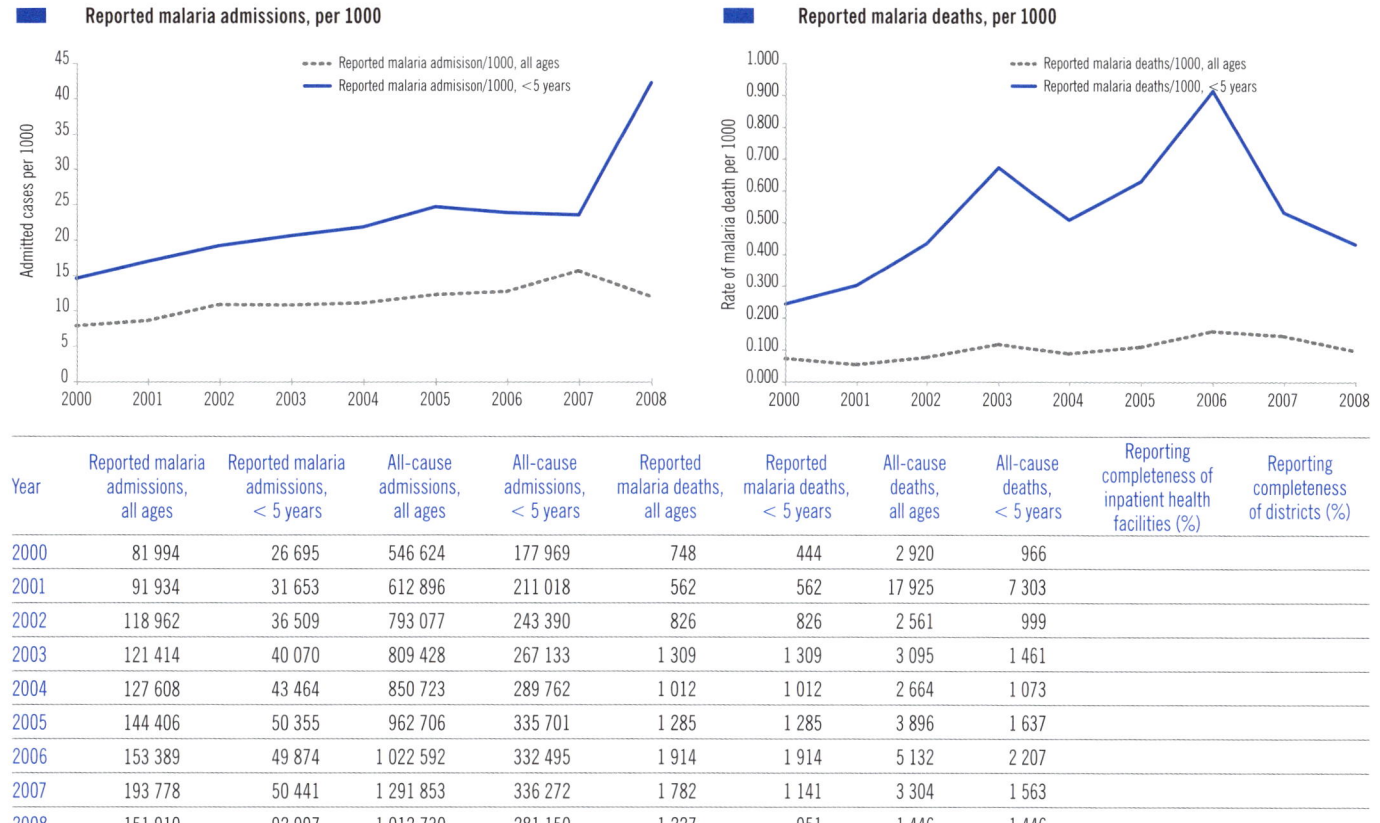

Year	Reported malaria admissions, all ages	Reported malaria admissions, < 5 years	All-cause admissions, all ages	All-cause admissions, < 5 years	Reported malaria deaths, all ages	Reported malaria deaths, < 5 years	All-cause deaths, all ages	All-cause deaths, < 5 years	Reporting completeness of inpatient health facilities (%)	Reporting completeness of districts (%)
2000	81 994	26 695	546 624	177 969	748	444	2 920	966		
2001	91 934	31 653	612 896	211 018	562	562	17 925	7 303		
2002	118 962	36 509	793 077	243 390	826	826	2 561	999		
2003	121 414	40 070	809 428	267 133	1 309	1 309	3 095	1 461		
2004	127 608	43 464	850 723	289 762	1 012	1 012	2 664	1 073		
2005	144 406	50 355	962 706	335 701	1 285	1 285	3 896	1 637		
2006	153 389	49 874	1 022 592	332 495	1 914	1 914	5 132	2 207		
2007	193 778	50 441	1 291 853	336 272	1 782	1 141	3 304	1 563		
2008	151 910	92 997	1 012 730	281 150	1 227	951	1 446	1 446		

II.   INTERVENTION POLICIES AND STRATEGIES

Intervention	WHO-RECOMMENDED POLICIES / STRATEGIES	Yes or No	Year adopted	OPTIONAL POLICIES / STRATEGIES	Yes or No	Year adoped
Insecticide-treated nets (ITN)	Distribution of ITN/LLINs – Free	Yes	2005	Distribution – Antenatal care	Yes	2006
	Targeting all age groups	No	–	Distribution – EPI routine and campaign	Yes	2005
				Targeting children < 5 years and pregnant women	Yes	2006
				ITN distribution is subsidized	Yes	2005
Indoor residual spraying (IRS)	IRS is a primary vector control intervention	Yes	2008	Insecticide-resistance management implemented	Yes	2000
	DDT is used for IRS (public health) only	No	–	Where IRS is conducted, other options are also implemented, e.g. ITN	Yes	2008
				IRS is used for prevention and control of epidemics	Yes	2005
Intermittent preventive treatment (IPT)	IPT used to prevent malaria during pregnancy	Yes	2003			
Case management	Oral artemisinin monotherapies banned (prohibited from registration or removed from the system)	No	–	Parasitological confirmation for patients ≥ 5 years only	No	–
	Parasitological confirmation for patients of all ages	Yes	2008	Malaria diagnosis is free of charge in the public sector	No	–
	ACT is free of charge for < 5 years old in the public sector	Yes	2006	ACT is free of charge for patients ≥ 5 years in the public sector	No	–
	Diagnosis of malaria of inpatients is based on parasitological confirmation	Yes	1997	ACT is delivered at community level through community agents (beyond the health facilities)	Yes	2005
	Pre-referral treatment with quinine or artemether IM or artesunate suppositories	Yes	2009	Uncomplicated malaria cases are admitted	No	–
	Oversight regulation of case management in the private sectors	No	–			
	RDTs used at community level	Yes	2005			

Antimalarial policy	Type of medicine	Year adopted	Results of therapeutic efficacy tests						
			Study year	No. of studies	Median	Minimum	Maximum	Percentiles: 25%	75%
First-line treatment of P. falciparum (unconfirmed)	AL	2004							
First-line treatment of P. falciparum (confirmed)	AL	2004							
Treatment failure of P. falciparum	AS+SP	2004							
Treatment of severe malaria	QN(7d)	2004							
Treatment of P. vivax	–	–							

III. IMPLEMENTING MALARIA CONTROL

Coverage of ITN: survey data

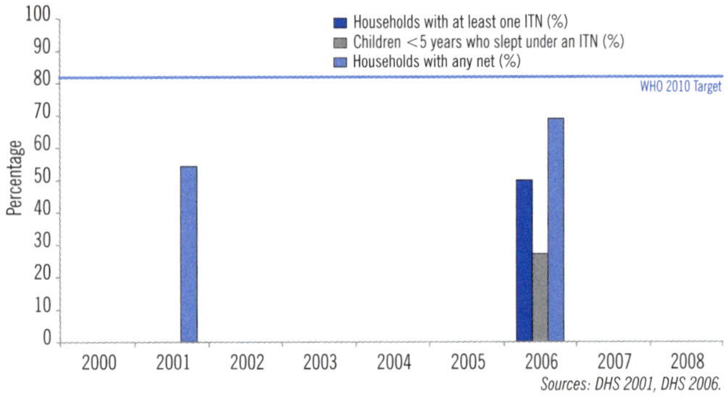

Percentage (y-axis 0–100)

Legend:
- Households with at least one ITN (%)
- Children <5 years who slept under an ITN (%)
- Households with any net (%)

WHO 2010 Target

Years: 2000–2008

Sources: DHS 2001, DHS 2006.

Coverage of IRS and ITN: programme data

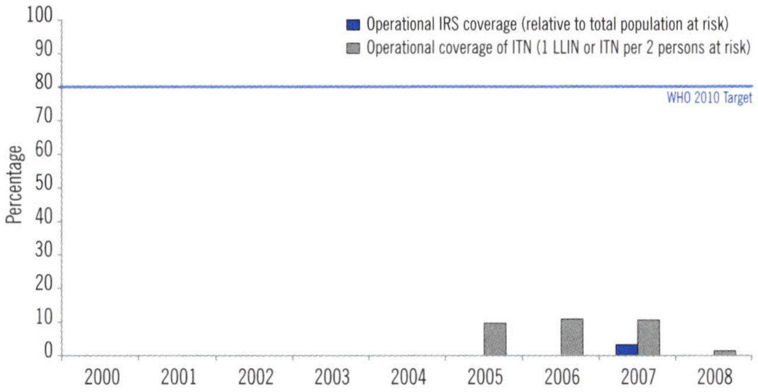

Percentage (y-axis 0–100)

Legend:
- Operational IRS coverage (relative to total population at risk)
- Operational coverage of ITN (1 LLIN or ITN per 2 persons at risk)

WHO 2010 Target

Years: 2000–2008

Access by febrile children to effective treatment: survey data

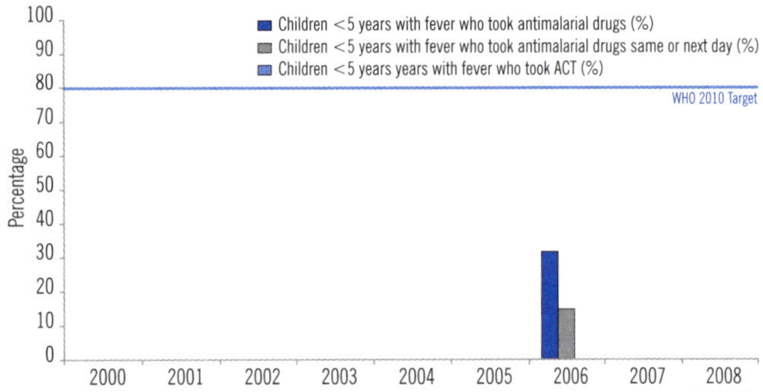

Percentage (y-axis 0–100)

Legend:
- Children <5 years with fever who took antimalarial drugs (%)
- Children <5 years with fever who took antimalarial drugs same or next day (%)
- Children <5 years years with fever who took ACT (%)

WHO 2010 Target

Years: 2000–2008

Sources: DHS 2006.

Access to effective treatment: programme data

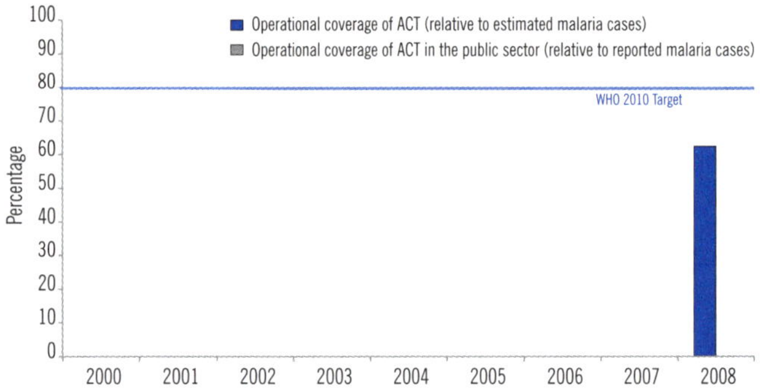

Percentage (y-axis 0–100)

Legend:
- Operational coverage of ACT (relative to estimated malaria cases)
- Operational coverage of ACT in the public sector (relative to reported malaria cases)

WHO 2010 Target

Years: 2000–2008

Year	Pregnant women who slept under any net (%)	Pregnant women who slept under an ITN (%)	Children < 5 years with fever (%)	Febrile children < 5 years who sought treatment in HF (%)	Number of households protected by IRS	Number of people protected by IRS	Number of ITNs and/or LLINs	Number of 1st-line treatment courses received	Number of ACT treatment courses received
2000									
2001			–	–					
2002									
2003									
2004									
2005							572 556		
2006		29	–	–			90 900		
2007					87 198	405 936	2 982 346		
2008							682 461		2 842 500

IV. FINANCING MALARIA CONTROL

Governmental and external financing

Funding by source ($m) (y-axis 0–30)

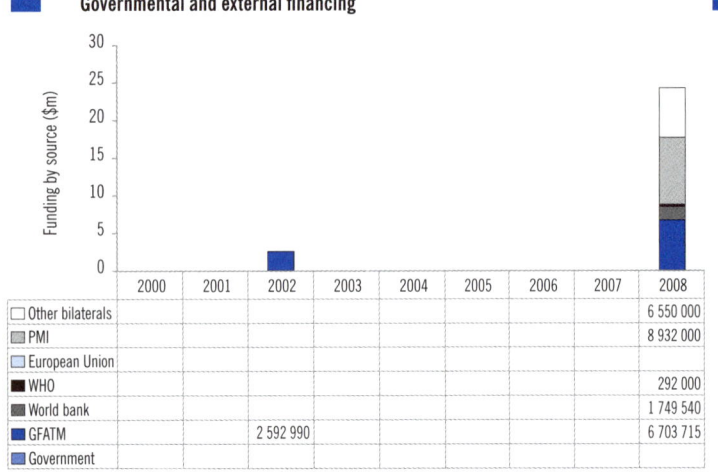

	2000	2001	2002	2003	2004	2005	2006	2007	2008
☐ Other bilaterals									6 550 000
▨ PMI									8 932 000
☐ European Union									
■ WHO									292 000
▨ World bank									1 749 540
■ GFATM			2 592 990						6 703 715
▨ Government									

Breakdown of expenditure by intervention in 2008

No data

V. SOURCE OF INFORMATION

PROGRAMME DATA		SURVEY AND OTHER DATA	
Reported cases	Surveillance data	Insecticide-treated nets (ITN)	DHS 2001, DHS 2006
Operational coverage of ITNs, IRS and access to medicines	Programme report	Treatment	DHS 2001, DHS 2006
Financial data	Programme report	Use of health services	DHS 2006

MOZAMBIQUE

Mozambique had an estimated 9.8 million malaria cases in 2006. Transmission is seasonal, mainly between November and July. Most cases are caused by *P. falciparum*, but most of the reported 4.8 million malaria cases in 2008 were not parasitologically tested. The inpatient data reported for 2001–2006 were inadequate to allow a trend analysis. IRS has been the principal method of mosquito control, covering 2 million households and protecting 6.5 million people at risk in 2008 (36% of people at risk). The national malaria control programme distributed about 4 million LLINs during 2006–2008, adequate to cover 44% of the population at risk. In the 2007 malaria indicator survey, 16% of households owned an ITN and only 7% of children under 5 had slept under an ITN the previous night. The programme delivered over 6.1 million ACT treatment courses in 2007 and 4.8 million in 2008, adequate to treat all reported cases in the public sector. The programme provided no information about funding, but the country has funding from Global Fund round 2 and 6 grants, amounting to US$ 65 million, from the World Bank and from other donors.

I. EPIDEMIOLOGICAL PROFILE

Population, endemicity and malaria burden

Population (in thousands)	2008	%
All age groups	22 383	
< 5 years	3 820	17
≥ 5 years	18 562	83

Population by malaria endemicity (in thousands)	2008	%
High transmission ≥ 1/1000	22 383	100
Low transmission (0–1/1000)	0	0
Malaria-free (0 cases)	0	0
Rural population	14 133	63

Vector and parasite profiles

Major *Anopheles* species	*gambiae, funestus, s.l, s.l.,*
Plasmodium species	*falciparum, vivax*

Stratification of burden (reported cases, per 1000)

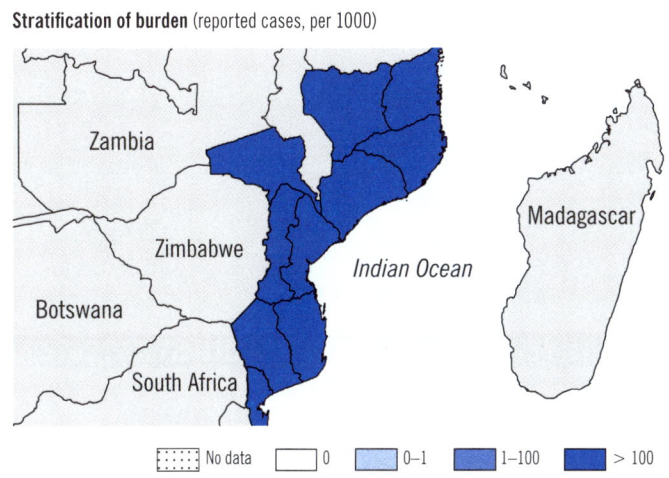

No data | 0 | 0–1 | 1–100 | > 100

Trends in malaria morbidity and mortality

Reported malaria cases, per 1000

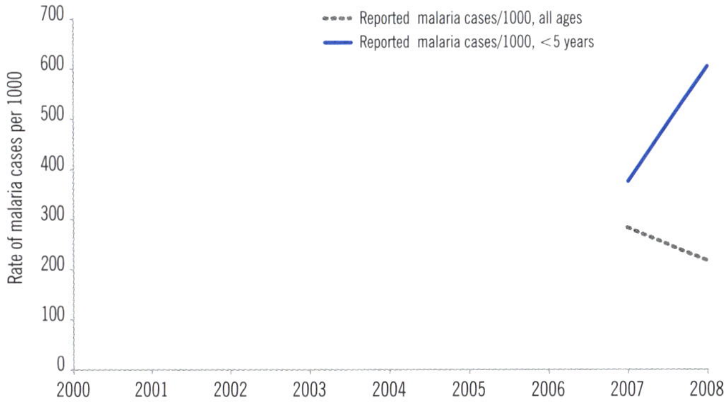

- - - Reported malaria cases/1000, all ages
—— Reported malaria cases/1000, < 5 years

Rate of examination, case confirmation, malaria test positivity, % of confirmed cases that are *P. falciparum*

No data

Year	Reported malaria cases, all ages	Reported malaria cases, < 5 years	All-cause outpatient consultations, all ages	All-cause outpatient consultations, < 5 years	Examined	Positive	*P. falciparum*	Reporting completeness of outpatient health facilities (%)	Reporting completeness of districts (%)
2000									
2001									
2002									
2003									
2004									
2005									
2006									
2007	6 155 082	1 419 774	21 720 674						
2008	4 831 491	2 304 974	21 266 935						

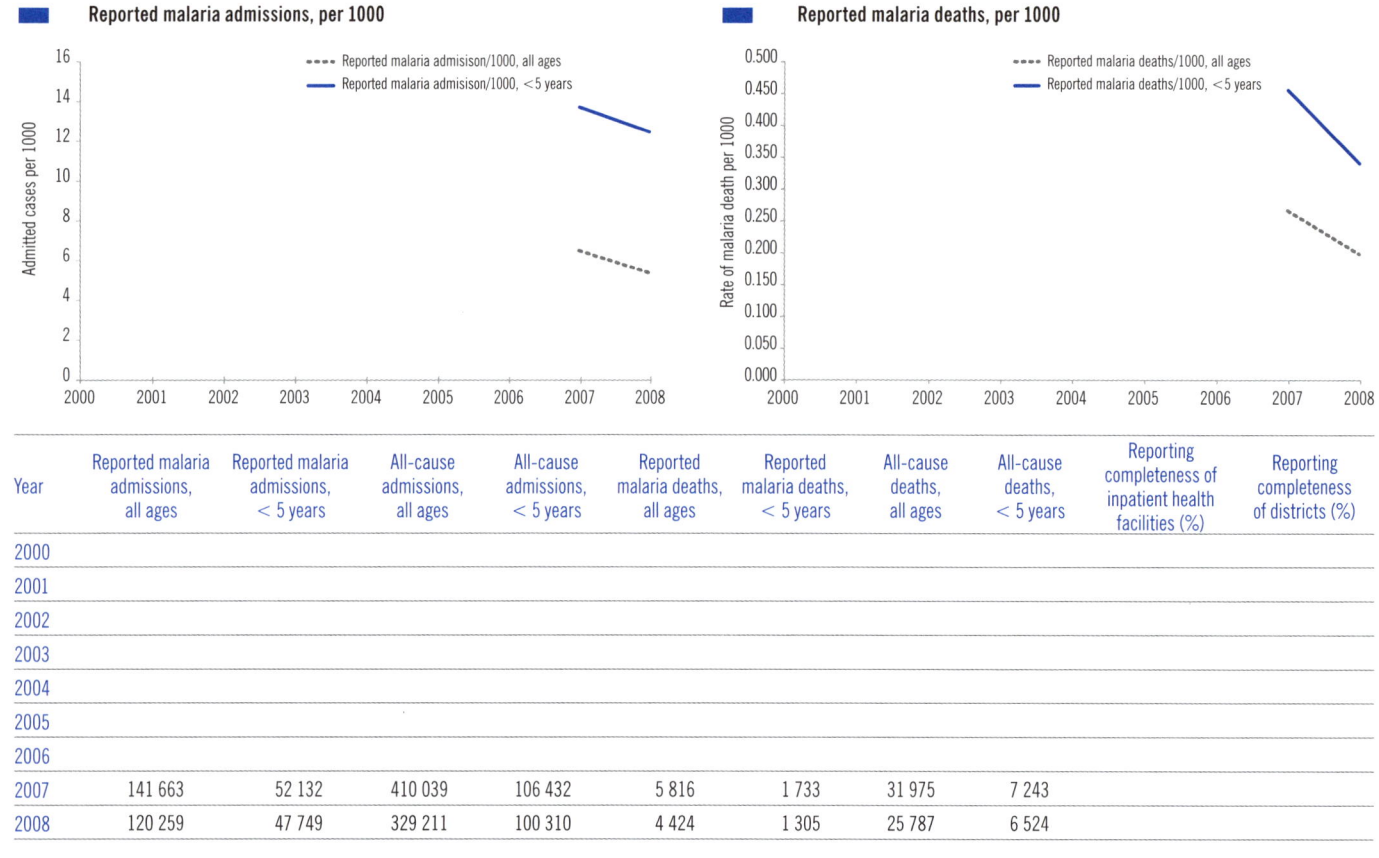

Year	Reported malaria admissions, all ages	Reported malaria admissions, < 5 years	All-cause admissions, all ages	All-cause admissions, < 5 years	Reported malaria deaths, all ages	Reported malaria deaths, < 5 years	All-cause deaths, all ages	All-cause deaths, < 5 years	Reporting completeness of inpatient health facilities (%)	Reporting completeness of districts (%)
2000										
2001										
2002										
2003										
2004										
2005										
2006										
2007	141 663	52 132	410 039	106 432	5 816	1 733	31 975	7 243		
2008	120 259	47 749	329 211	100 310	4 424	1 305	25 787	6 524		

II. INTERVENTION POLICIES AND STRATEGIES

Intervention	WHO-RECOMMENDED POLICIES / STRATEGIES	Yes or No	Year adopted	OPTIONAL POLICIES / STRATEGIES	Yes or No	Year adoped
Insecticide-treated nets (ITN)	Distribution of ITN/LLINs – Free	Yes	2003	Distribution – Antenatal care	Yes	2003
	Targeting all age groups	Yes	2009	Distribution – EPI routine and campaign	No	–
				Targeting children < 5 years and pregnant women	Yes	2003
				ITN distribution is subsidized	No	–
Indoor residual spraying (IRS)	IRS is a primary vector control intervention	Yes	–	Insecticide-resistance management implemented	Yes	2007
	DDT is used for IRS (public health) only	Yes	2005	Where IRS is conducted, other options are also implemented, e.g. ITN	Yes	2003
				IRS is used for prevention and control of epidemics	Yes	–
Intermittent preventive treatment (IPT)	IPT used to prevent malaria during pregnancy	Yes	2006			
Case management	Oral artemisinin monotherapies banned (prohibited from registration or removed from the system)	Yes	2004	Parasitological confirmation for patients ≥ 5 years only	–	–
	Parasitological confirmation for patients of all ages	Yes	2009	Malaria diagnosis is free of charge in the public sector	Yes	–
	ACT is free of charge for < 5 years old in the public sector	Yes	2005	ACT is free of charge for patients ≥ 5 years in the public sector	Yes	–
	Diagnosis of malaria of inpatients is based on parasitological confirmation	Yes	–	ACT is delivered at community level through community agents (beyond the health facilities)	Yes	2005
	Pre-referral treatment with quinine or artemether IM or artesunate suppositories	Yes	–	Uncomplicated malaria cases are admitted	No	–
	Oversight regulation of case management in the private sectors	–	–			
	RDTs used at community level	Yes	2007			

Antimalarial policy	Type of medicine	Year adopted	Results of therapeutic efficacy tests						
			Study year	No. of studies	Median	Minimum	Maximum	Percentiles: 25%	75%
First-line treatment of *P. falciparum* (unconfirmed)	AL	2004	2006–2008	3	0	0	2	0	2
First-line treatment of *P. falciparum* (confirmed)	AL	2004							
Treatment failure of *P. falciparum*	AS+AQ	2004							
Treatment of severe malaria	QN(7d)	2004							
Treatment of *P. vivax*	–	–							

III. IMPLEMENTING MALARIA CONTROL

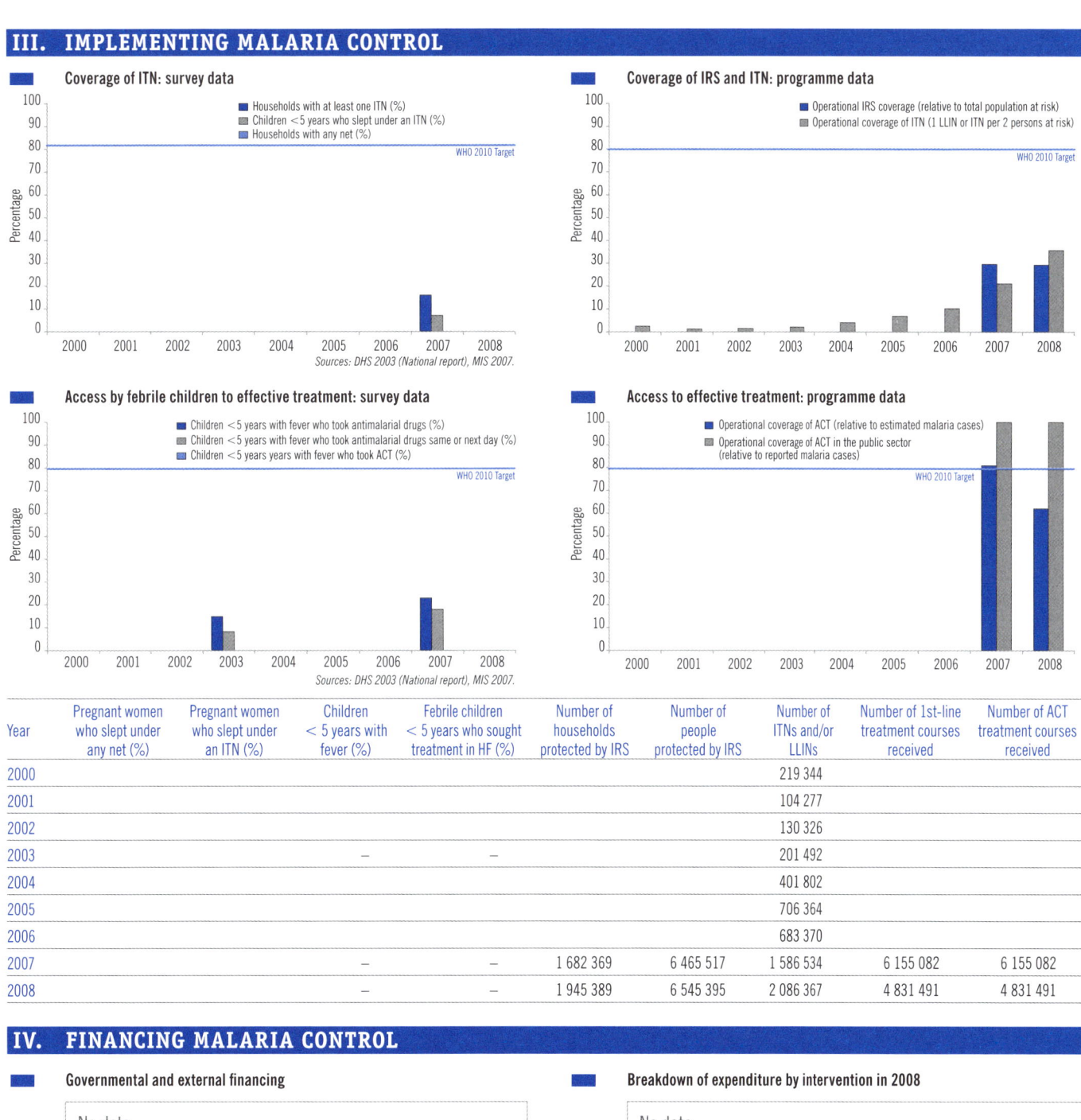

Coverage of ITN: survey data

Households with at least one ITN (%)
Children <5 years who slept under an ITN (%)
Households with any net (%)

WHO 2010 Target

Sources: DHS 2003 (National report), MIS 2007.

Coverage of IRS and ITN: programme data

Operational IRS coverage (relative to total population at risk)
Operational coverage of ITN (1 LLIN or ITN per 2 persons at risk)

WHO 2010 Target

Access by febrile children to effective treatment: survey data

Children <5 years with fever who took antimalarial drugs (%)
Children <5 years with fever who took antimalarial drugs same or next day (%)
Children <5 years years with fever who took ACT (%)

WHO 2010 Target

Sources: DHS 2003 (National report), MIS 2007.

Access to effective treatment: programme data

Operational coverage of ACT (relative to estimated malaria cases)
Operational coverage of ACT in the public sector (relative to reported malaria cases)

WHO 2010 Target

Year	Pregnant women who slept under any net (%)	Pregnant women who slept under an ITN (%)	Children < 5 years with fever (%)	Febrile children < 5 years who sought treatment in HF (%)	Number of households protected by IRS	Number of people protected by IRS	Number of ITNs and/or LLINs	Number of 1st-line treatment courses received	Number of ACT treatment courses received
2000							219 344		
2001							104 277		
2002							130 326		
2003			–	–			201 492		
2004							401 802		
2005							706 364		
2006							683 370		
2007		–		–	1 682 369	6 465 517	1 586 534	6 155 082	6 155 082
2008		–		–	1 945 389	6 545 395	2 086 367	4 831 491	4 831 491

IV. FINANCING MALARIA CONTROL

Governmental and external financing

No data

Breakdown of expenditure by intervention in 2008

No data

V. SOURCE OF INFORMATION

PROGRAMME DATA		SURVEY AND OTHER DATA	
Reported cases	Surveillance data	Insecticide-treated nets (ITN)	DHS 2003 (National report), MIS 2007
Operational coverage of ITNs, IRS and access to medicines	Programme report	Treatment	DHS 2003 (National report), MIS 2007
Financial data	Programme report	Use of health services	DHS 2003

MYANMAR

Although much of the population is at risk for malaria, the most vulnerable segment consists of non-immune migrant workers involved in gem-mining in forests, logging, agriculture and construction. The number of reported cases increased from 245 000 in 2000 to 566 000 in 2008, but most reported cases are not examined by microscopy or RDT. The number of cases confirmed by microscopy increased from 120 029 in 2000 to 411 494 in 2008. The increase was associated with a 20% increase in the number of slides examined and an increase in the slide positivity rate, from 31% to 45%. The introduction of RDTs added a further 187 289 confirmed cases in 2008. The percentage of cases due to *P. falciparum* was approximately 75% in 2008. The number of malaria admissions decreased from 85 409 in 2000 to 47 553 in 2008, and the number of deaths decreased from 2756 to 1088. Malaria represented 6% of all admissions in 2008 as compared with 16% in 2000 and 11% of recorded deaths in 2008 as compared with 19% in 2000. About 694 000 ITNs were delivered in 2008, of which 113 000 were LLINs. An additional 11 000 people were protected by IRS.

I.   EPIDEMIOLOGICAL PROFILE

Population, endemicity and malaria burden

Population (in thousands)	2008	%
All age groups	49 563	
< 5 years	4 629	9
≥ 5 years	44 934	91

Population by malaria endemicity (in thousands)	2008	%
High transmission ≥ 1/1000	25 011	50
Low transmission (0–1/1000)	9 038	18
Malaria-free (0 cases)	15 514	31
Rural population	33 418	67

Vector and parasite profiles

Major *Anopheles* species	*dirus, minimus, sundaicus*
Plasmodium species	*falciparum, vivax*

Stratification of burden (reported cases, per 1000)

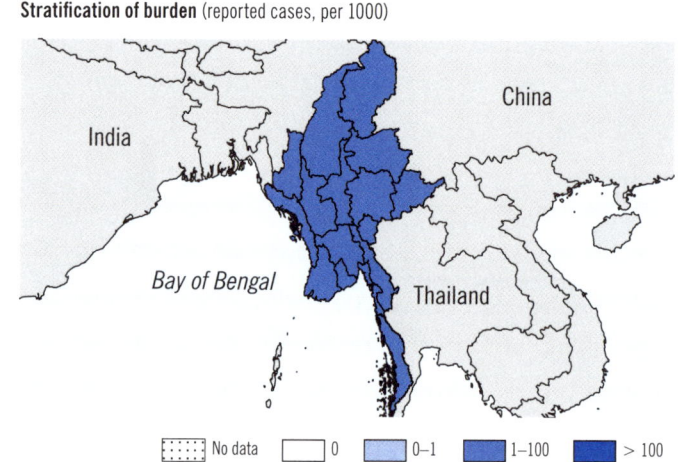

No data   0   0–1   1–100   > 100

Trends in malaria morbidity and mortality

Reported malaria cases, per 1000

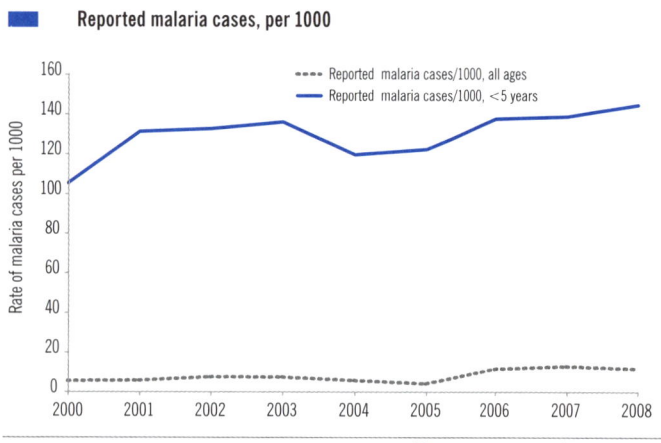

- - - Reported malaria cases/1000, all ages
—— Reported malaria cases/1000, <5 years

Rate of examination, case confirmation, malaria test positivity, % of confirmed cases that are *P. falciparum*

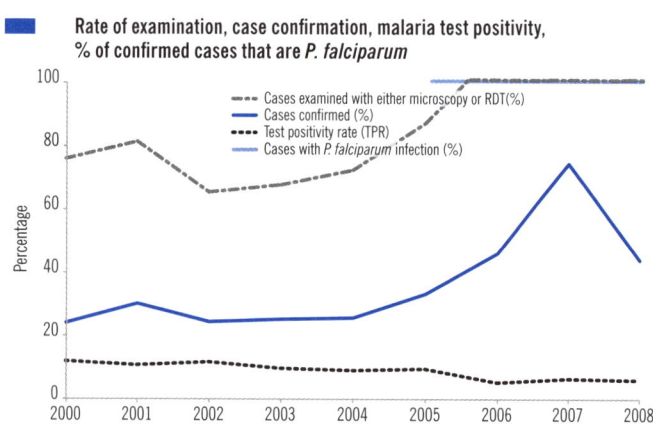

- - - Cases examined with either microscopy or RDT(%)
—— Cases confirmed (%)
· · · Test positivity rate (TPR)
—— Cases with *P. falciparum* infection (%)

Year	Reported malaria cases, all ages	Reported malaria cases, < 5 years	All-cause outpatient consultations, all ages	All-cause outpatient consultations, < 5 years	Examined	Positive	*P. falciparum*	Reporting completeness of outpatient health facilities (%)	Reporting completeness of districts (%)
2000	245 355	477 108	4 828 170		381 619	120 029			
2001	254 660	593 223	5 182 738		463 194	170 502			
2002	344 791	601 038	5 243 515		467 851	173 096			
2003	340 311	619 389	5 250 160		481 201	177 530			
2004	263 731	547 104	5 195 966		432 581	152 070			
2005	184 986	562 031	5 406 736		437 387	165 737			
2006	551 537	634 650	5 222 385		522 187	216 470			
2007	630 385	641 117	6 345 263		838 660	332 056			
2008	566 204	668 697	6 288 374		948 937	411 494			

Reported malaria admissions, per 1000

- ···· Reported malaria admision/1000, all ages
- —— Reported malaria admision/1000, <5 years

Reported malaria deaths, per 1000

- ···· Reported malaria deaths/1000, all ages
- —— Reported malaria deaths/1000, <5 years

Year	Reported malaria admissions, all ages	Reported malaria admissions, < 5 years	All-cause admissions, all ages	All-cause admissions, < 5 years	Reported malaria deaths, all ages	Reported malaria deaths, < 5 years	All-cause deaths, all ages	All-cause deaths, < 5 years	Reporting completeness of inpatient health facilities (%)	Reporting completeness of districts (%)
2000	85 409	8 259	529 464	46 908	2 756	347	14 212	2 007		
2001	87 111	9 301	591 546	61 296	2 814	398	15 382	1 791		
2002	82 193	10 610	612 823	70 639	2 634	383	14 583	2 546		
2003	72 824	7 470	602 178	63 738	2 476	320	14 269	1 969		
2004	58 641	8 615	600 939	76 002	1 982	326	13 183	1 995		
2005	59 405	9 147	650 417	81 201	1 707	286	13 560	1 734		
2006	62 813	7 974	643 594	80 138	1 647	242	12 473	1 674		
2007	53 220	8 516	723 380	83 279	1 265	194	12 682	1 669		
2008	47 553	6 701	740 930	96 135	1 088	137	9 676	1 356		

II.   INTERVENTION POLICIES AND STRATEGIES

Intervention	WHO-RECOMMENDED POLICIES / STRATEGIES	Yes or No	Year adopted	OPTIONAL POLICIES / STRATEGIES	Yes or No	Year adoped
Insecticide-treated nets (ITN)	Distribution of ITN/LLINs – Free	Yes	2003	Distribution – Antenatal care	No	–
	Targeting all age groups	Yes	2003	Distribution – EPI routine and campaign	No	–
				Targeting children < 5 years and pregnant women	No	–
				ITN distribution is subsidized	No	–
Indoor residual spraying (IRS)	IRS is a primary vector control intervention	Yes	–	Insecticide-resistance management implemented	Yes	–
	DDT is used for IRS (public health) only	Yes	–	Where IRS is conducted, other options are also implemented, e.g. ITN	Yes	–
				IRS is used for prevention and control of epidemics	Yes	–
Intermittent preventive treatment (IPT)	IPT used to prevent malaria during pregnancy	No	–			
Case management	Oral artemisinin monotherapies banned (prohibited from registration or removed from the system)	No	–	Parasitological confirmation for patients ≥ 5 years only	No	–
	Parasitological confirmation for patients of all ages	Yes	–	Malaria diagnosis is free of charge in the public sector	Yes	–
	ACT is free of charge for < 5 years old in the public sector	Yes	2002	ACT is free of charge for patients ≥ 5 years in the public sector	Yes	–
	Diagnosis of malaria of inpatients is based on parasitological confirmation	Yes	2002	ACT is delivered at community level through community agents (beyond the health facilities)	Yes	2008
	Pre-referral treatment with quinine or artemether IM or artesunate suppositories	Yes	2002	Uncomplicated malaria cases are admitted	No	–
	Oversight regulation of case management in the private sectors	No	–			
	RDTs used at community level	Yes	–			

Antimalarial policy	Type of medicine	Year adopted	Study year	No. of studies	Median	Minimum	Maximum	Percentiles: 25%	75%
					Results of therapeutic efficacy tests				
First-line treatment of P. falciparum (unconfirmed)	CQ	2002	2000–2006	9	1.8	0	8.9	0	6.55
First-line treatment of P. falciparum (confirmed)	DHA-PPQ, AL, AS+MQ	2008	2003–2008	5	0	0	5	0	2.85
Treatment failure of P. falciparum	DHA-PPQ, AS+AM, AL	2008							
Treatment of severe malaria	AM inj, QN and ACT*, AS inj	2008							
Treatment of P. vivax	CQ+PQ(14d)	2008							

* if patient can tolerate oral treatment

III. IMPLEMENTING MALARIA CONTROL

Coverage of ITN: survey data

No data

Coverage of IRS and ITN: programme data

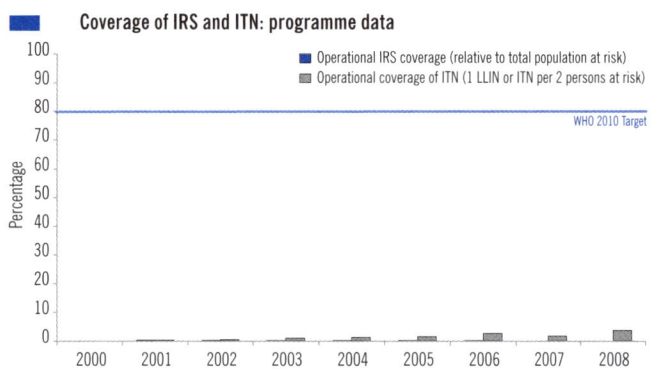

Access by febrile children to effective treatment: survey data

No data

Access to effective treatment: programme data

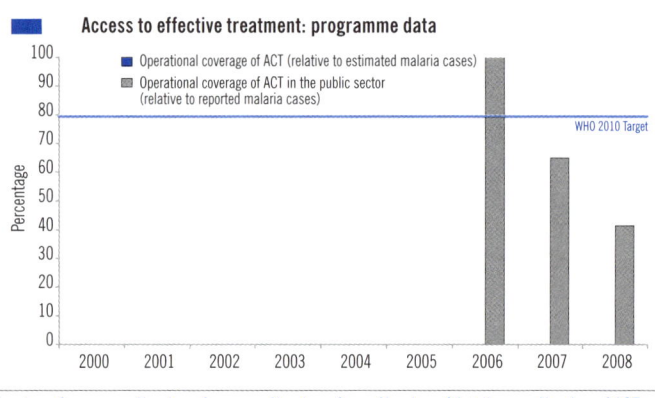

Year	Pregnant women who slept under any net (%)	Pregnant women who slept under an ITN (%)	Children < 5 years with fever (%)	Febrile children < 5 years who sought treatment in HF (%)	Number of households protected by IRS	Number of people protected by IRS	Number of ITNs and/or LLINs	Number of 1st-line treatment courses received	Number of ACT treatment courses received
2000									
2001					20 437	95 795	46 903		
2002					12 445	63 015	47 329		
2003					7 932	44 075	137 695		
2004					4 165	19 764	181 072		
2005					4 934	32 840	222 886		
2006					6 116	33 391	538 436		326 188
2007					3 098	10 479	298 579		226 397
2008					2 902	11 284	693 858		187 102

IV. FINANCING MALARIA CONTROL

Governmental and external financing

No data

Breakdown of expenditure by intervention in 2008

No data

V. SOURCE OF INFORMATION

PROGRAMME DATA		SURVEY AND OTHER DATA	
Reported cases	Surveillance data	Insecticide-treated nets (ITN)	No surveys
Operational coverage of ITNs, IRS and access to medicines	Programme report	Treatment	No surveys
Financial data	Programme report	Use of health services	MICS 2000

NIGER

Malaria transmission is more intensive in the south, occurring seasonally between January and April. The desert areas in the north are malaria-free. Almost all cases are caused by *P. falciparum*, but only a fraction of the suspected cases are parasitologically tested. The numbers of reported cases and deaths fluctuated over the period 2001–2008, mostly showing increasing trends, probably due to better reporting. During 2006–2008, the national malaria control programme delivered nearly 4 million LLINs, of which 1.7 million were delivered during a mass campaign in 2007. The 2006 demographic and health survey reported that 69% of households owned a mosquito net and 43% an ITN, but only 7% of children under 5 years slept under an ITN. After the adoption of ACTs as first-line treatment in 2005, the programme delivered 1.4 million ACT treatment courses in 2007 and 1.6 million in 2008, adequate to treat about 80% of the reported suspected malaria cases in the public sector. In the survey, only one third of children with fever were given antimalarial medicine. The programme provided little information about funding in recent years but reported a major award from the Global Fund in 2004.

I. EPIDEMIOLOGICAL PROFILE

Population, endemicity and malaria burden

Population (in thousands)	2008	%
All age groups	14 704	
< 5 years	3 121	21
≥ 5 years	11 584	79

Population by malaria endemicity (in thousands)	2008	%
High transmission ≥ 1/1000	10 146	69
Low transmission (0–1/1000)	4 558	31
Malaria-free (0 cases)	0	0
Rural population	12 283	84

Vector and parasite profiles

Major *Anopheles* species	*gambiae, arabiensis, funestus, coustani, moucheti, moucheti, nili, pharoensis*
Plasmodium species	*falciparum, vivax*

Stratification of burden (reported cases, per 1000)

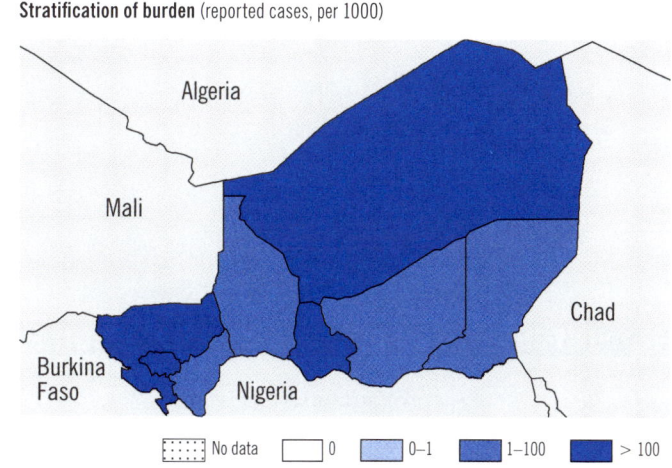

No data | 0 | 0–1 | 1–100 | > 100

Trends in malaria morbidity and mortality

Reported malaria cases, per 1000

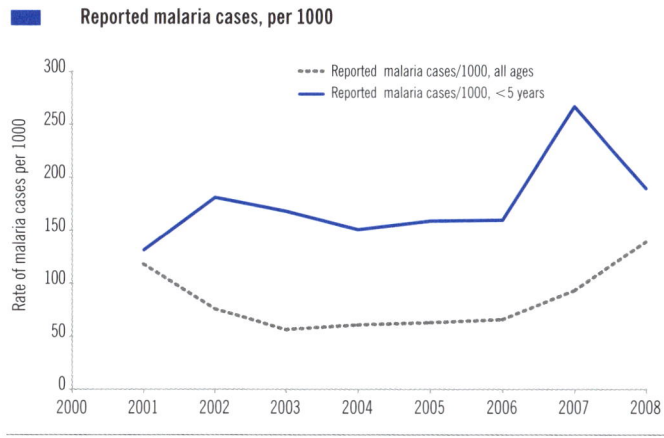

Rate of examination, case confirmation, malaria test positivity, % of confirmed cases that are *P. falciparum*

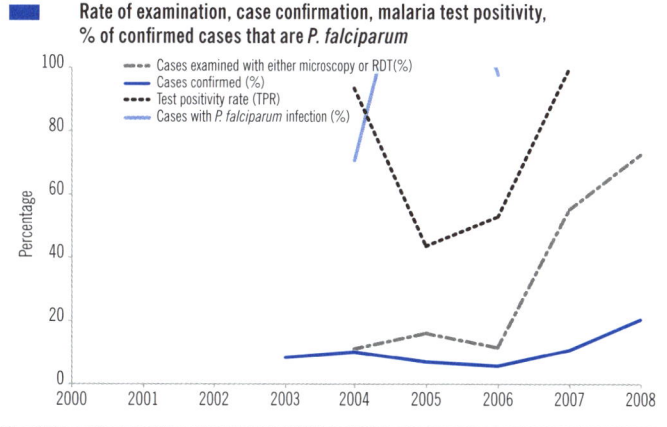

Year	Reported malaria cases, all ages	Reported malaria cases, < 5 years	All-cause outpatient consultations, all ages	All-cause outpatient consultations, < 5 years	Examined	Positive	*P. falciparum*	Reporting completeness of outpatient health facilities (%)	Reporting completeness of districts (%)
2000									100
2001	1 340 142	304 032	4 989 176	2 137 498					100
2002	888 345	431 710	4 827 380	2 080 927					100
2003	681 783	414 284	3 996 584	1 847 222		56 460			100
2004	760 718	385 674	1 663 367	731 299	81 814	76 030	53 637		100
2005	817 707	424 691	2 595 771	833 437	128 322	56 043	74 129		100
2006	886 531	449 044	3 458 631	1 627 033	99 670	49 624	44 612		100
2007	1 308 234	790 448	5 119 076	1 957 624	718 215	138 902			100
2008	2 033 971	593 153			1 466 095	413 252			100

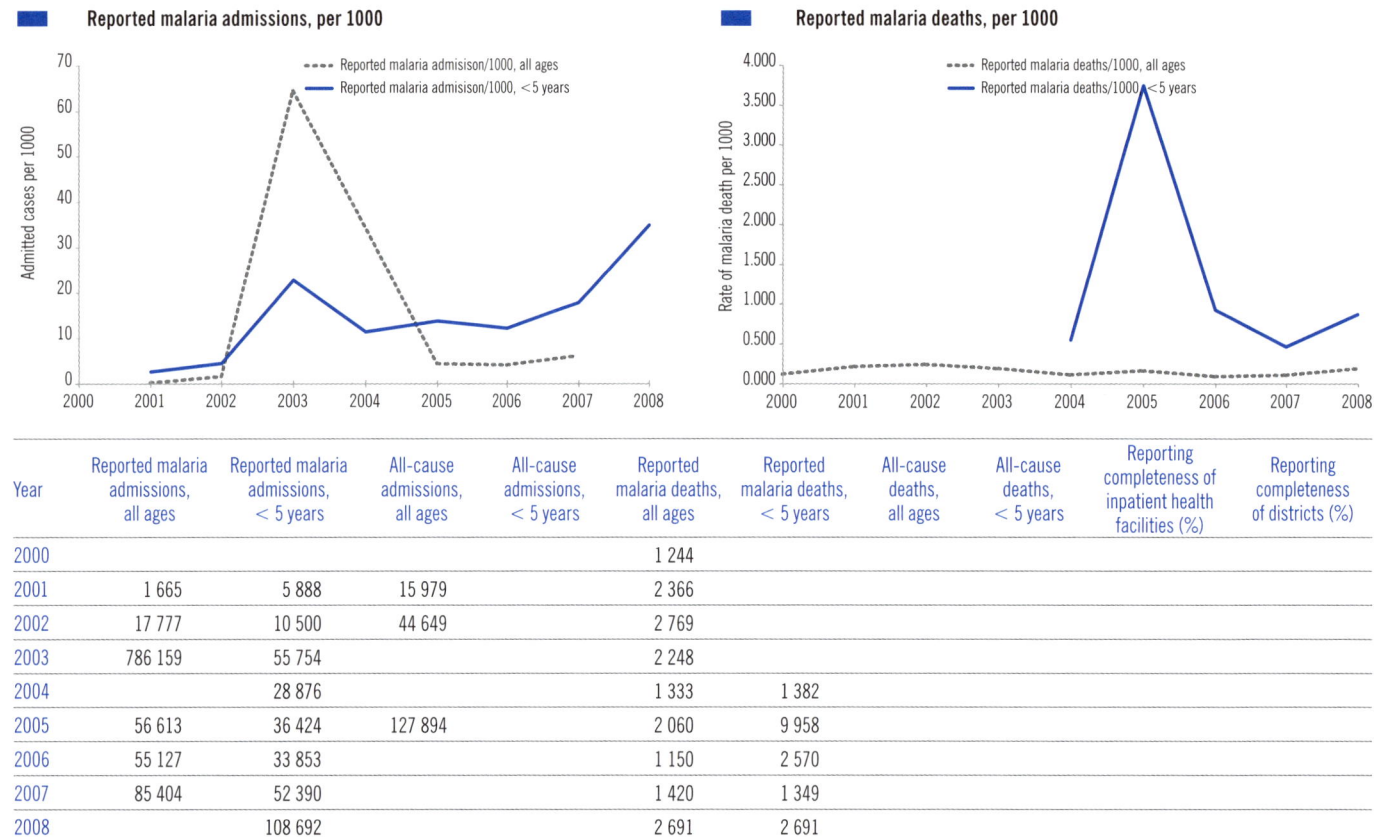

Reported malaria admissions, per 1000 — Reported malaria admision/1000, all ages; Reported malaria admision/1000, <5 years

Reported malaria deaths, per 1000 — Reported malaria deaths/1000, all ages; Reported malaria deaths/1000,<5 years

Year	Reported malaria admissions, all ages	Reported malaria admissions, < 5 years	All-cause admissions, all ages	All-cause admissions, < 5 years	Reported malaria deaths, all ages	Reported malaria deaths, < 5 years	All-cause deaths, all ages	All-cause deaths, < 5 years	Reporting completeness of inpatient health facilities (%)	Reporting completeness of districts (%)
2000					1 244					
2001	1 665	5 888	15 979		2 366					
2002	17 777	10 500	44 649		2 769					
2003	786 159	55 754			2 248					
2004		28 876			1 333	1 382				
2005	56 613	36 424	127 894		2 060	9 958				
2006	55 127	33 853			1 150	2 570				
2007	85 404	52 390			1 420	1 349				
2008		108 692			2 691	2 691				

II. INTERVENTION POLICIES AND STRATEGIES

Intervention	WHO-RECOMMENDED POLICIES / STRATEGIES	Yes or No	Year adopted	OPTIONAL POLICIES / STRATEGIES	Yes or No	Year adoped
Insecticide-treated nets (ITN)	Distribution of ITN/LLINs – Free	Yes	2005	Distribution – Antenatal care	Yes	2004
	Targeting all age groups	No	–	Distribution – EPI routine and campaign	Yes	2005
				Targeting children < 5 years and pregnant women	Yes	1998
				ITN distribution is subsidized	Yes	2003
Indoor residual spraying (IRS)	IRS is a primary vector control intervention	No	–	Insecticide-resistance management implemented	Yes	1998
	DDT is used for IRS (public health) only	No	–	Where IRS is conducted, other options are also implemented, e.g. ITN	Yes	2003
				IRS is used for prevention and control of epidemics	Yes	2000
Intermittent preventive treatment (IPT)	IPT used to prevent malaria during pregnancy	Yes	2005			
Case management	Oral artemisinin monotherapies banned (prohibited from registration or removed from the system)	Yes	2006	Parasitological confirmation for patients ≥ 5 years only	No	–
	Parasitological confirmation for patients of all ages	No	–	Malaria diagnosis is free of charge in the public sector	No	–
	ACT is free of charge for < 5 years old in the public sector	Yes	2005	ACT is free of charge for patients ≥ 5 years in the public sector	No	–
	Diagnosis of malaria of inpatients is based on parasitological confirmation	No	–	ACT is delivered at community level through community agents (beyond the health facilities)	Yes	2005
	Pre-referral treatment with quinine or artemether IM or artesunate suppositories	Yes	1998	Uncomplicated malaria cases are admitted	No	–
	Oversight regulation of case management in the private sectors	Yes	2000			
	RDTs used at community level	Yes	2006			

				Results of therapeutic efficacy tests					
Antimalarial policy	Type of medicine	Year adopted	Study year	No. of studies	Median	Minimum	Maximum	Percentiles: 25%	75%
First-line treatment of *P. falciparum* (unconfirmed)	AL	2005	2006	1	4.4	4.4	4.4	4.4	4.4
First-line treatment of *P. falciparum* (confirmed)	AL	2005							
Treatment failure of *P. falciparum*	QN(7d)	2005							
Treatment of severe malaria	QN(7d)	2005							
Treatment of *P. vivax*	–	–							

III. IMPLEMENTING MALARIA CONTROL

Coverage of ITN: survey data

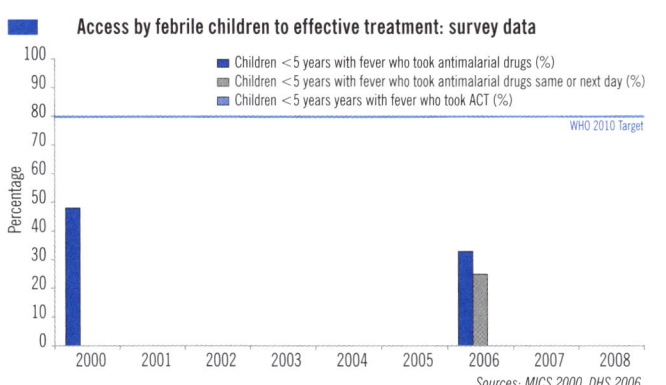

Legend:
- Households with at least one ITN (%)
- Children <5 years who slept under an ITN (%)
- Households with any net (%)

WHO 2010 Target

Sources: MICS 2000, DHS 2006.

Coverage of IRS and ITN: programme data

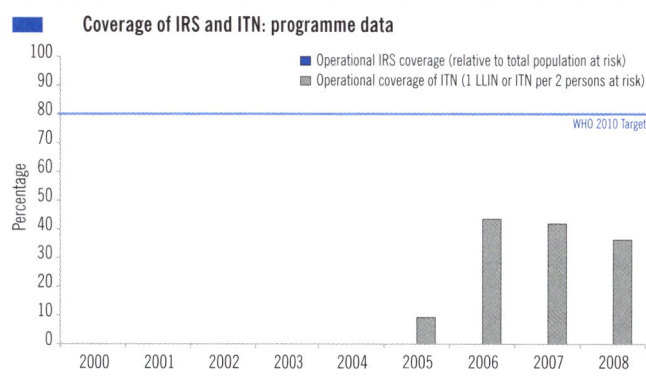

Legend:
- Operational IRS coverage (relative to total population at risk)
- Operational coverage of ITN (1 LLIN or ITN per 2 persons at risk)

WHO 2010 Target

Access by febrile children to effective treatment: survey data

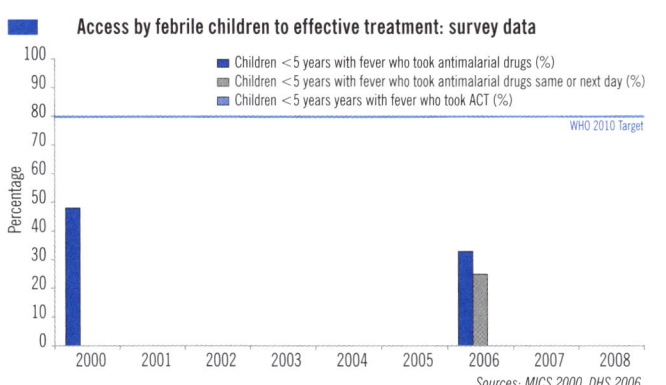

Legend:
- Children <5 years with fever who took antimalarial drugs (%)
- Children <5 years with fever who took antimalarial drugs same or next day (%)
- Children <5 years years with fever who took ACT (%)

WHO 2010 Target

Sources: MICS 2000, DHS 2006.

Access to effective treatment: programme data

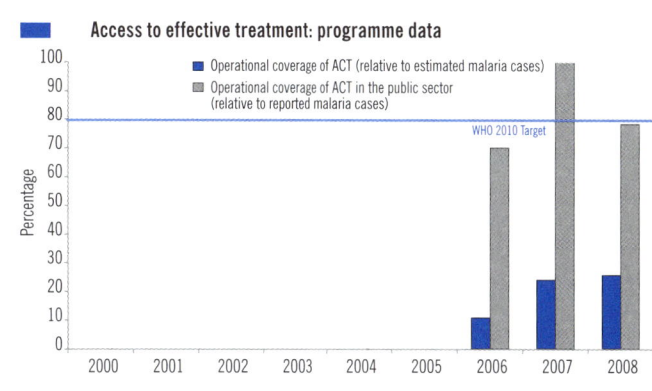

Legend:
- Operational coverage of ACT (relative to estimated malaria cases)
- Operational coverage of ACT in the public sector (relative to reported malaria cases)

WHO 2010 Target

Year	Pregnant women who slept under any net (%)	Pregnant women who slept under an ITN (%)	Children < 5 years with fever (%)	Febrile children < 5 years who sought treatment in HF (%)	Number of households protected by IRS	Number of people protected by IRS	Number of ITNs and/or LLINs	Number of 1st-line treatment courses received	Number of ACT treatment courses received
2000			–	–				592 334	
2001								938 268	
2002								1 323 335	
2003								888 345	
2004								681 783	
2005							300 000	764 443	
2006	13	7	–	–			2 665 000	622 127	622 127
2007							710 000	1 162 636	1 431 358
2008							700 000	2 033 971	1 593 782

IV. FINANCING MALARIA CONTROL

Governmental and external financing

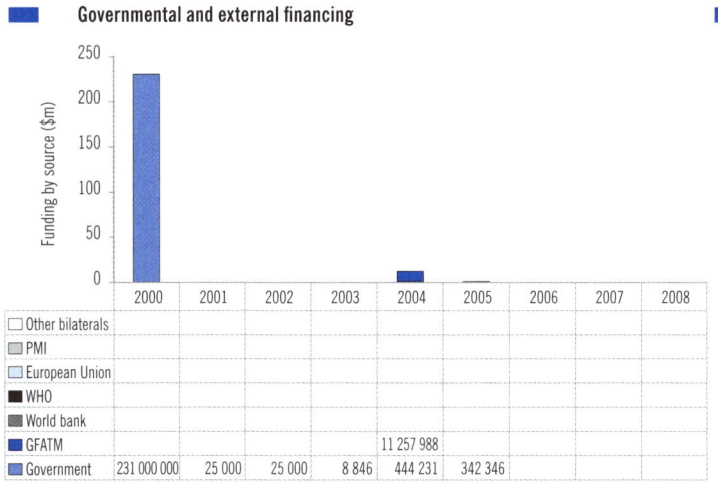

	2000	2001	2002	2003	2004	2005	2006	2007	2008
Other bilaterals									
PMI									
European Union									
WHO									
World bank									
GFATM					11 257 988				
Government	231 000 000	25 000	25 000	8 846	444 231	342 346			

Breakdown of expenditure by intervention in 2008

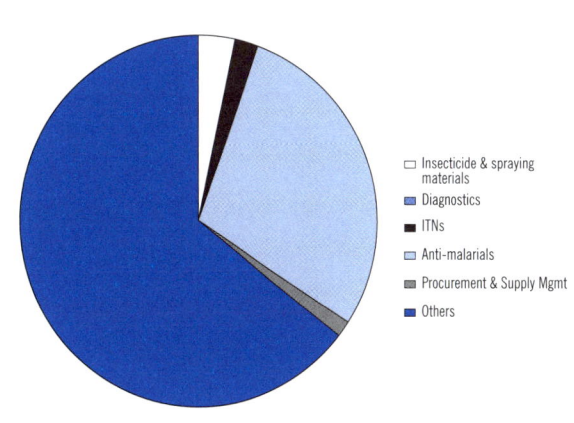

Legend:
- Insecticide & spraying materials
- Diagnostics
- ITNs
- Anti-malarials
- Procurement & Supply Mgmt
- Others

V. SOURCE OF INFORMATION

PROGRAMME DATA		SURVEY AND OTHER DATA	
Reported cases	Surveillance data	Insecticide-treated nets (ITN)	No surveys
Operational coverage of ITNs, IRS and access to medicines	Programme report	Treatment	No surveys
Financial data	Programme report	Use of health services	MICS 2000

NIGERIA

Nigeria accounted for one fourth of all estimated malaria cases in the WHO African Region in 2006. Transmission occurs all year round in the south but is more seasonal in the north. Almost all cases are caused by *P. falciparum*, but only a small fraction are parasitologically tested. The surveillance data show neither the true magnitude of the malaria burden nor evidence of a systematic decrease, because of inconsistent and incomplete reporting. IRS was piloted in some project areas in 2008. The national malaria control programme delivered about 11.5 LLINs and 7.3 million ITNs during 2006–2008 (7.7 million LLINs were delivered in 2007 and 2008), covering only 5% of the population at risk. The programme delivered about 8 million ACT treatment courses in 2006 and 12 million in 2008, far fewer (10%) than the estimated treatment needs. Funding for malaria control was reported to have increased from US$ 17 million in 2005 to over US$ 82 million in 2008, provided mainly by the Government, the Global Fund and the World Bank. This amount is unlikely to be sufficient to reach the national targets for prevention and cure.

I. EPIDEMIOLOGICAL PROFILE

Population, endemicity and malaria burden

Population (in thousands)	2008	%
All age groups	151 212	
< 5 years	25 020	17
≥ 5 years	126 193	83

Population by malaria endemicity (in thousands)	2008	%
High transmission ≥ 1/1000	151 212	100
Low transmission (0–1/1000)	0	0
Malaria-free (0 cases)	0	0
Rural population	78 089	52

Vector and parasite profiles

Major *Anopheles* species	*gambiae, arabiensis, funestus, brochieri, coustani, flavicosta, hancocki, hargreavesi, melas, moucheti, moucheti, nili, paludis, pharoensis*
Plasmodium species	*falciparum, vivax*

Stratification of burden (reported cases, per 1000)

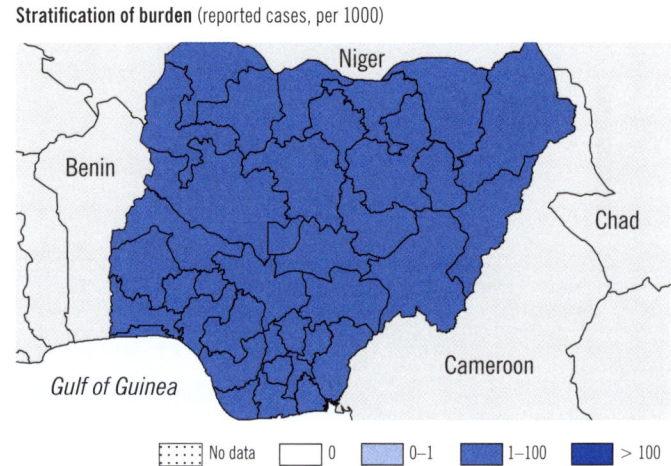

No data   0   0–1   1–100   > 100

Trends in malaria morbidity and mortality

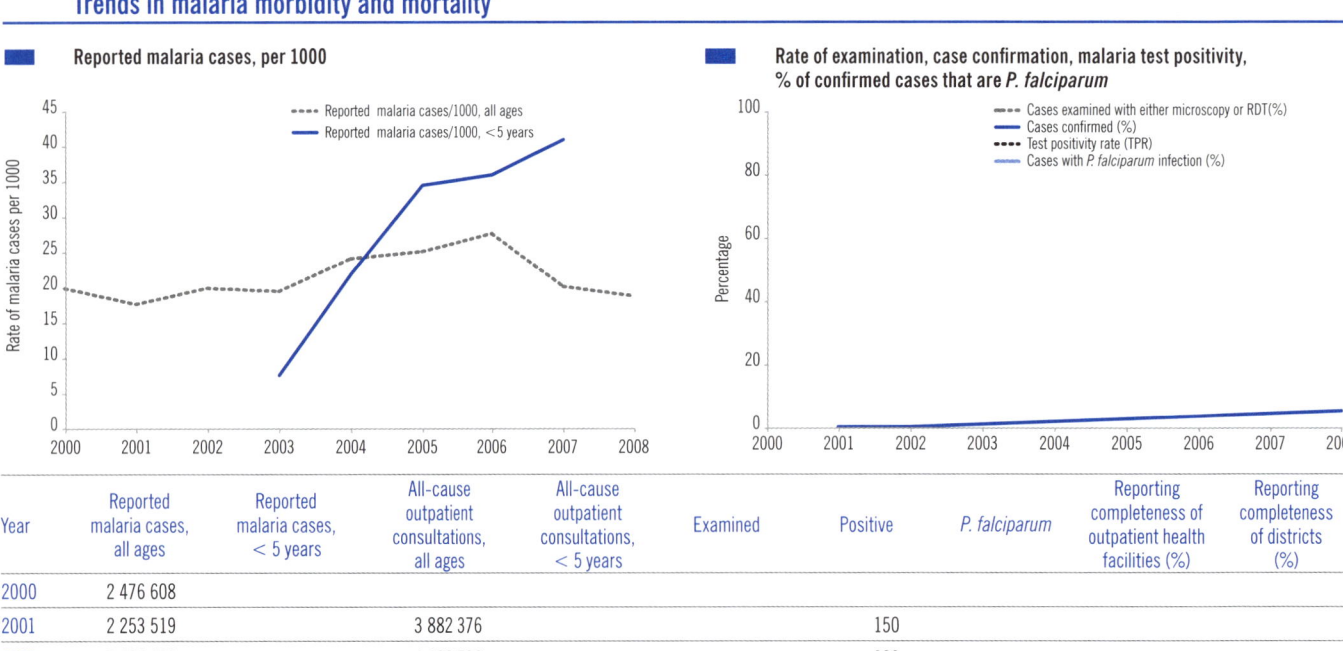

Reported malaria cases, per 1000
- Reported malaria cases/1000, all ages
- Reported malaria cases/1000, <5 years

Rate of examination, case confirmation, malaria test positivity, % of confirmed cases that are *P. falciparum*
- Cases examined with either microscopy or RDT(%)
- Cases confirmed (%)
- Test positivity rate (TPR)
- Cases with *P. falciparum* infection (%)

Year	Reported malaria cases, all ages	Reported malaria cases, < 5 years	All-cause outpatient consultations, all ages	All-cause outpatient consultations, < 5 years	Examined	Positive	*P. falciparum*	Reporting completeness of outpatient health facilities (%)	Reporting completeness of districts (%)
2000	2 476 608								
2001	2 253 519		3 882 376			150			
2002	2 605 381		4 488 796			380			
2003	2 608 479	171 812	4 237 566						
2004	3 310 229	507 173	4 970 109						
2005	3 532 108	814 274	5 302 576						
2006	3 982 372	865 374	5 633 088						
2007	2 969 950	1 004 392							
2008	2 834 174		6 305 973			143 079		92	

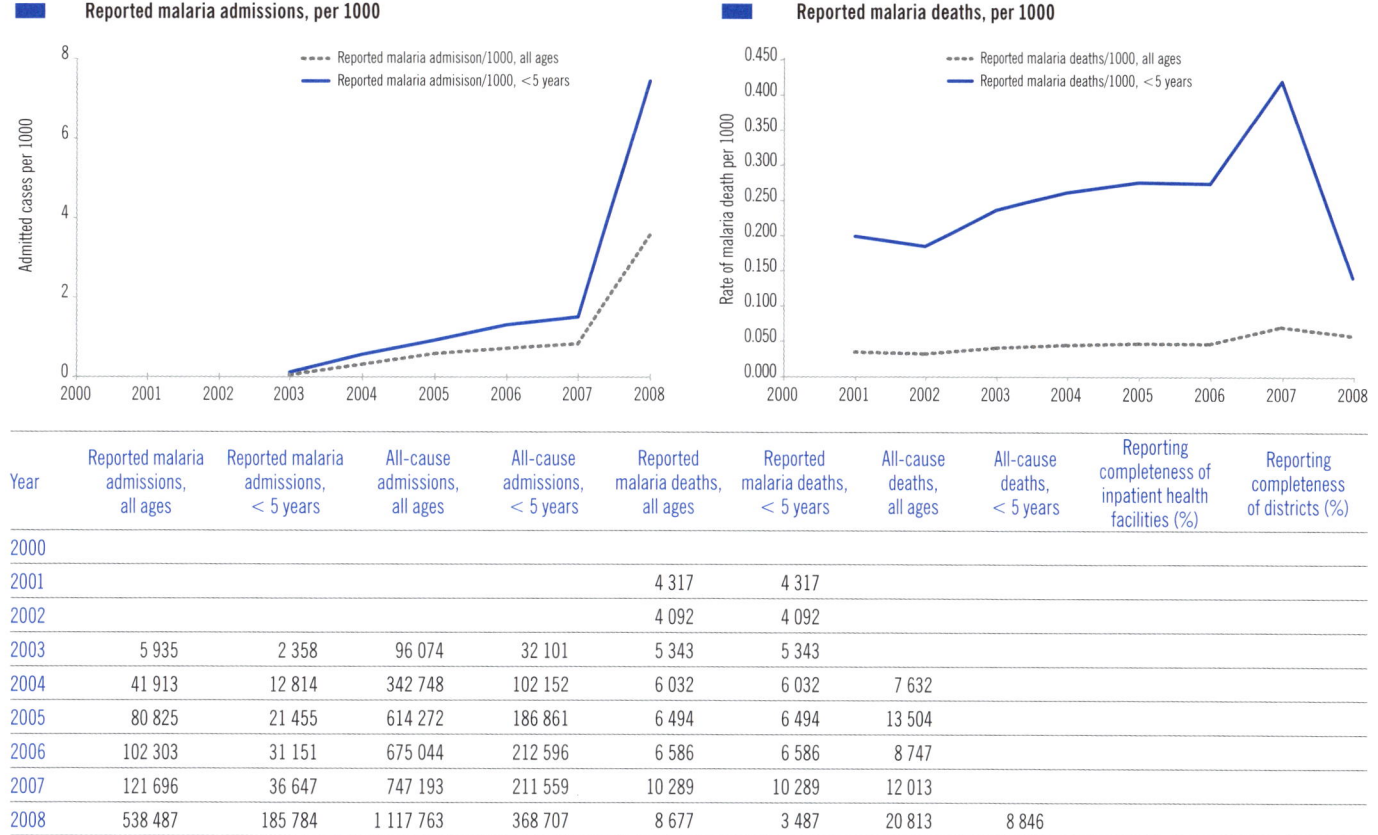

Reported malaria admissions, per 1000

- Reported malaria admission/1000, all ages
- Reported malaria admission/1000, <5 years

Reported malaria deaths, per 1000

- Reported malaria deaths/1000, all ages
- Reported malaria deaths/1000, <5 years

Year	Reported malaria admissions, all ages	Reported malaria admissions, < 5 years	All-cause admissions, all ages	All-cause admissions, < 5 years	Reported malaria deaths, all ages	Reported malaria deaths, < 5 years	All-cause deaths, all ages	All-cause deaths, < 5 years	Reporting completeness of inpatient health facilities (%)	Reporting completeness of districts (%)
2000										
2001					4 317	4 317				
2002					4 092	4 092				
2003	5 935	2 358	96 074	32 101	5 343	5 343				
2004	41 913	12 814	342 748	102 152	6 032	6 032	7 632			
2005	80 825	21 455	614 272	186 861	6 494	6 494	13 504			
2006	102 303	31 151	675 044	212 596	6 586	6 586	8 747			
2007	121 696	36 647	747 193	211 559	10 289	10 289	12 013			
2008	538 487	185 784	1 117 763	368 707	8 677	3 487	20 813	8 846		

II. INTERVENTION POLICIES AND STRATEGIES

Intervention	WHO-RECOMMENDED POLICIES / STRATEGIES	Yes or No	Year adopted	OPTIONAL POLICIES / STRATEGIES	Yes or No	Year adoped
Insecticide-treated nets (ITN)	Distribution of ITN/LLINs – Free	Yes	2001	Distribution – Antenatal care	Yes	2001
	Targeting all age groups	Yes	2009	Distribution – EPI routine and campaign	Yes	2006
				Targeting children < 5 years and pregnant women	Yes	2001
				ITN distribution is subsidized	Yes	2004
Indoor residual spraying (IRS)	IRS is a primary vector control intervention	No	–	Insecticide-resistance management implemented	No	–
	DDT is used for IRS (public health) only	No	–	Where IRS is conducted, other options are also implemented, e.g. ITN	Yes	2007
				IRS is used for prevention and control of epidemics	No	–
Intermittent preventive treatment (IPT)	IPT used to prevent malaria during pregnancy	Yes	2004			
Case management	Oral artemisinin monotherapies banned (prohibited from registration or removed from the system)	Yes	2006	Parasitological confirmation for patients ≥ 5 years only	No	–
	Parasitological confirmation for patients of all ages	Yes	2006	Malaria diagnosis is free of charge in the public sector	No	–
	ACT is free of charge for < 5 years old in the public sector	Yes	2006	ACT is free of charge for patients ≥ 5 years in the public sector	Yes	2009
	Diagnosis of malaria of inpatients is based on parasitological confirmation	Yes	1997	ACT is delivered at community level through community agents (beyond the health facilities)	Yes	–
	Pre-referral treatment with quinine or artemether IM or artesunate suppositories	Yes	2006	Uncomplicated malaria cases are admitted	No	–
	Oversight regulation of case management in the private sectors	Yes	1997			
	RDTs used at community level	No	–			

Antimalarial policy	Type of medicine	Year adopted	Study year	No. of studies	Median	Minimum	Maximum	Percentiles: 25%	75%
							Results of therapeutic efficacy tests		
First-line treatment of P. falciparum (unconfirmed)	AS+AQ, AL	2004							
First-line treatment of P. falciparum (confirmed)	AS+AQ, AL	2004							
Treatment failure of P. falciparum	QN(7d)	2004							
Treatment of severe malaria	QN(7d)	2004							
Treatment of P. vivax	–	–							

III. IMPLEMENTING MALARIA CONTROL

Coverage of ITN: survey data

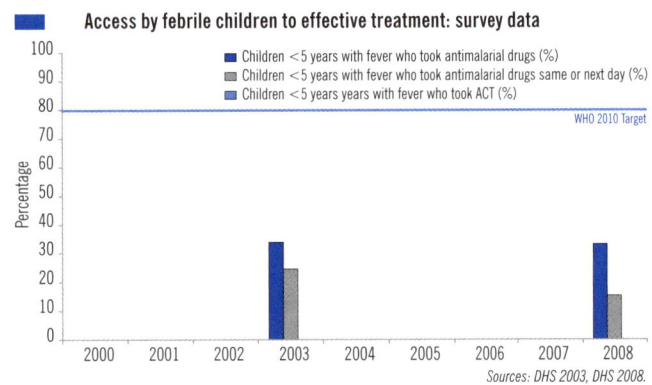

Households with at least one ITN (%)
Children <5 years who slept under an ITN (%)
Households with any net (%)

WHO 2010 Target

Sources: DHS 2003, DHS 2008.

Coverage of IRS and ITN: programme data

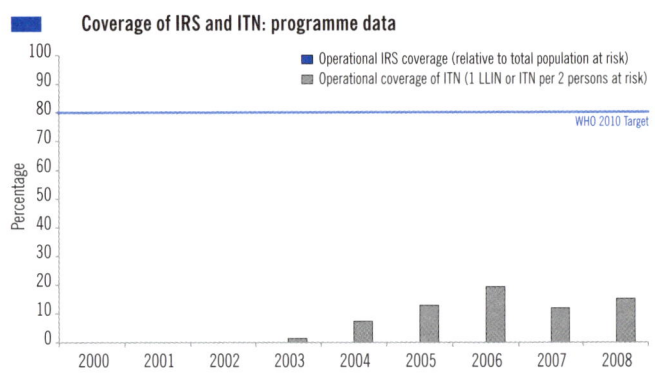

Operational IRS coverage (relative to total population at risk)
Operational coverage of ITN (1 LLIN or ITN per 2 persons at risk)

WHO 2010 Target

Access by febrile children to effective treatment: survey data

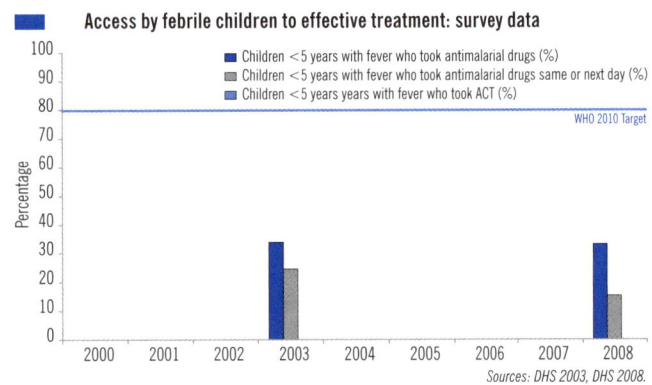

Children <5 years with fever who took antimalarial drugs (%)
Children <5 years with fever who took antimalarial drugs same or next day (%)
Children <5 years years with fever who took ACT (%)

WHO 2010 Target

Sources: DHS 2003, DHS 2008.

Access to effective treatment: programme data

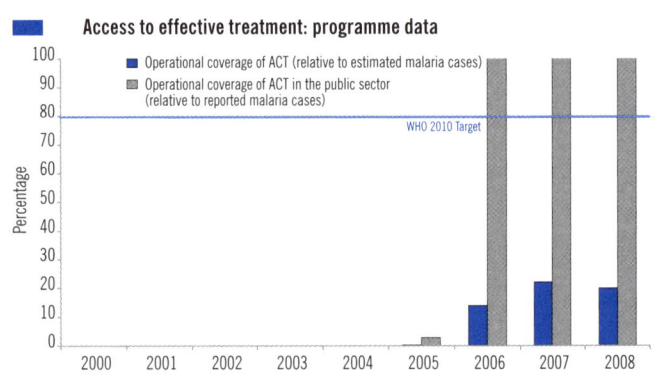

Operational coverage of ACT (relative to estimated malaria cases)
Operational coverage of ACT in the public sector (relative to reported malaria cases)

WHO 2010 Target

Year	Pregnant women who slept under any net (%)	Pregnant women who slept under an ITN (%)	Children < 5 years with fever (%)	Febrile children < 5 years who sought treatment in HF (%)	Number of households protected by IRS	Number of people protected by IRS	Number of ITNs and/or LLINs	Number of 1st-line treatment courses received	Number of ACT treatment courses received
2000									
2001							200 000	2 253 519	
2002							218 900	2 605 381	
2003	5	1	–	–			917 964	2 608 479	
2004							4 324 230	3 310 229	726
2005							5 086 934	3 532 108	100 000
2006					900	4 500	8 853 589	8 512 480	8 000 000
2007			–	–	600	3 000	3 225 594	13 019 950	13 000 000
2008			–	–			6 700 000	12 000 000	12 000 000

IV. FINANCING MALARIA CONTROL

Governmental and external financing

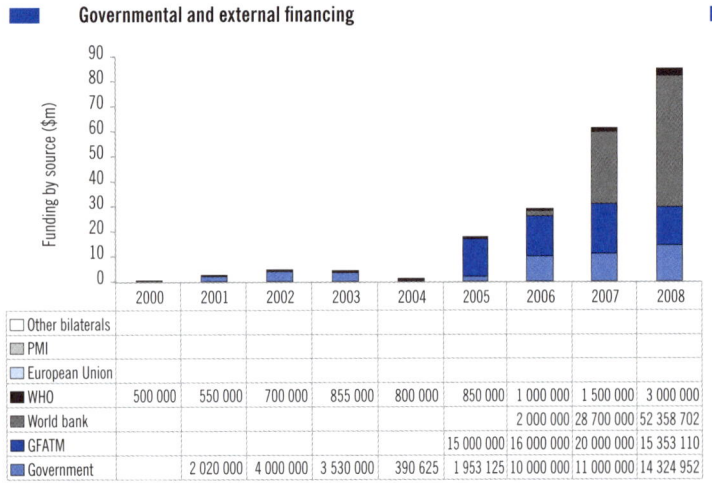

	2000	2001	2002	2003	2004	2005	2006	2007	2008
Other bilaterals									
PMI									
European Union									
WHO	500 000	550 000	700 000	855 000	800 000	850 000	1 000 000	1 500 000	3 000 000
World bank							2 000 000	28 700 000	52 358 702
GFATM						15 000 000	16 000 000	20 000 000	15 353 110
Government		2 020 000	4 000 000	3 530 000	390 625	1 953 125	10 000 000	11 000 000	14 324 952

Breakdown of expenditure by intervention in 2008

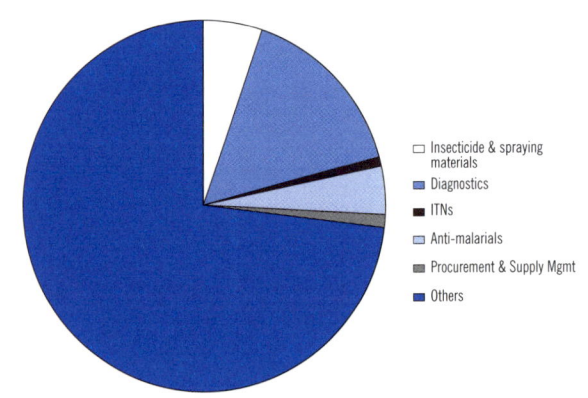

☐ Insecticide & spraying materials
■ Diagnostics
■ ITNs
▨ Anti-malarials
■ Procurement & Supply Mgmt
■ Others

V. SOURCE OF INFORMATION

PROGRAMME DATA		SURVEY AND OTHER DATA	
Reported cases	Surveillance data	Insecticide-treated nets (ITN)	DHS 2003, DHS 2008
Operational coverage of ITNs, IRS and access to medicines	Programme report	Treatment	DHS 2003, DHS 2008
Financial data	Programme report	Use of health services	DHS 2003

PAKISTAN

A total of 4.5 million suspected malaria cases were reported in 2008, comprising 6% of all outpatient attendances and 18% of admissions; only 59 284 confirmed cases were reported in 2008, 40% of which originated in Balochistan province. About 30% of the confirmed cases are due to *P. falciparum*. IRS has been used selectively, covering about 600 000 households and protecting 4.9 million people at risk in 2008. Between 2006 and 2008, the programme delivered 300 000 LLINs, far fewer than the number needed to protect the population at risk. Information about the provision of ACT in 2008 was not provided by the programme, although delivery of 6.8 million doses of antimalarial medicine was reported. With a decrease in the number of malaria cases in Punjab, the malaria programme is considering a pre-elimination project in that province. Government funding for malaria control has been approximately US$ 1 million annually since 2002, while Global Fund disbursements between 2003 and 2008 totalled US$ 12 million.

I. EPIDEMIOLOGICAL PROFILE

Population, endemicity and malaria burden

Population (in thousands)	2008	%
All age groups	176 952	
< 5 years	23 778	13
≥ 5 years	153 174	87

Population by malaria endemicity (in thousands)	2008	%
High transmission ≥ 1/1000	26 173	15
Low transmission (0–1/1000)	143 129	81
Malaria-free (0 cases)	7 649	4
Rural population	113 048	64

Vector and parasite profiles

Major *Anopheles* species	*culicifacies*
Plasmodium species	*falciparum, vivax*

Stratification of burden (reported cases, per 1000)

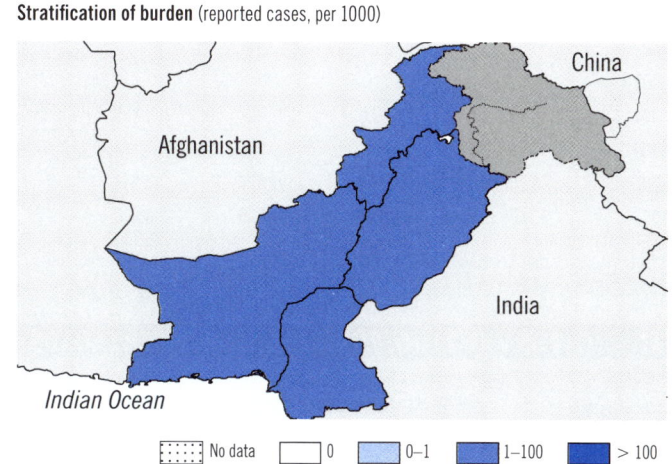

Trends in malaria morbidity and mortality

■ **Reported malaria cases, per 1000**

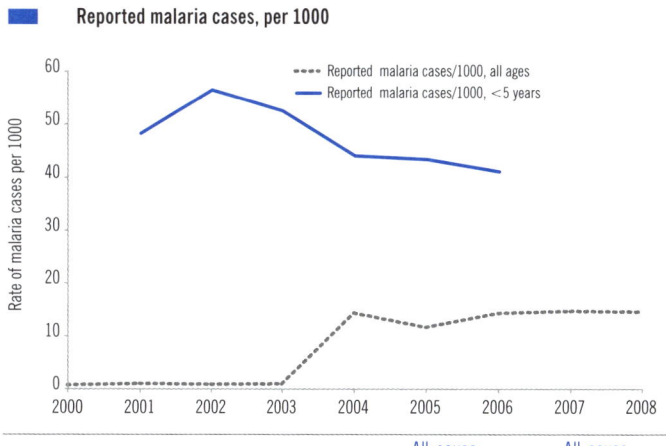

■ **Rate of examination, case confirmation, malaria test positivity, % of confirmed cases that are *P. falciparum***

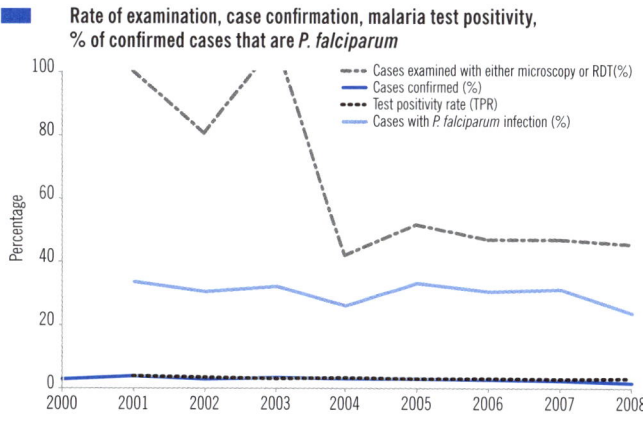

Year	Reported malaria cases, all ages	Reported malaria cases, < 5 years	All-cause outpatient consultations, all ages	All-cause outpatient consultations, < 5 years	Examined	Positive	*P. falciparum*	Reporting completeness of outpatient health facilities (%)	Reporting completeness of districts (%)
2000	82 526		55 762 741			82 526			
2001	125 292	1 048 071	62 367 045		3 572 425	125 292	41 771		
2002	107 666	1 240 606	70 175 717		3 399 524	107 666	32 591		
2003	125 152	1 167 377	70 444 716		4 577 037	125 152	39 944		
2004	2 304 920	990 248	67 360 844		1 574 181	101 640	32 761		
2005	1 914 607	988 624	73 067 297		1 918 977	97 049	42 056		
2006	2 404 055	948 337	74 045 571		2 011 538	100 956	37 837		
2007	2 523 696		75 466 786		2 123 007	92 971	39 856		
2008	2 558 998		76 890 457		2 054 533	59 284	24 550		

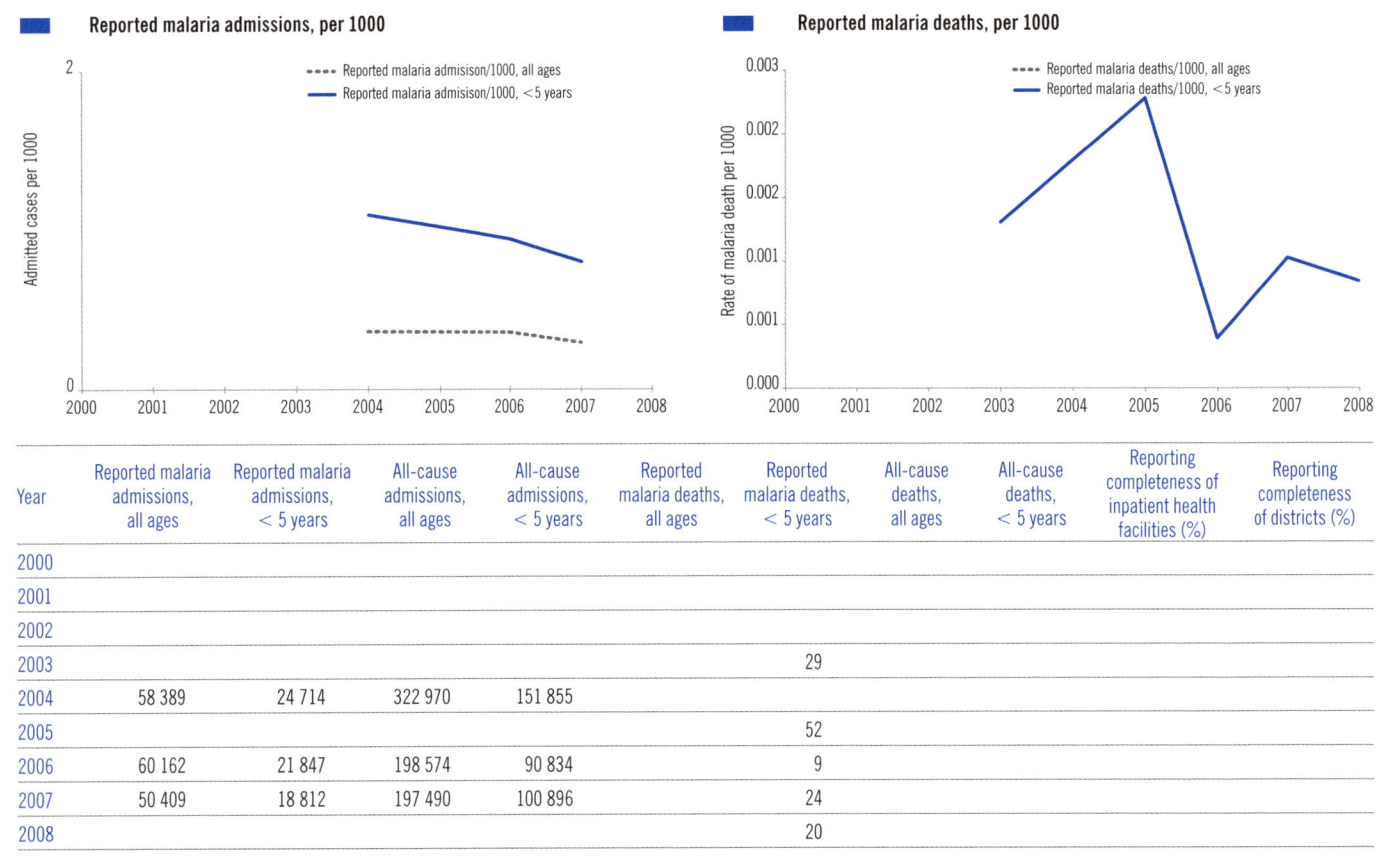

Reported malaria admissions, per 1000

- ···· Reported malaria admisison/1000, all ages
- —— Reported malaria admisison/1000, <5 years

Reported malaria deaths, per 1000

- ···· Reported malaria deaths/1000, all ages
- —— Reported malaria deaths/1000, <5 years

Year	Reported malaria admissions, all ages	Reported malaria admissions, < 5 years	All-cause admissions, all ages	All-cause admissions, < 5 years	Reported malaria deaths, all ages	Reported malaria deaths, < 5 years	All-cause deaths, all ages	All-cause deaths, < 5 years	Reporting completeness of inpatient health facilities (%)	Reporting completeness of districts (%)
2000										
2001										
2002										
2003					29					
2004	58 389	24 714	322 970	151 855						
2005					52					
2006	60 162	21 847	198 574	90 834	9					
2007	50 409	18 812	197 490	100 896	24					
2008					20					

II. INTERVENTION POLICIES AND STRATEGIES

Intervention	WHO-RECOMMENDED POLICIES / STRATEGIES	Yes or No	Year adopted	OPTIONAL POLICIES / STRATEGIES	Yes or No	Year adoped
Insecticide-treated nets (ITN)	Distribution of ITN/LLINs – Free	Yes	2008	Distribution – Antenatal care	Yes	2008
	Targeting all age groups	No	–	Distribution – EPI routine and campaign	No	–
				Targeting children < 5 years and pregnant women	Yes	2008
				ITN distribution is subsidized	No	–
Indoor residual spraying (IRS)	IRS is a primary vector control intervention	Yes	1998	Insecticide-resistance management implemented	Yes	2005
	DDT is used for IRS (public health) only	No	–	Where IRS is conducted, other options are also implemented, e.g. ITN	No	–
				IRS is used for prevention and control of epidemics	Yes	1998
Intermittent preventive treatment (IPT)	IPT used to prevent malaria during pregnancy	No	–			
Case management	Oral artemisinin monotherapies banned (prohibited from registration or removed from the system)	Yes	2007	Parasitological confirmation for patients ≥ 5 years only	No	–
	Parasitological confirmation for patients of all ages	Yes	2009	Malaria diagnosis is free of charge in the public sector	Yes	2000
	ACT is free of charge for < 5 years old in the public sector	Yes	2007	ACT is free of charge for patients ≥ 5 years in the public sector	Yes	2009
	Diagnosis of malaria of inpatients is based on parasitological confirmation	Yes	2000	ACT is delivered at community level through community agents (beyond the health facilities)	No	–
	Pre-referral treatment with quinine or artemether IM or artesunate suppositories	Yes	1998	Uncomplicated malaria cases are admitted	No	–
	Oversight regulation of case management in the private sectors	No	–			
	RDTs used at community level	No	–			

				Results of therapeutic efficacy tests						
Antimalarial policy	Type of medicine	Year adopted	Study year	No. of studies	Median	Minimum	Maximum	Percentiles:	25%	75%
First-line treatment of *P. falciparum* (unconfirmed)	AS+SP	–								
First-line treatment of *P. falciparum* (confirmed)	AS+SP	–								
Treatment failure of *P. falciparum*	QN	–								
Treatment of severe malaria	AM, QN	–								
Treatment of *P. vivax*	CQ+PQ(5d)	–								

III. IMPLEMENTING MALARIA CONTROL

Coverage of ITN: survey data

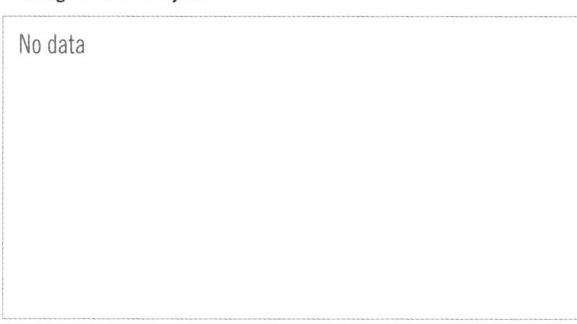

No data

Coverage of IRS and ITN: programme data

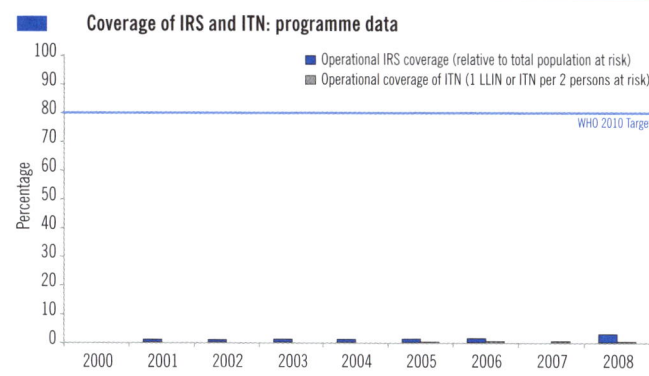

Access by febrile children to effective treatment: survey data

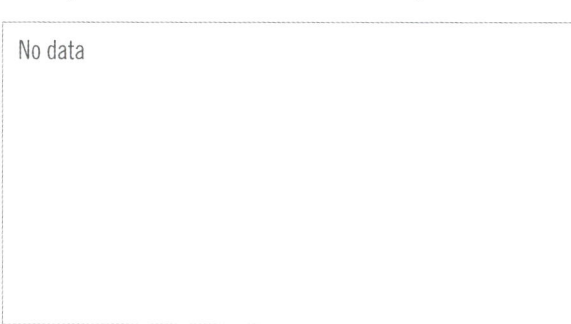

No data

Access to effective treatment: programme data

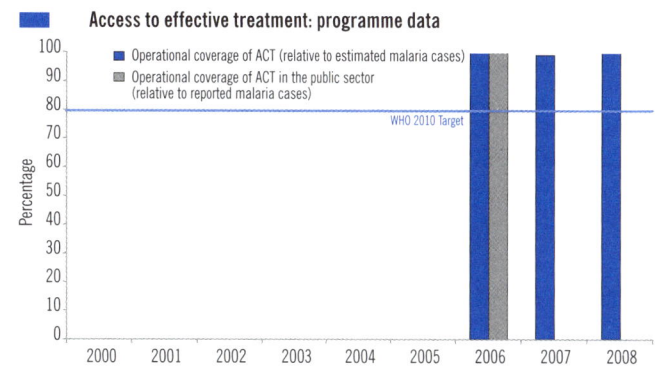

Year	Pregnant women who slept under any net (%)	Pregnant women who slept under an ITN (%)	Children < 5 years with fever (%)	Febrile children < 5 years who sought treatment in HF (%)	Number of households protected by IRS	Number of people protected by IRS	Number of ITNs and/or LLINs	Number of 1st-line treatment courses received	Number of ACT treatment courses received
2000									
2001					277 704	1 369 032			
2002					234 691	1 339 800	20 000		
2003					229 680	1 696 380			
2004					289 829	1 690 668	2 000		
2005					325 886	1 901 004	140 000		
2006					319 920	2 291 520	240 000	8 097 000	39 856
2007							90 000	4 513 876	
2008					602 314	4 938 975	41 400	6 762 058	

IV. FINANCING MALARIA CONTROL

Governmental and external financing

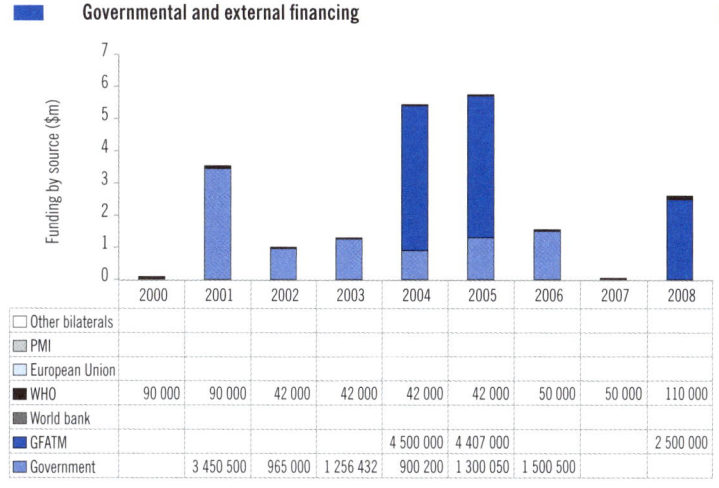

Breakdown of expenditure by intervention in 2008

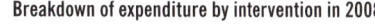
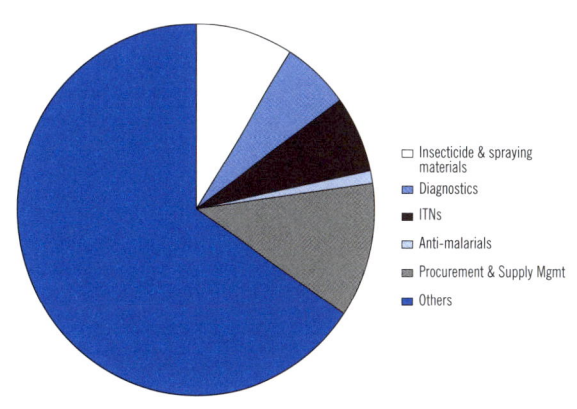

V. SOURCE OF INFORMATION

PROGRAMME DATA		SURVEY AND OTHER DATA	
Reported cases	Surveillance data	Insecticide-treated nets (ITN)	No surveys
Operational coverage of ITNs, IRS and access to medicines	Programme report	Treatment	No surveys
Financial data	Programme report	Use of health services	DHS 1990

PAPUA NEW GUINEA

Malaria is highly endemic and comparatively stable in coastal areas; it is less stable in the highlands, which are prone to epidemics with many fatalities. Between 70% and 80% of infections are due to *P. falciparum*. Malaria is among the leading causes of hospital admissions and among the most important causes of death in children. There was no evidence of a systematic decrease in the numbers of cases of suspected malaria, severe cases and deaths during the period 2001–2008. About 15% of suspected cases attending health centres and hospitals are confirmed parasitologically. IRS is implemented in limited areas in the highlands, protecting just 25 000 people at risk in 2007. The programme delivered about 1 million LLINs between 2006 and 2008. The 2006 demographic and health survey estimated that 33% of households owned at least one ITN, while 17% of children under 5 and 17% of pregnant women had slept under an ITN the previous night. The use of ACTs for treatment of *P. falciparum* malaria has been adopted as policy but is not yet implemented. Before 2003, investment in malaria control was limited, but the funds disbursed by the Global Fund exceeded US$ 15 million between 2003 and 2008, and Papua New Guinea was successful in obtaining US$ 147 million from the Global Fund in round 8 to cover the period 2009–2014, the highest award outside Africa, corresponding to more than US$ 25 per person at risk for malaria.

I.   EPIDEMIOLOGICAL PROFILE

Population, endemicity and malaria burden

Population (in thousands)	2008	%
All age groups	6 577	
< 5 years	950	14
≥ 5 years	5 626	86

Population by malaria endemicity (in thousands)	2008	%
High transmission ≥ 1/1000	6 182	94
Low transmission (0–1/1000)	395	6
Malaria-free (0 cases)	0	0
Rural population	5 756	88

Vector and parasite profiles

Major *Anopheles* species	*farauti, farauti4, hinesorum koliensis, punctulatus*
Plasmodium species	*falciparum, vivax*

Stratification of burden (reported cases, per 1000)

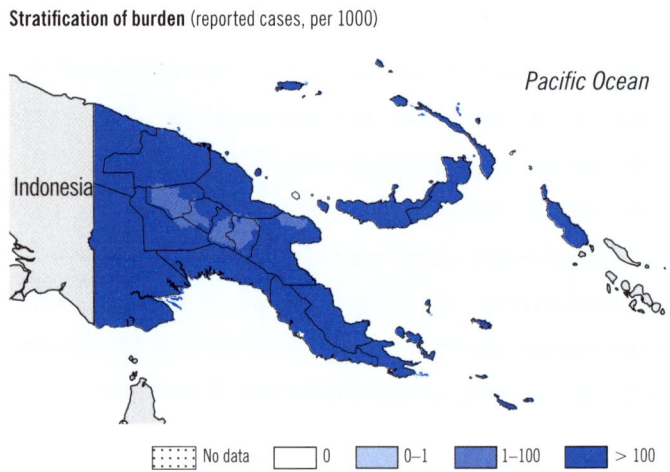

Trends in malaria morbidity and mortality

Reported malaria cases, per 1000

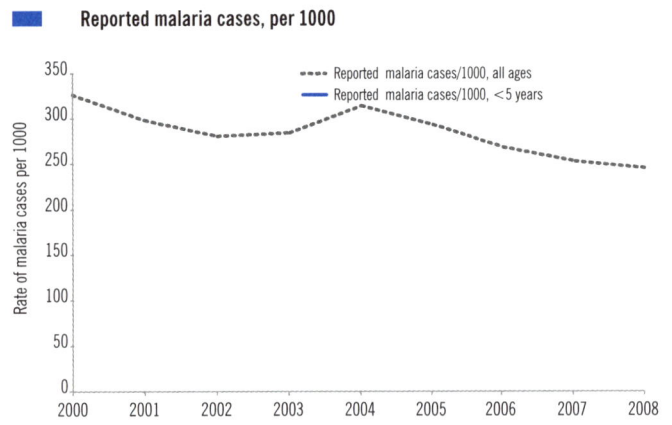

Rate of examination, case confirmation, malaria test positivity, % of confirmed cases that are *P. falciparum*

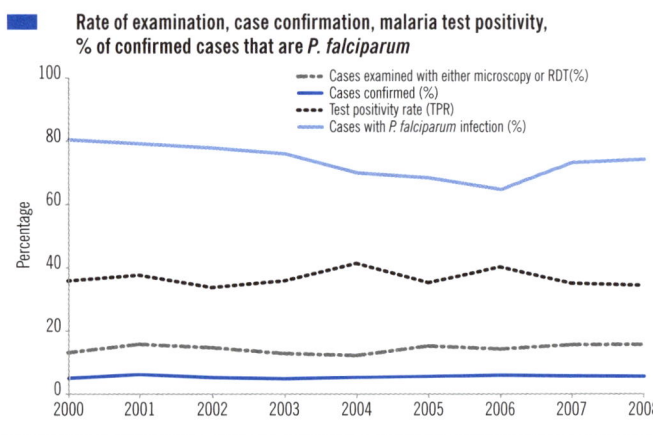

Year	Reported malaria cases, all ages	Reported malaria cases, < 5 years	All-cause outpatient consultations, all ages	All-cause outpatient consultations, < 5 years	Examined	Positive	P. falciparum	Reporting completeness of outpatient health facilities (%)	Reporting completeness of districts (%)
2000	1 751 883		5 466 222		225 535	79 839	63 591	87	
2001	1 643 075		5 592 434		254 266	94 484	74 117	88	
2002	1 587 580		5 351 135		228 665	75 748	58 403	89	
2003	1 650 662		5 448 841		207 901	72 620	54 653	89	
2004	1 868 413		5 855 904		222 904	91 055	63 053	88	
2005	1 788 318		5 659 581		267 123	92 957	62 926	90	
2006	1 676 681		5 469 413		234 220	93 938	56 917	90	
2007	1 618 699		5 543 155		247 465	86 912	60 129	90	
2008	1 606 843		8 838 540		246 641	84 452	60 000	89	

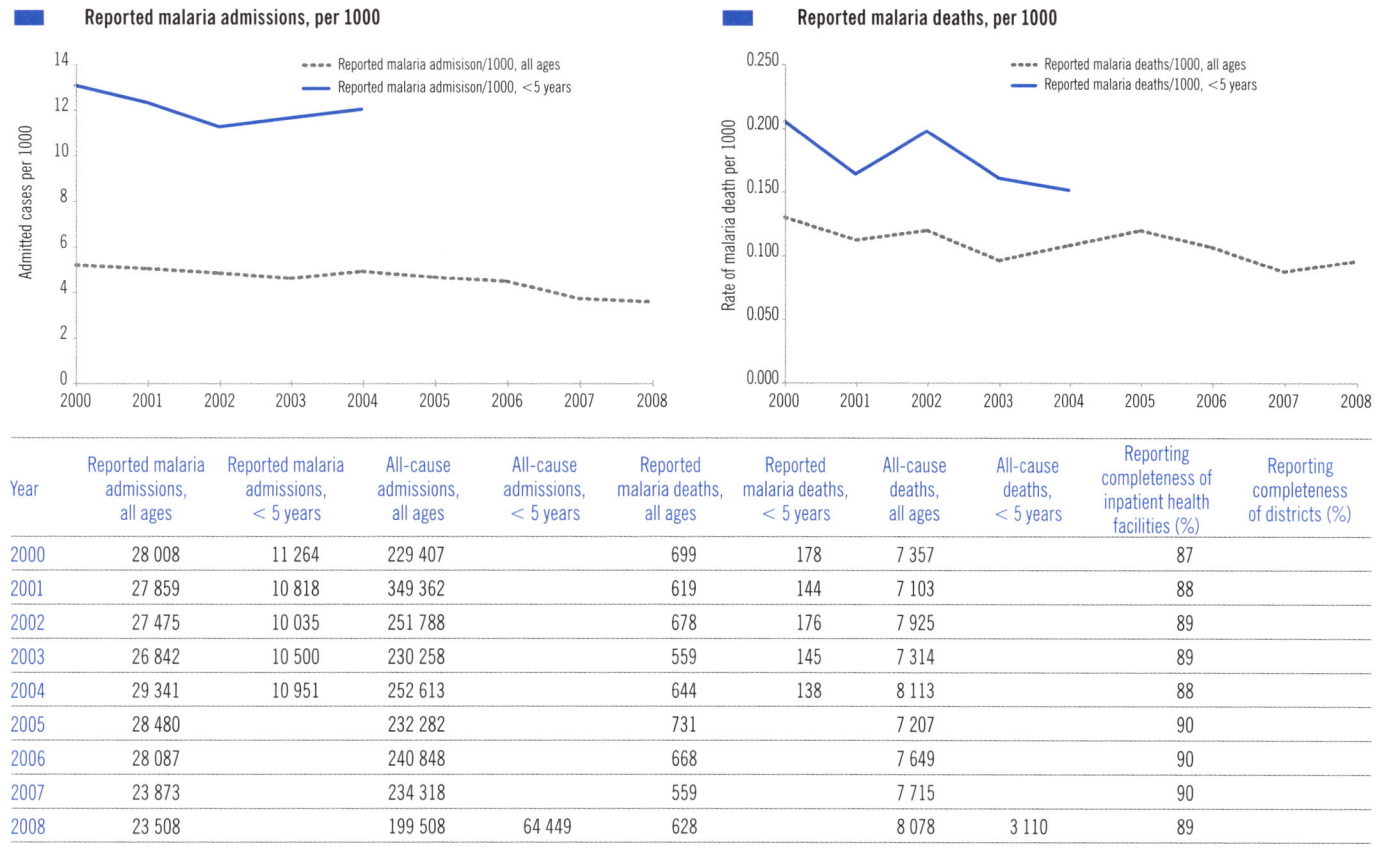

Reported malaria admissions, per 1000

- ---- Reported malaria admission/1000, all ages
- —— Reported malaria admission/1000, <5 years

Admitted cases per 1000 (y-axis: 0–14)
(x-axis: 2000–2008)

Reported malaria deaths, per 1000

- ---- Reported malaria deaths/1000, all ages
- —— Reported malaria deaths/1000, <5 years

Rate of malaria death per 1000 (y-axis: 0.000–0.250)
(x-axis: 2000–2008)

Year	Reported malaria admissions, all ages	Reported malaria admissions, < 5 years	All-cause admissions, all ages	All-cause admissions, < 5 years	Reported malaria deaths, all ages	Reported malaria deaths, < 5 years	All-cause deaths, all ages	All-cause deaths, < 5 years	Reporting completeness of inpatient health facilities (%)	Reporting completeness of districts (%)
2000	28 008	11 264	229 407		699	178	7 357		87	
2001	27 859	10 818	349 362		619	144	7 103		88	
2002	27 475	10 035	251 788		678	176	7 925		89	
2003	26 842	10 500	230 258		559	145	7 314		89	
2004	29 341	10 951	252 613		644	138	8 113		88	
2005	28 480		232 282		731		7 207		90	
2006	28 087		240 848		668		7 649		90	
2007	23 873		234 318		559		7 715		90	
2008	23 508		199 508	64 449	628		8 078	3 110	89	

II. INTERVENTION POLICIES AND STRATEGIES

Intervention	WHO-RECOMMENDED POLICIES / STRATEGIES	Yes or No	Year adopted	OPTIONAL POLICIES / STRATEGIES	Yes or No	Year adoped
Insecticide-treated nets (ITN)	Distribution of ITN/LLINs — Free	Yes	2004	Distribution — Antenatal care	No	–
	Targeting all age groups	Yes	2000	Distribution — EPI routine and campaign	No	–
				Targeting children < 5 years and pregnant women	No	–
				ITN distribution is subsidized	Yes	2004
Indoor residual spraying (IRS)	IRS is a primary vector control intervention	Yes	2000	Insecticide-resistance management implemented	No	–
	DDT is used for IRS (public health) only	Yes	2000	Where IRS is conducted, other options are also implemented, e.g. ITN	Yes	2000
				IRS is used for prevention and control of epidemics	Yes	2000
Intermittent preventive treatment (IPT)	IPT used to prevent malaria during pregnancy	Yes	2009			
Case management	Oral artemisinin monotherapies banned (prohibited from registration or removed from the system)	Yes	2000	Parasitological confirmation for patients ≥ 5 years only	No	–
	Parasitological confirmation for patients of all ages	No	–	Malaria diagnosis is free of charge in the public sector	Yes	2004
	ACT is free of charge for < 5 years old in the public sector	Yes	2004	ACT is free of charge for patients ≥ 5 years in the public sector	Yes	2004
	Diagnosis of malaria of inpatients is based on parasitological confirmation	Yes	2000	ACT is delivered at community level through community agents (beyond the health facilities)	No	–
	Pre-referral treatment with quinine or artemether IM or artesunate suppositories	Yes	2000	Uncomplicated malaria cases are admitted	No	–
	Oversight regulation of case management in the private sectors	No	–			
	RDTs used at community level	No	–			

				Results of therapeutic efficacy tests					
Antimalarial policy	Type of medicine	Year adopted	Study year	No. of studies	Median	Minimum	Maximum	Percentiles: 25%	75%
First-line treatment of *P. falciparum* (unconfirmed)	AL	2008							
First-line treatment of *P. falciparum* (confirmed)	AL	2008							
Treatment failure of *P. falciparum*	QN(7d)	2008							
Treatment of severe malaria	AM, AS	2008							
Treatment of *P. vivax*	CQ+PQ(14d)	2008							

III. IMPLEMENTING MALARIA CONTROL

Coverage of ITN: survey data

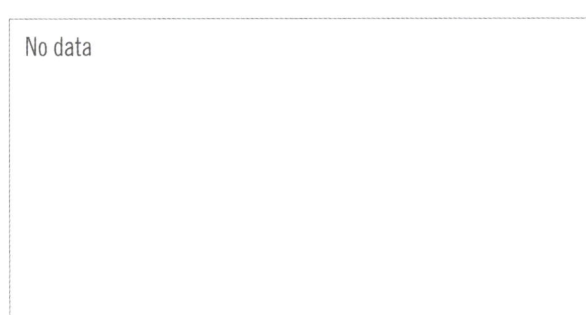

- Households with at least one ITN (%)
- Households with any net (%)
- Children <5 years who slept under an ITN (%)
- Children <5 years who slept under any net (%)

Sources: DHS 2008.

Coverage of IRS and ITN: programme data

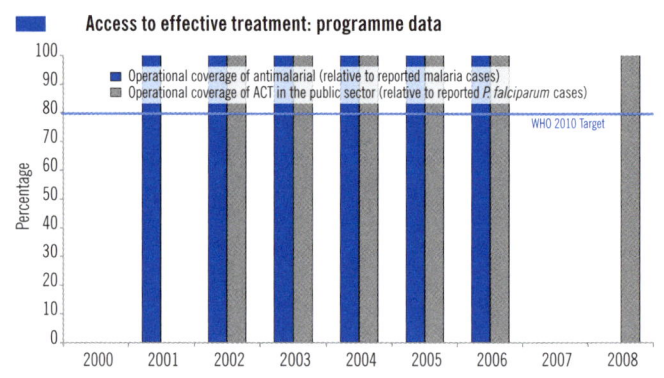

- Operational IRS coverage (relative to total population at risk)
- Operational coverage of ITN (1 LLIN or ITN per 2 persons at risk)

Access by febrile children to effective treatment: survey data

No data

Access to effective treatment: programme data

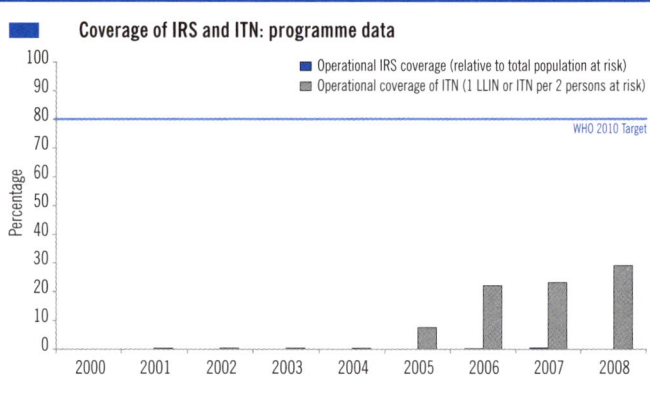

- Operational coverage of antimalarial (relative to reported malaria cases)
- Operational coverage of ACT in the public sector (relative to reported *P. falciparum* cases)

Year	Pregnant women who slept under any net (%)	Pregnant women who slept under an ITN (%)	Children < 5 years with fever (%)	Febrile children < 5 years who sought treatment in HF (%)	Number of households protected by IRS	Number of people protected by IRS	Number of ITNs and/or LLINs	Number of 1st-line treatment courses received	Number of ACT treatment courses received
2000									
2001							6 606	3 719 444	
2002							8 708	9 407 778	89 545
2003							9 154	1 729 167	62 620
2004							8 418	7 958 122	362 071
2005							228 421	3 896 627	321 296
2006	17		–	–	2 000	10 000	461 231	4 822 368	395 185
2007						24 699	53 500		
2008							438 441		110 000

IV. FINANCING MALARIA CONTROL

Governmental and external financing

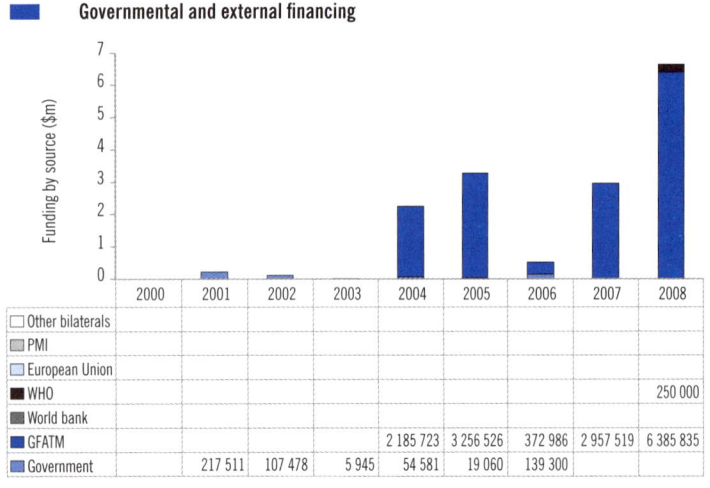

	2000	2001	2002	2003	2004	2005	2006	2007	2008
Other bilaterals									
PMI									
European Union									
WHO									250 000
World bank									
GFATM					2 185 723	3 256 526	372 986	2 957 519	6 385 835
Government		217 511	107 478	5 945	54 581	19 060	139 300		

Breakdown of expenditure by intervention in 2008

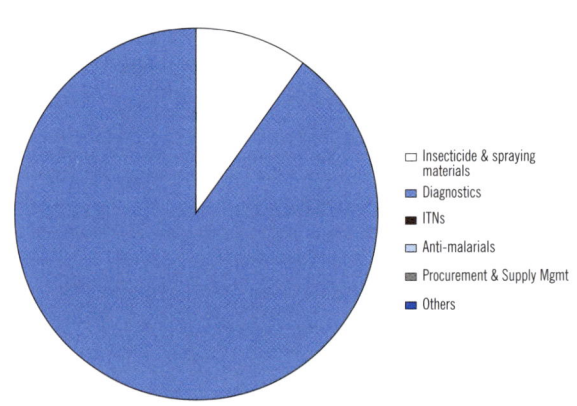

- Insecticide & spraying materials
- Diagnostics
- ITNs
- Anti-malarials
- Procurement & Supply Mgmt
- Others

V. SOURCE OF INFORMATION

PROGRAMME DATA		SURVEY AND OTHER DATA	
Reported cases	Surveillance data	Insecticide-treated nets (ITN)	No surveys
Operational coverage of ITNs, IRS and access to medicines	Programme report	Treatment	No surveys
Financial data	Programme report	Use of health services	DHS 1996

SENEGAL

Malaria is endemic throughout the country, and transmission occurs seasonally from June to November. Almost all cases are *P. falciparum*, and, with the introduction of RDTs in 2007, nearly 72% of the suspected cases were parasitologically tested. As a result, the trend in the number of malaria cases decreased from an average of 1.2 million during 2000–2006 to 701 460 cases in 2008 (42% decrease). The numbers of malaria inpatient cases and deaths in children under 5 years decreased by 59% (from 9147 to 3881) and 47% (from 581 to 306), respectively, during the same period. While these decreases must be interpreted with caution (with 94% completeness of reporting in districts in 2008), the recent scale-up of interventions appears to have had a significant impact. The national malaria control programme delivered 340 000 LLINs in 2006 and 1.6 million in 2008 (half of which were distributed during a mass campaign). Over 233 000 households were sprayed in 2008, protecting nearly 635 000 people at risk (5%). In the 2008 malaria indicator survey, 63% of households had an ITN, 46% of children under 5 had slept under an ITN the previous night and 4.6% of febrile children received an ACT. The programme delivered about 990 000 treatment courses of ACT in 2007 and 320 000 in 2008, adequate to treat roughly half the reported cases in the public sector. There is some evidence, from routine surveillance that the numbers of malaria inpatient cases and deaths are falling; however, this report should be interpreted with caution, because of possible effects of the introduction of diagnostics and a probable change in case definition. While funding has increased (from the Government, the Global Fund, the United States President's Malaria Initiative and other agencies), the national malaria control programme reported that US$ 23 million were spent on malaria during 2005–2008.

I. EPIDEMIOLOGICAL PROFILE

Population, endemicity and malaria burden

Population (in thousands)	2008	%
All age groups	12 211	
< 5 years	2 046	17
≥ 5 years	10 165	83

Population by malaria endemicity (in thousands)	2008	%
High transmission ≥ 1/1000	11 703	96
Low transmission (0–1/1000)	509	4
Malaria-free (0 cases)	0	0
Rural population	7 046	58

Vector and parasite profiles

Major *Anopheles* species	*gambiae, arabiensis, funestus, brochieri, coustani, flavicosta, hancocki, melas, nili, pharoensis*
Plasmodium species	*falciparum, vivax*

Stratification of burden (reported cases, per 1000)

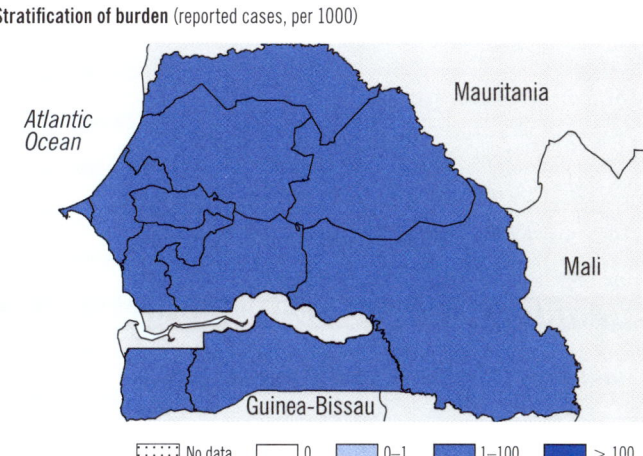

No data — 0 — 0–1 — 1–100 — > 100

Trends in malaria morbidity and mortality

Reported malaria cases, per 1000

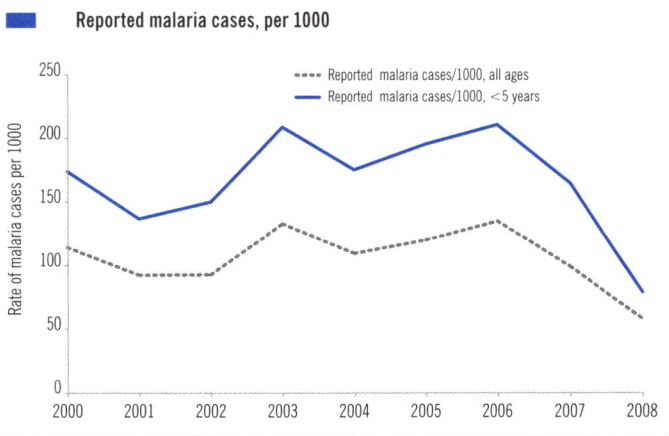

- Reported malaria cases/1000, all ages
- Reported malaria cases/1000, <5 years

Rate of examination, case confirmation, malaria test positivity, % of confirmed cases that are *P. falciparum*

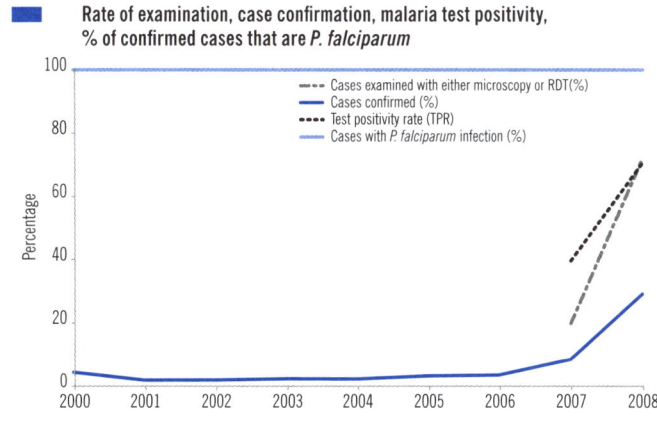

- Cases examined with either microscopy or RDT(%)
- Cases confirmed (%)
- Test positivity rate (TPR)
- Cases with *P. falciparum* infection (%)

Year	Reported malaria cases, all ages	Reported malaria cases, < 5 years	All-cause outpatient consultations, all ages	All-cause outpatient consultations, < 5 years	Examined	Positive	P. falciparum	Reporting completeness of outpatient health facilities (%)	Reporting completeness of districts (%)
2000	1 123 377	299 210	3 463 849	1 096 685		44 959	44 959	84	
2001	931 682	239 508	2 608 245	712 816		14 261	14 261	72	
2002	960 478	267 341	2 878 312	813 345		15 261	15 261	75	
2003	1 414 383	379 339	3 671 650	968 408		28 272	28 272	85	
2004	1 195 402	324 620	3 744 390	985 149		23 171	23 171	87	
2005	1 346 158	370 061	4 064 305	1 059 420		38 746	38 746	95	
2006	1 555 310	408 588	4 632 716	1 191 498		49 366	49 366	97	
2007	1 170 234	327 867	5 260 160	1 380 054	230 186	95 169	95 169	98	
2008	701 460	160 657	4 909 307	1 214 122	505 045	202 466	202 466	94	

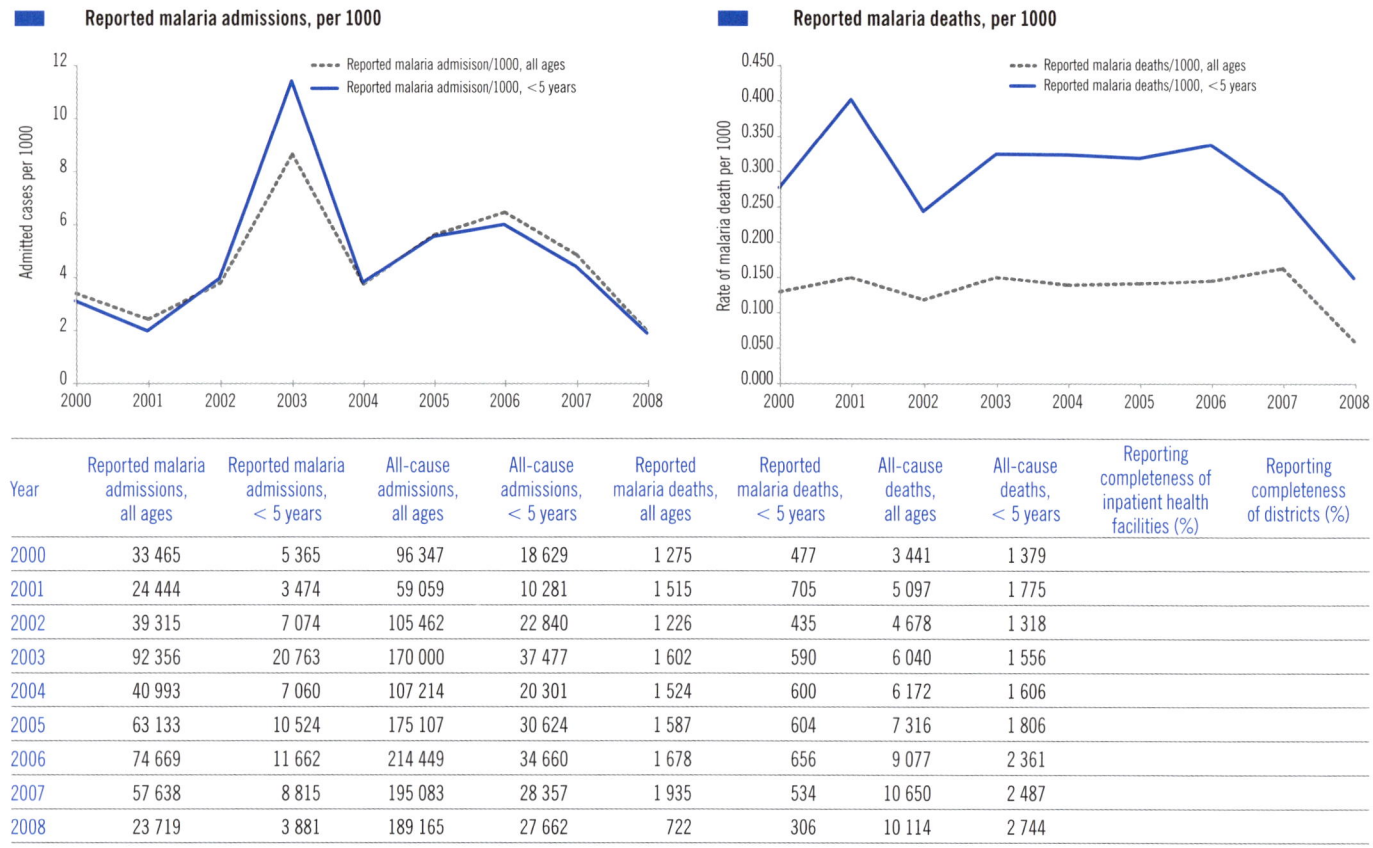

Reported malaria admissions, per 1000

Legend: Reported malaria admission/1000, all ages; Reported malaria admission/1000, <5 years

Reported malaria deaths, per 1000

Legend: Reported malaria deaths/1000, all ages; Reported malaria deaths/1000, <5 years

Year	Reported malaria admissions, all ages	Reported malaria admissions, < 5 years	All-cause admissions, all ages	All-cause admissions, < 5 years	Reported malaria deaths, all ages	Reported malaria deaths, < 5 years	All-cause deaths, all ages	All-cause deaths, < 5 years	Reporting completeness of inpatient health facilities (%)	Reporting completeness of districts (%)
2000	33 465	5 365	96 347	18 629	1 275	477	3 441	1 379		
2001	24 444	3 474	59 059	10 281	1 515	705	5 097	1 775		
2002	39 315	7 074	105 462	22 840	1 226	435	4 678	1 318		
2003	92 356	20 763	170 000	37 477	1 602	590	6 040	1 556		
2004	40 993	7 060	107 214	20 301	1 524	600	6 172	1 606		
2005	63 133	10 524	175 107	30 624	1 587	604	7 316	1 806		
2006	74 669	11 662	214 449	34 660	1 678	656	9 077	2 361		
2007	57 638	8 815	195 083	28 357	1 935	534	10 650	2 487		
2008	23 719	3 881	189 165	27 662	722	306	10 114	2 744		

II. INTERVENTION POLICIES AND STRATEGIES

Intervention	WHO-RECOMMENDED POLICIES / STRATEGIES	Yes or No	Year adopted	OPTIONAL POLICIES / STRATEGIES	Yes or No	Year adoped
Insecticide-treated nets (ITN)	Distribution of ITN/LLINs – Free	Yes	1998	Distribution – Antenatal care	Yes	2005
	Targeting all age groups	Yes	1998	Distribution – EPI routine and campaign	Yes	–
				Targeting children < 5 years and pregnant women	Yes	1998
				ITN distribution is subsidized	Yes	2000
Indoor residual spraying (IRS)	IRS is a primary vector control intervention	Yes	2007	Insecticide-resistance management implemented	Yes	2000
	DDT is used for IRS (public health) only	No	–	Where IRS is conducted, other options are also implemented, e.g. ITN	Yes	2007
				IRS is used for prevention and control of epidemics	No	–
Intermittent preventive treatment (IPT)	IPT used to prevent malaria during pregnancy	Yes	2004			
Case management	Oral artemisinin monotherapies banned (prohibited from registration or removed from the system)	No	–	Parasitological confirmation for patients ≥ 5 years only	No	–
	Parasitological confirmation for patients of all ages	Yes	2007	Malaria diagnosis is free of charge in the public sector	Yes	2007
	ACT is free of charge for < 5 years old in the public sector	No	–	ACT is free of charge for patients ≥ 5 years in the public sector	No	–
	Diagnosis of malaria of inpatients is based on parasitological confirmation	Yes	2007	ACT is delivered at community level through community agents (beyond the health facilities)	Yes	2007
	Pre-referral treatment with quinine or artemether IM or artesunate suppositories	Yes	2005	Uncomplicated malaria cases are admitted	No	–
	Oversight regulation of case management in the private sectors	No	–			
	RDTs used at community level	Yes	2008			

Antimalarial policy	Type of medicine	Year adopted	Study year	Results of therapeutic efficacy tests					
				No. of studies	Median	Minimum	Maximum	Percentiles: 25%	75%
First-line treatment of *P. falciparum* (unconfirmed)	AS + AQ	2005							
First-line treatment of *P. falciparum* (confirmed)	AL, AS + AQ	2005							
Treatment failure of *P. falciparum*	–	–							
Treatment of severe malaria	QN(7d)	2005							
Treatment of *P. vivax*	–	–							

III. IMPLEMENTING MALARIA CONTROL

Coverage of ITN: survey data

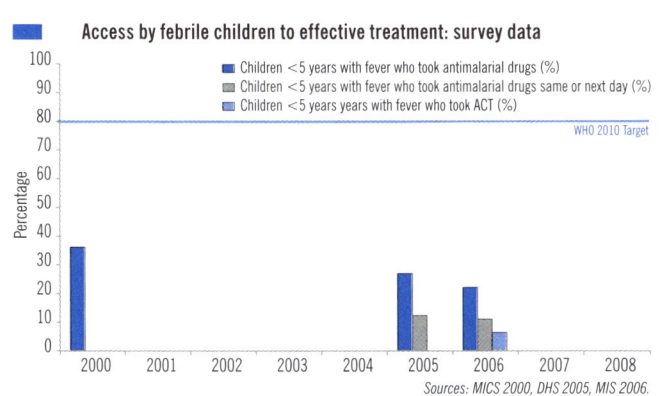

Legend:
- Households with at least one ITN (%)
- Children <5 years who slept under an ITN (%)
- Households with any net (%)

WHO 2010 Target

Sources: MICS 2000, DHS 2005, MIS 2006, MIS 2008.

Coverage of IRS and ITN: programme data

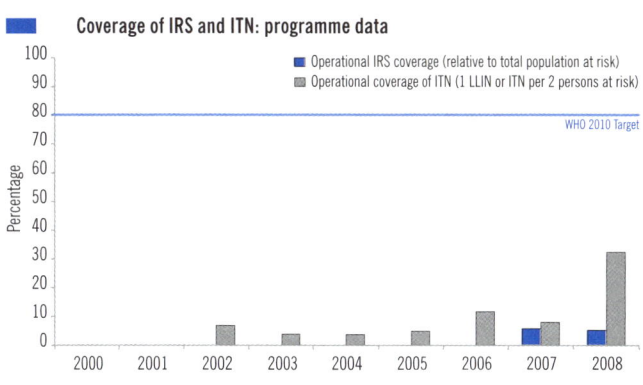

Legend:
- Operational IRS coverage (relative to total population at risk)
- Operational coverage of ITN (1 LLIN or ITN per 2 persons at risk)

WHO 2010 Target

Access by febrile children to effective treatment: survey data

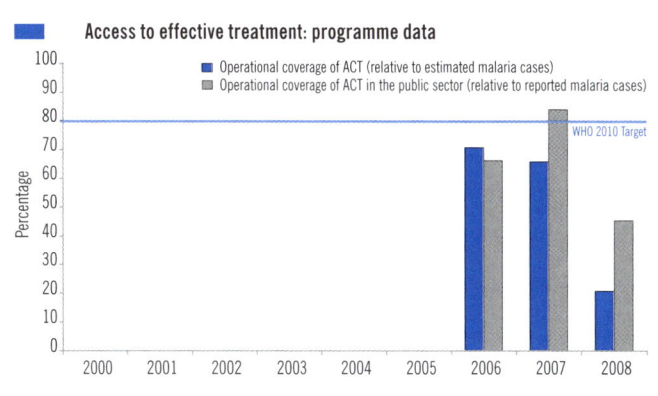

Legend:
- Children <5 years with fever who took antimalarial drugs (%)
- Children <5 years with fever who took antimalarial drugs same or next day (%)
- Children <5 years years with fever who took ACT (%)

WHO 2010 Target

Sources: MICS 2000, DHS 2005, MIS 2006.

Access to effective treatment: programme data

Legend:
- Operational coverage of ACT (relative to estimated malaria cases)
- Operational coverage of ACT in the public sector (relative to reported malaria cases)

WHO 2010 Target

Year	Pregnant women who slept under any net (%)	Pregnant women who slept under an ITN (%)	Children < 5 years with fever (%)	Febrile children < 5 years who sought treatment in HF (%)	Number of households protected by IRS	Number of people protected by IRS	Number of ITNs and/or LLINs	Number of 1st-line treatment courses received	Number of ACT treatment courses received
2000			–	–					
2001								931 682	
2002							350 000	960 478	
2003							125 409	1 414 383	
2004							223 731	1 195 402	
2005	14	9	–	–			402 706	1 346 158	
2006		17	–	–			342 328	1 555 310	1 036 872
2007						678 971		990 141	990 141
2008			–	–		635 666	1 572 261	320 335	320 335

IV. FINANCING MALARIA CONTROL

Governmental and external financing

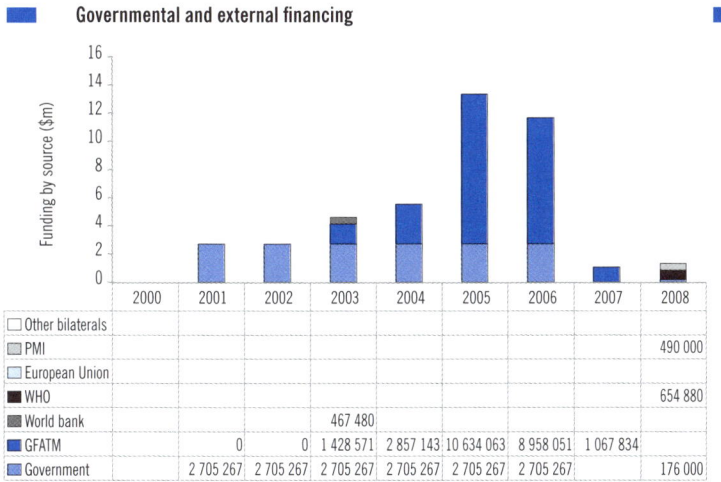

	2000	2001	2002	2003	2004	2005	2006	2007	2008
Other bilaterals									
PMI									490 000
European Union									
WHO									654 880
World bank				467 480					
GFATM		0	0	1 428 571	2 857 143	10 634 063	8 958 051	1 067 834	
Government		2 705 267	2 705 267	2 705 267	2 705 267	2 705 267	2 705 267		176 000

Breakdown of expenditure by intervention in 2008

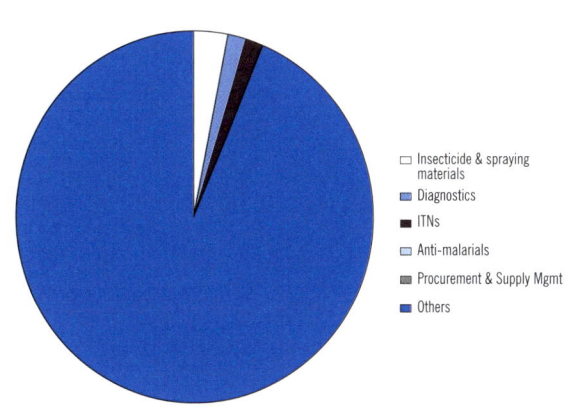

Legend:
- Insecticide & spraying materials
- Diagnostics
- ITNs
- Anti-malarials
- Procurement & Supply Mgmt
- Others

V. SOURCE OF INFORMATION

PROGRAMME DATA		SURVEY AND OTHER DATA	
Reported cases	Surveillance data	Insecticide-treated nets (ITN)	MICS 2000, DHS 2005, MIS 2006, MIS 2008
Operational coverage of ITNs, IRS and access to medicines	Programme report	Treatment	MICS 2000, DHS 2005, MIS 2006
Financial data	Programme report	Use of health services	DHS 2005

SUDAN

Malaria transmission in the northern, eastern and western states of Sudan is low-to-moderate, highly seasonal and occasionally epidemic. In the southern, malaria transmission is generally perennial with moderate-to-high intensity. The data presented in this report are from 15 states in the north, east and west of the country as the information from the southern states was incomplete. In the northern, eastern and western states, in 2008, there were 3 073 966 reported malaria cases and 1 125 deaths. In the states from which information is complete, more than 95% of malaria cases are due to *P. falciparum*. In these areas, the malaria control programme distributed over 3.3 million long-lasting insecticide-impregnated nets between 2006 and 2008. About 90% of public heath facilities provide ACTs free of charge; in 2008, about 3 million treatment courses were delivered, enough to treat all reported cases. During the past 5 years, the Government has allocated more than US$ 31 million for malaria control, complemented by more than US$ 69 million from the Global Fund.

I. EPIDEMIOLOGICAL PROFILE

Population, endemicity and malaria burden

Population (in thousands)	2008	%
All age groups	41 348	
< 5 years	5 836	14
≥ 5 years	35 511	86

Population by malaria endemicity (in thousands)	2008	%
High transmission ≥ 1/1000	6 808	16
Low transmission (0–1/1000)	34 501	83
Malaria-free (0 cases)	40	0
Rural population	23 372	57

Vector and parasite profiles

Major *Anopheles* species	*arabiensis*
Plasmodium species	*falciparum, vivax*

Stratification of burden (reported cases, per 1000)

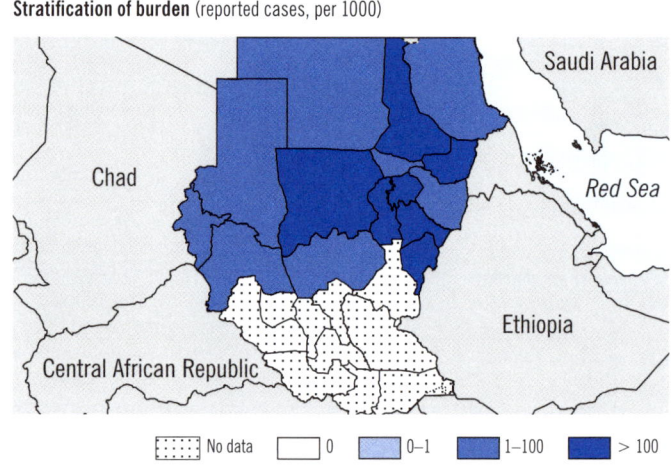

No data | 0 | 0–1 | 1–100 | > 100

Trends in malaria morbidity and mortality

Reported malaria cases, per 1000

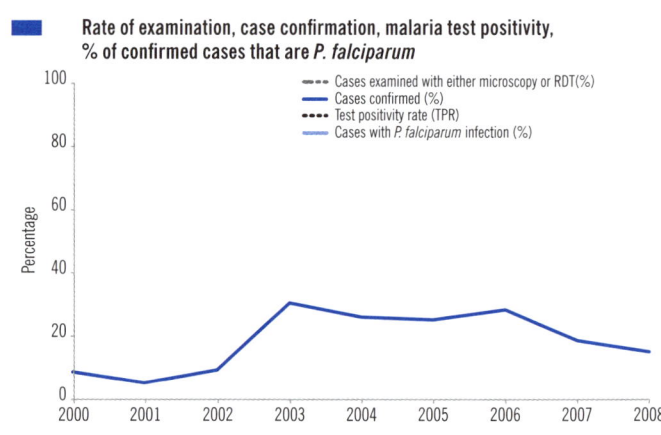

- - - Reported malaria cases/1000, all ages
—— Reported malaria cases/1000, <5 years

Rate of examination, case confirmation, malaria test positivity, % of confirmed cases that are *P. falciparum*

- - - Cases examined with either microscopy or RDT(%)
—— Cases confirmed (%)
···· Test positivity rate (TPR)
—— Cases with *P. falciparum* infection (%)

Year	Reported malaria cases, all ages	Reported malaria cases, < 5 years	All-cause outpatient consultations, all ages	All-cause outpatient consultations, < 5 years	Examined	Positive	*P. falciparum*	Reporting completeness of outpatient health facilities (%)	Reporting completeness of districts (%)
2000	4 428 277	1 159 328	25 151 371	6 255 772		464 007			
2001	4 105 613	868 893	20 337 398	5 700 642		323 402			
2002	3 167 456	760 572	20 486 801	5 058 783		393 606			
2003	3 237 006	676 525	19 628 283	4 499 077		1 085 953			
2004	2 214 296	547 011	18 285 220	4 401 768		668 484			
2005	2 648 310	654 044	17 462 890	4 347 518		761 034			
2006	2 243 064	379 172	8 703 556	1 760 093		721 233			
2007	3 166 661	771 419	13 988 723	2 879 177		686 908		81	
2008	3 185 930	886 294	13 745 635	3 205 353		569 296		83	

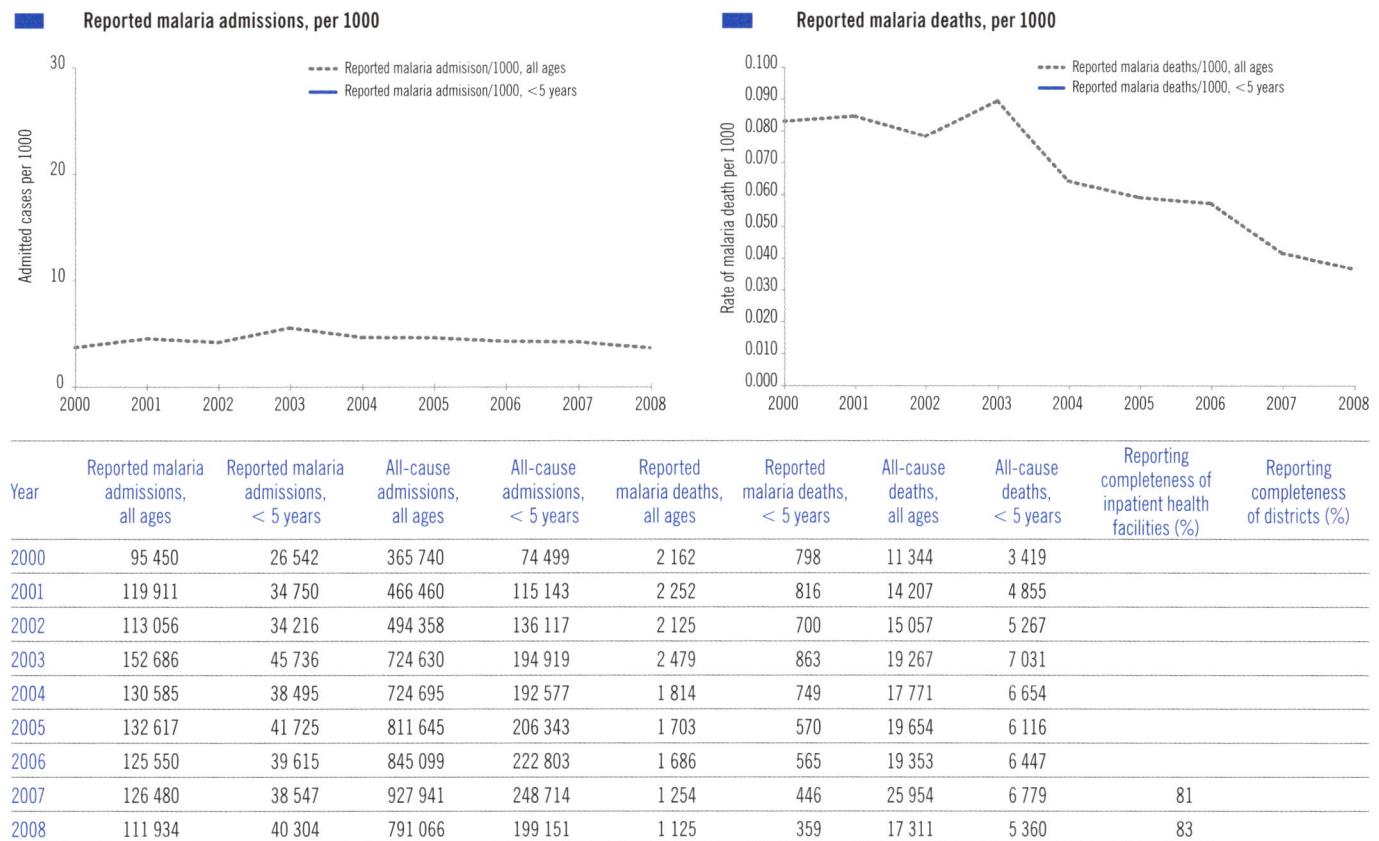

Reported malaria admissions, per 1000

- - - Reported malaria admission/1000, all ages
—— Reported malaria admission/1000, <5 years

Reported malaria deaths, per 1000

- - - Reported malaria deaths/1000, all ages
—— Reported malaria deaths/1000, <5 years

Year	Reported malaria admissions, all ages	Reported malaria admissions, < 5 years	All-cause admissions, all ages	All-cause admissions, < 5 years	Reported malaria deaths, all ages	Reported malaria deaths, < 5 years	All-cause deaths, all ages	All-cause deaths, < 5 years	Reporting completeness of inpatient health facilities (%)	Reporting completeness of districts (%)
2000	95 450	26 542	365 740	74 499	2 162	798	11 344	3 419		
2001	119 911	34 750	466 460	115 143	2 252	816	14 207	4 855		
2002	113 056	34 216	494 358	136 117	2 125	700	15 057	5 267		
2003	152 686	45 736	724 630	194 919	2 479	863	19 267	7 031		
2004	130 585	38 495	724 695	192 577	1 814	749	17 771	6 654		
2005	132 617	41 725	811 645	206 343	1 703	570	19 654	6 116		
2006	125 550	39 615	845 099	222 803	1 686	565	19 353	6 447		
2007	126 480	38 547	927 941	248 714	1 254	446	25 954	6 779	81	
2008	111 934	40 304	791 066	199 151	1 125	359	17 311	5 360	83	

II. INTERVENTION POLICIES AND STRATEGIES

Intervention	WHO-RECOMMENDED POLICIES / STRATEGIES	Yes or No	Year adopted	OPTIONAL POLICIES / STRATEGIES	Yes or No	Year adoped
Insecticide-treated nets (ITN)	Distribution of ITN/LLINs – Free	Yes	2001	Distribution – Antenatal care	Yes	2007
	Targeting all age groups	Yes	2006	Distribution – EPI routine and campaign	Yes	2008
				Targeting children < 5 years and pregnant women	Yes	2001
				ITN distribution is subsidized	Yes	2002
Indoor residual spraying (IRS)	IRS is a primary vector control intervention	No	–	Insecticide-resistance management implemented	Yes	1999
	DDT is used for IRS (public health) only	No	–	Where IRS is conducted, other options are also implemented, e.g. ITN	Yes	2003
				IRS is used for prevention and control of epidemics	Yes	1998
Intermittent preventive treatment (IPT)	IPT used to prevent malaria during pregnancy	Yes	2005			
Case management	Oral artemisinin monotherapies banned (prohibited from registration or removed from the system)	Yes	2004	Parasitological confirmation for patients ≥ 5 years only	Yes	2000
	Parasitological confirmation for patients of all ages	Yes	2000	Malaria diagnosis is free of charge in the public sector	No	–
	ACT is free of charge for < 5 years old in the public sector	Yes	2005	ACT is free of charge for patients ≥ 5 years in the public sector	Yes	2004
	Diagnosis of malaria of inpatients is based on parasitological confirmation	Yes	2001	ACT is delivered at community level through community agents (beyond the health facilities)	Yes	2007
	Pre-referral treatment with quinine or artemether IM or artesunate suppositories	Yes	2004	Uncomplicated malaria cases are admitted	No	–
	Oversight regulation of case management in the private sectors	Yes	2004			
	RDTs used at community level	Yes	2005			

Antimalarial policy	Type of medicine	Year adopted	Results of therapeutic efficacy tests					
			Study year	No. of studies	Median	Minimum	Maximum	Percentiles: 25% 75%
First-line treatment of *P. falciparum* (unconfirmed)	AS + SP	2004						
First-line treatment of *P. falciparum* (confirmed)	AS + SP	2004						
Treatment failure of *P. falciparum*	AL	2004						
Treatment of severe malaria	QN (7d), AM (7d), AM (3d) + AS+SP	2004						
Treatment of *P. vivax*	CQ + PQ(14d)	2004						

III. IMPLEMENTING MALARIA CONTROL

Coverage of ITN: survey data

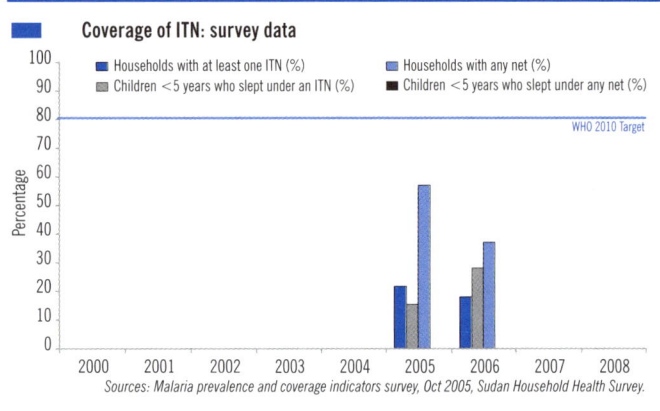

Sources: Malaria prevalence and coverage indicators survey, Oct 2005, Sudan Household Health Survey.

Coverage of IRS and ITN: programme data

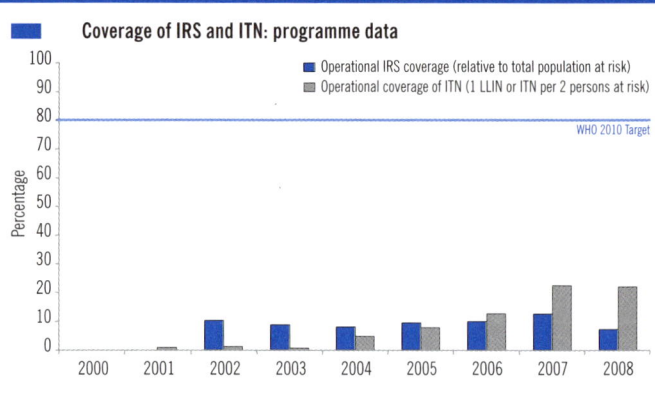

Access by febrile children to effective treatment: survey data

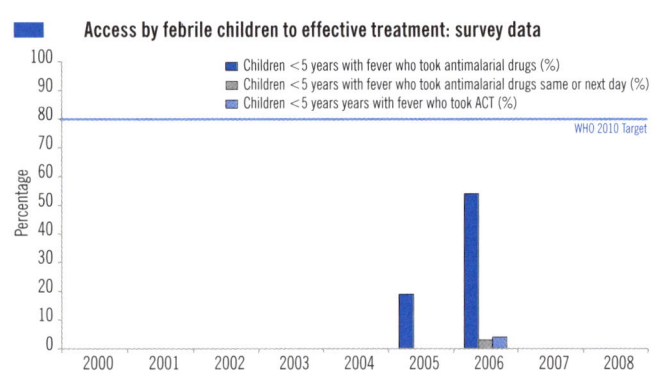

Access to effective treatment: programme data

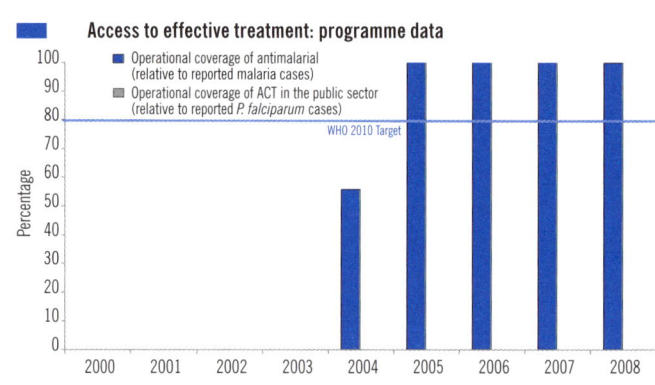

Year	Pregnant women who slept under any net (%)	Pregnant women who slept under an ITN (%)	Children < 5 years with fever (%)	Febrile children < 5 years who sought treatment in HF (%)	Number of households protected by IRS	Number of people protected by IRS	Number of ITNs and/or LLINs	Number of 1st-line treatment courses received	Number of ACT treatment courses received
2000									
2001							135 000		
2002					565 605	2 828 025	160 600		
2003					494 795	2 473 973	76 500		
2004					465 454	2 327 272	665 400	1 165 019	
2005	13		–	–	555 311	2 776 555	752 900	3 613 133	
2006			–	–	595 486	2 977 432	796 199	2 888 943	2 814 000
2007					641 123	3 846 738	1 910 000	3 337 103	2 677 199
2008					456 337	2 281 687	1 806 540	3 073 996	3 073 996

IV. FINANCING MALARIA CONTROL

Governmental and external financing

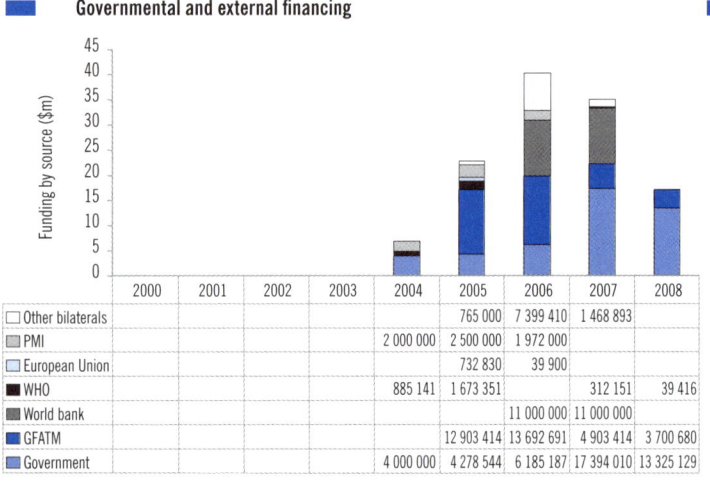

	2000	2001	2002	2003	2004	2005	2006	2007	2008
Other bilaterals						765 000	7 399 410	1 468 893	
PMI					2 000 000	2 500 000	1 972 000		
European Union						732 830	39 900		
WHO					885 141	1 673 351		312 151	39 416
World bank							11 000 000	11 000 000	
GFATM						12 903 414	13 692 691	4 903 414	3 700 680
Government					4 000 000	4 278 544	6 185 187	17 394 010	13 325 129

Breakdown of expenditure by intervention in 2008

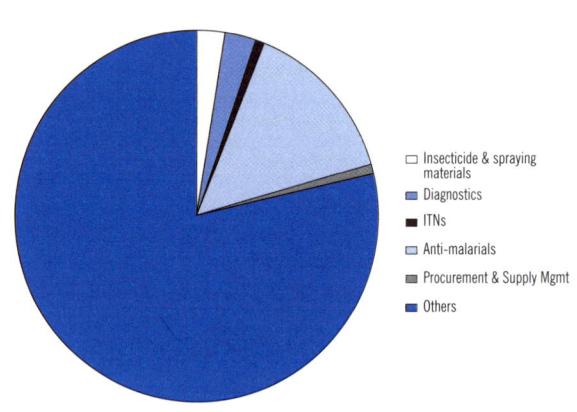

- Insecticide & spraying materials
- Diagnostics
- ITNs
- Anti-malarials
- Procurement & Supply Mgmt
- Others

V. SOURCE OF INFORMATION

PROGRAMME DATA		SURVEY AND OTHER DATA	
Reported cases	Surveillance data	Insecticide-treated nets (ITN)	Malaria prevalence and coverage indicators survey, Oct 2005, Sudan Household Health Survey
Operational coverage of ITNs, IRS and access to medicines	Programme report	Treatment	
Financial data	Programme report	Use of health services	0

TAJIKISTAN

Malaria transmission due to *P. vivax* and *P. falciparum* is seasonal, from June to October, with areas below 2500 m most at risk. The number of malaria cases has decreased significantly, from over 19 000 cases in 2000 to only 318 cases in 2008, including two *P. falciparum* cases reported in the southern and central parts of the country. Tajikistan shows a strong political commitment to the Tashkent Declaration and has cross-border collaboration with Afghanistan and other countries of Central Asia. IRS is the principal method of mosquito control, covering over 630 000 people at risk in 2008 in focal areas. Additionally, about 19 000 LLINs were distributed, and the Gambusia fish was introduced into 795 ha of water reservoirs. All malaria cases are treated with full doses of chloroquine and primaquine. While malaria control is funded primarily by the Government, the country recently secured a Global Fund grant of US$ 5.4 million to interrupt *P. vivax* transmission by 2015.

I. EPIDEMIOLOGICAL PROFILE

Population, endemicity and malaria burden

Population (in thousands)	2008	%
All age groups	6 836	
< 5 years	871	13
≥ 5 years	5 965	87

Population by malaria endemicity (in thousands)	2008	%
High transmission ≥ 1/1000	195	3
Low transmission (0–1/1000)	5 007	73
Malaria-free (0 cases)	1 634	24
Rural population	5 031	74

Vector and parasite profiles

Major *Anopheles* species	*hyrcanus, maculipennis, martinius, pulcherimus, superpictus*
Plasmodium species	*falciparum, vivax*

Stratification of burden (reported cases, per 1000)

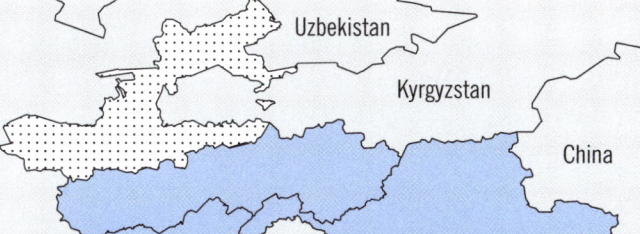

No data | 0 | 0–1 | 1–100 | > 100

Trends in malaria morbidity and mortality

Reported malaria cases, per 1000

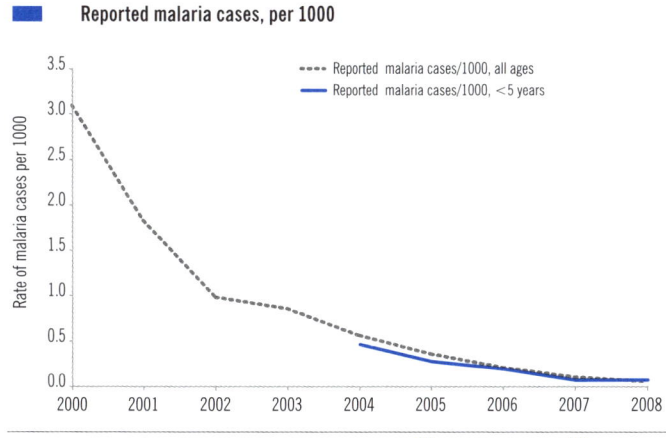

- Reported malaria cases/1000, all ages
- Reported malaria cases/1000, <5 years

Rate of examination, case confirmation, malaria test positivity, % of confirmed cases that are *P. falciparum*

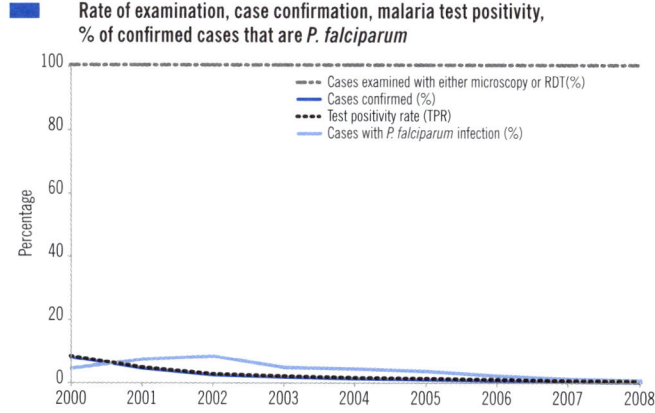

- Cases examined with either microscopy or RDT(%)
- Cases confirmed (%)
- Test positivity rate (TPR)
- Cases with *P. falciparum* infection (%)

Year	Reported malaria cases, all ages	Reported malaria cases, < 5 years	All-cause outpatient consultations, all ages	All-cause outpatient consultations, < 5 years	Examined	Positive	*P. falciparum*	Reporting completeness of outpatient health facilities (%)	Reporting completeness of districts (%)
2000	19 064				233 785	19 064	831	100	100
2001	11 387				248 565	11 387	826	100	100
2002	6 160				244 632	6 160	509	100	100
2003	5 428				296 123	5 428	252	100	100
2004	3 588	392			272 743	3 588	151	100	100
2005	2 309	231			216 197	2 309	81	100	100
2006	1 344	159			175 894	1 344	28	100	100
2007	635	53	19 420 525		159 232	635	7	100	100
2008	318	56	29 043 834		158 068	318	2	100	100

Reported malaria admissions, per 1000

No data

Reported malaria deaths, per 1000

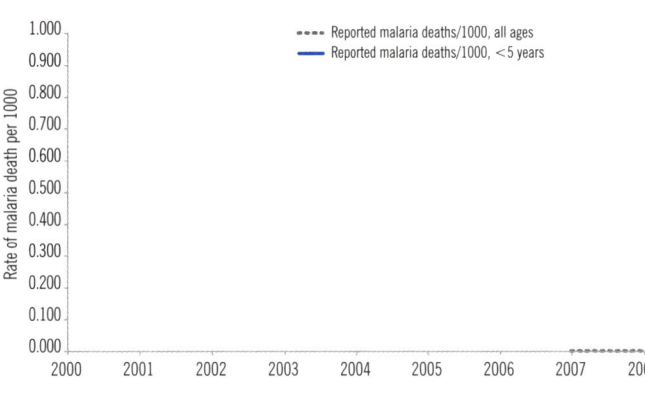

Year	Reported malaria admissions, all ages	Reported malaria admissions, < 5 years	All-cause admissions, all ages	All-cause admissions, < 5 years	Reported malaria deaths, all ages	Reported malaria deaths, < 5 years	All-cause deaths, all ages	All-cause deaths, < 5 years	Reporting completeness of inpatient health facilities (%)	Reporting completeness of districts (%)
2000									100	100
2001									100	100
2002									100	100
2003									100	100
2004									100	100
2005									100	100
2006									100	100
2007			740 502						100	100
2008			830 394						100	100

II.   INTERVENTION POLICIES AND STRATEGIES

Intervention	WHO-RECOMMENDED POLICIES / STRATEGIES	Yes or No	Year adopted	OPTIONAL POLICIES / STRATEGIES	Yes or No	Year adoped
Insecticide-treated nets (ITN)	Distribution of ITN/LLINs – Free	Yes	1997	Distribution – Antenatal care	No	–
	Targeting all age groups	Yes	1997	Distribution – EPI routine and campaign	No	–
				Targeting children < 5 years and pregnant women	Yes	1997
				ITN distribution is subsidized	No	–
Indoor residual spraying (IRS)	IRS is a primary vector control intervention	Yes	1997	Insecticide-resistance management implemented	Yes	2000
	DDT is used for IRS (public health) only	No	–	Where IRS is conducted, other options are also implemented, e.g. ITN	Yes	1997
				IRS is used for prevention and control of epidemics	Yes	1997
Intermittent preventive treatment (IPT)	IPT used to prevent malaria during pregnancy	No	–			
Case management	Oral artemisinin monotherapies banned (prohibited from registration or removed from the system)	Yes	2004	Parasitological confirmation for patients ≥ 5 years only	No	–
	Parasitological confirmation for patients of all ages	Yes	1997	Malaria diagnosis is free of charge in the public sector	Yes	2000
	ACT is free of charge for < 5 years old in the public sector	Yes	2004	ACT is free of charge for patients ≥ 5 years in the public sector	Yes	2004
	Diagnosis of malaria of inpatients is based on parasitological confirmation	Yes	2000	ACT is delivered at community level through community agents (beyond the health facilities)	No	–
	Pre-referral treatment with quinine or artemether IM or artesunate suppositories	No	–	Uncomplicated malaria cases are admitted	Yes	2000
	Oversight regulation of case management in the private sectors	Yes	2000			
	RDTs used at community level	No	–			

Antimalarial policy	Type of medicine	Year adopted	Results of therapeutic efficacy tests						
			Study year	No. of studies	Median	Minimum	Maximum	Percentiles: 25%	75%
First-line treatment of *P. falciparum* (unconfirmed)	–	–							
First-line treatment of *P. falciparum* (confirmed)	AL, AS+SP	2008							
Treatment failure of *P. falciparum*	QN(7d)	2004							
Treatment of severe malaria	QN(7d)	2004							
Treatment of *P. vivax*	CQ+PQ(14d)	2004							

III. IMPLEMENTING MALARIA CONTROL

Coverage of ITN: survey data

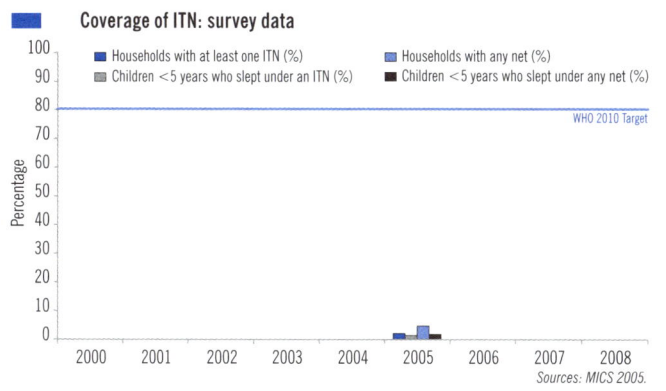

Sources: MICS 2005.

Coverage of IRS and ITN: programme data

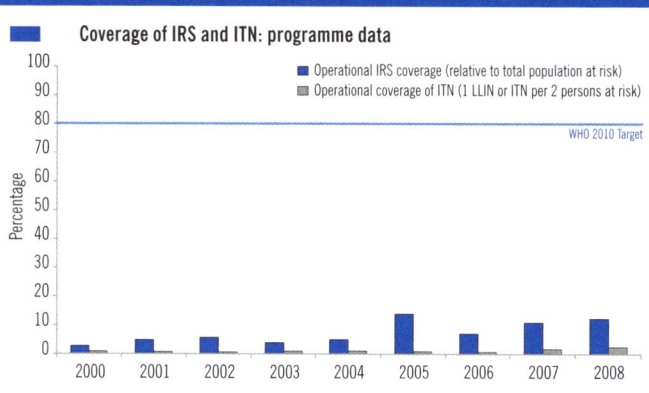

Access by febrile children to effective treatment: survey data

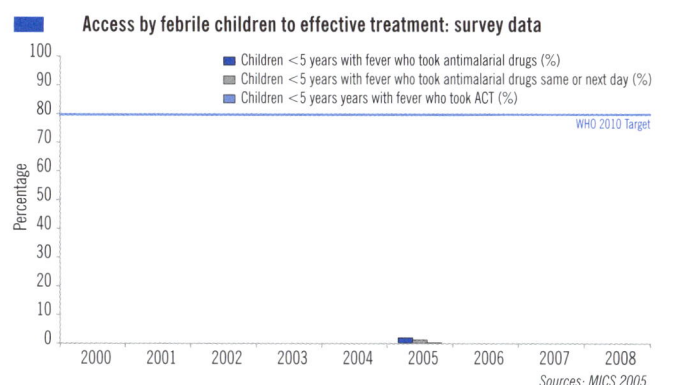

Sources: MICS 2005.

Access to effective treatment: programme data

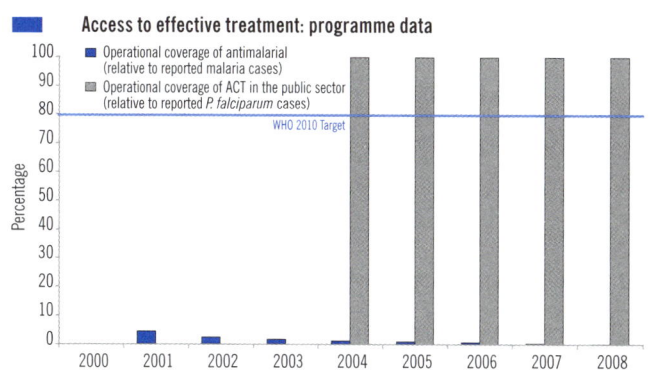

Year	Pregnant women who slept under any net (%)	Pregnant women who slept under an ITN (%)	Children < 5 years with fever (%)	Febrile children < 5 years who sought treatment in HF (%)	Number of households protected by IRS	Number of people protected by IRS	Number of ITNs and/or LLINs	Number of 1st-line treatment courses received	Number of ACT treatment courses received
2000					20 450	122 700	16 779	13	
2001					37 580	221 480	14 188	11 387	
2002					51 800	264 240	10 625	6 160	
2003					30 323	183 280	19 986	5 428	
2004					81 950	238 651	22 952	3 588	151
2005			–	–	71 454	685 130	19 993	2 309	81
2006					58 410	350 460	15 150	1 344	28
2007					183 464	552 912	26 438	635	7
2008					624 000	632 622	19 494	318	2

IV. FINANCING MALARIA CONTROL

Governmental and external financing

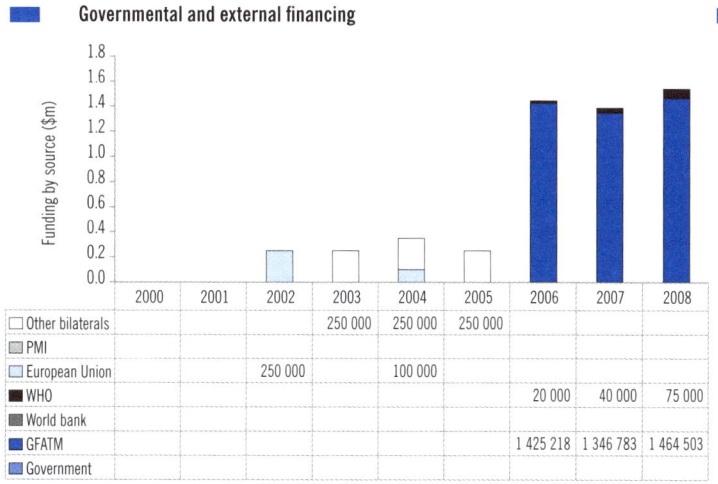

Breakdown of expenditure by intervention in 2008

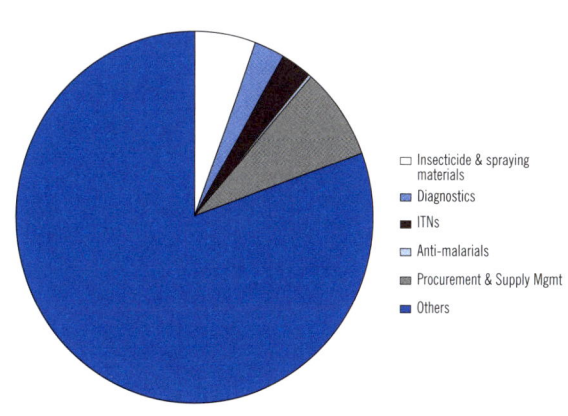

V. SOURCE OF INFORMATION

PROGRAMME DATA		SURVEY AND OTHER DATA	
Reported cases	Surveillance data	Insecticide-treated nets (ITN)	MICS 2005
Operational coverage of ITNs, IRS and access to medicines	Programme report	Treatment	MICS 2005
Financial data	Programme report	Use of health services	MICS 2005

TURKEY

Before the 1970s, *P. falciparum* was the dominant parasite; however, since implementation of control activities, malaria transmission is now due exclusively to *P. vivax* and is seasonal, occurring from June to October. The number of malaria cases decreased from over 9 465 in 2000 to only 136 in 2008, of which 49 were imported. Although the number of malaria cases and their foci have decreased dramatically, transmission continues in new and residual foci in five south-eastern provinces of the country, on a seasonal basis. In 2008, all the local cases were found in five provinces (Diyarkabir, Siirt, Mardin, Sanliurfa and Batman), and the case rate was 0.003–0.005 per 1000. Turkey shows a strong political commitment to the Tashkent Declaration, endorsed in 2005, and malaria surveillance activities have been intensified all over the country, with priority given to the provinces in south-eastern Anatolia. All foci of malaria are determined and totally covered by IRS. Malaria elimination activities are supported by the Ministry of Health, other Government entities and WHO. In 2008, 624 000 households were sprayed, and 632 000 people living at risk for malaria were protected by IRS. A national malaria elimination strategy and a relevant plan of action with the goal of interrupting transmission by 2012 and eliminating the disease by 2105 have been prepared and are to be launched.

I. EPIDEMIOLOGICAL PROFILE

Population, endemicity and malaria burden

Population (in thousands)	2008	%
All age groups	73 914	
< 5 years	6 543	9
≥ 5 years	67 372	91

Population by malaria endemicity (in thousands)	2008	%
High transmission ≥ 1/1000	0	0
Low transmission (0–1/1000)	4 757	6
Malaria-free (0 cases)	69 157	94
Rural population	23 120	31

Vector and parasite profiles

Major *Anopheles* species	*sacharovi*
Plasmodium species	*vivax risk only*

Stratification of burden (reported cases, per 1000)

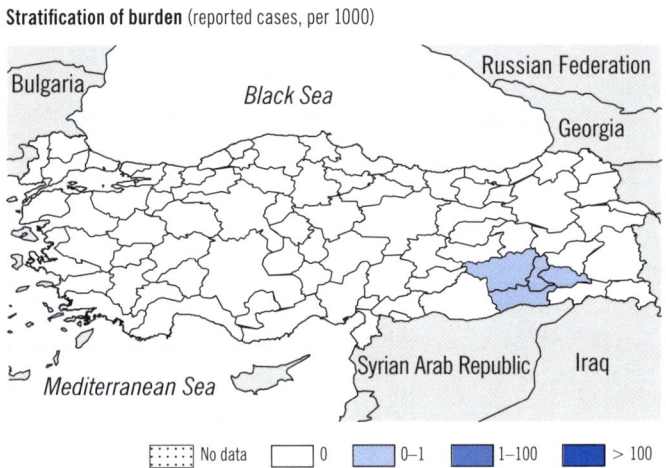

No data · 0 · 0–1 · 1–100 · > 100

Trends in malaria morbidity and mortality

Reported malaria cases, per 1000

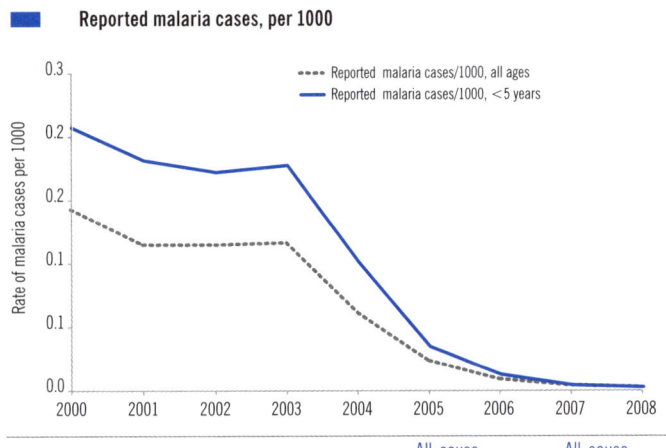

- Reported malaria cases/1000, all ages
- Reported malaria cases/1000, <5 years

Rate of examination, case confirmation, malaria test positivity, % of confirmed cases that are *P. falciparum*

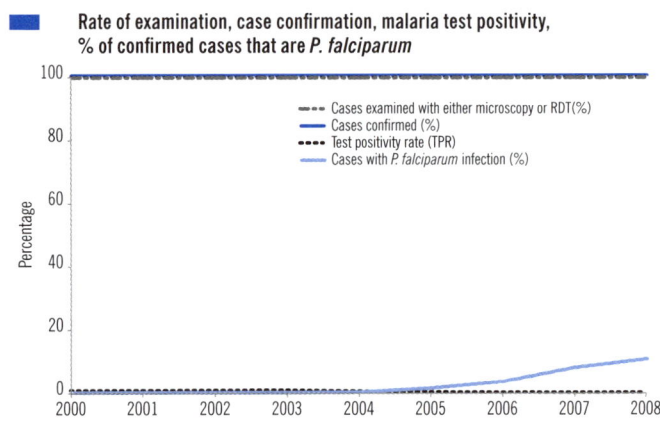

- Cases examined with either microscopy or RDT(%)
- Cases confirmed (%)
- Test positivity rate (TPR)
- Cases with *P. falciparum* infection (%)

Year	Reported malaria cases, all ages	Reported malaria cases, < 5 years	All-cause outpatient consultations, all ages	All-cause outpatient consultations, < 5 years	Examined	Positive	P. falciparum	Reporting completeness of outpatient health facilities (%)	Reporting completeness of districts (%)
2000	9 465	1 433	161 051 503		253 562	9 465	7		675
2001	7 710	1 243	182 177 063		234 250	7 710	11		675
2002	7 814	1 165	184 238 055		193 970	7 814	12		675
2003	8 025	1 185	201 112 942		183 748	8 025	12		675
2004	4 278	666	232 906 560		169 592	4 278	13		675
2005	1 627	224	295 860 209		143 899	1 627	32		675
2006	605	80	341 676 429		134 146	605	29		675
2007	250	24	398 121 987		96 938	250	29		675
2008	136	13	444 606 049		55 856	136	23		675

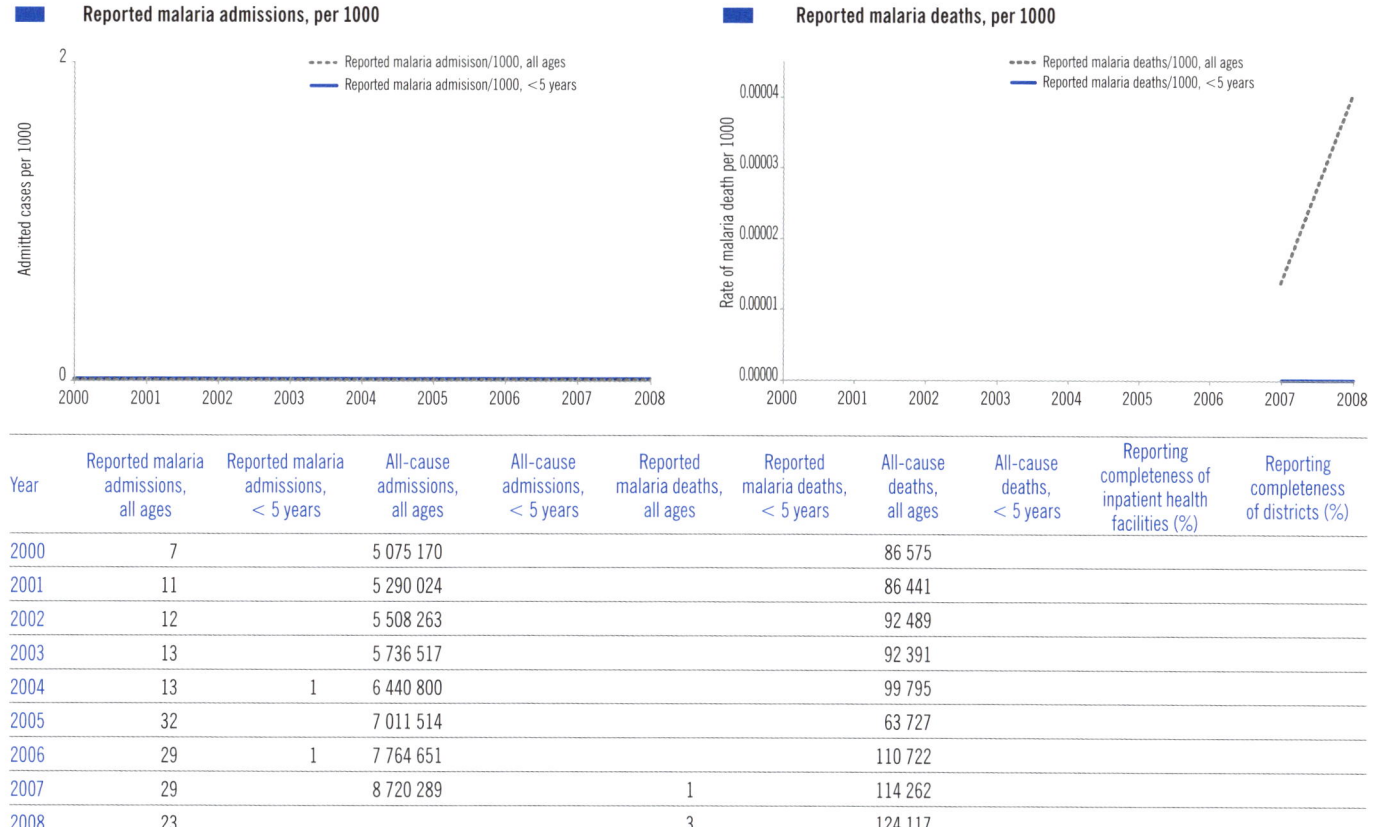

Reported malaria admissions, per 1000

- - - - Reported malaria admisison/1000, all ages
——— Reported malaria admisison/1000, <5 years

Reported malaria deaths, per 1000

- - - - Reported malaria deaths/1000, all ages
——— Reported malaria deaths/1000, <5 years

Year	Reported malaria admissions, all ages	Reported malaria admissions, < 5 years	All-cause admissions, all ages	All-cause admissions, < 5 years	Reported malaria deaths, all ages	Reported malaria deaths, < 5 years	All-cause deaths, all ages	All-cause deaths, < 5 years	Reporting completeness of inpatient health facilities (%)	Reporting completeness of districts (%)
2000	7		5 075 170				86 575			
2001	11		5 290 024				86 441			
2002	12		5 508 263				92 489			
2003	13		5 736 517				92 391			
2004	13	1	6 440 800				99 795			
2005	32		7 011 514				63 727			
2006	29	1	7 764 651				110 722			
2007	29		8 720 289		1		114 262			
2008	23				3		124 117			

II. INTERVENTION POLICIES AND STRATEGIES

Intervention	WHO-RECOMMENDED POLICIES / STRATEGIES	Yes or No	Year adopted	OPTIONAL POLICIES / STRATEGIES	Yes or No	Year adoped
Insecticide-treated nets (ITN)	Distribution of ITN/LLINs – Free	No	–	Distribution – Antenatal care	No	–
	Targeting all age groups	No	–	Distribution – EPI routine and campaign	No	–
				Targeting children < 5 years and pregnant women	No	–
				ITN distribution is subsidized	No	–
Indoor residual spraying (IRS)	IRS is a primary vector control intervention	Yes	2000	Insecticide-resistance management implemented	Yes	2000
	DDT is used for IRS (public health) only	No	–	Where IRS is conducted, other options are also implemented, e.g. ITN	No	–
				IRS is used for prevention and control of epidemics	Yes	2000
Intermittent preventive treatment (IPT)	IPT used to prevent malaria during pregnancy	No	–			
Case management	Oral artemisinin monotherapies banned (prohibited from registration or removed from the system)	No	–	Parasitological confirmation for patients ≥ 5 years only	No	–
	Parasitological confirmation for patients of all ages	Yes	2000	Malaria diagnosis is free of charge in the public sector	Yes	2000
	ACT is free of charge for < 5 years old in the public sector	Yes	2009	ACT is free of charge for patients ≥ 5 years in the public sector	Yes	2009
	Diagnosis of malaria of inpatients is based on parasitological confirmation	Yes	2000	ACT is delivered at community level through community agents (beyond the health facilities)	No	–
	Pre-referral treatment with quinine or artemether IM or artesunate suppositories	No	–	Uncomplicated malaria cases are admitted	No	–
	Oversight regulation of case management in the private sectors	Yes	2000			
	RDTs used at community level	No	–			

Antimalarial policy	Type of medicine	Year adopted	Study year	No. of studies	Median	Minimum	Maximum	Percentiles: 25%	75%
				Results of therapeutic efficacy tests					
First-line treatment of *P. falciparum* (unconfirmed)	–	–							
First-line treatment of *P. falciparum* (confirmed)	–	–							
Treatment failure of *P. falciparum*	–	–							
Treatment of severe malaria	–	–							
Treatment of *P. vivax*	CQ+PQ(14d)	–							

III. IMPLEMENTING MALARIA CONTROL

Coverage of ITN: survey data

No data

Coverage of IRS and ITN: programme data

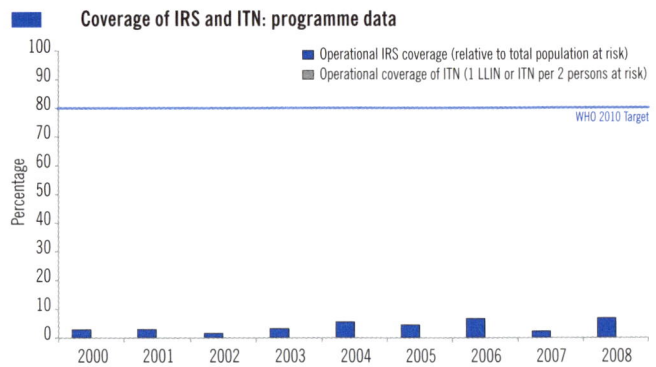

Access by febrile children to effective treatment: survey data

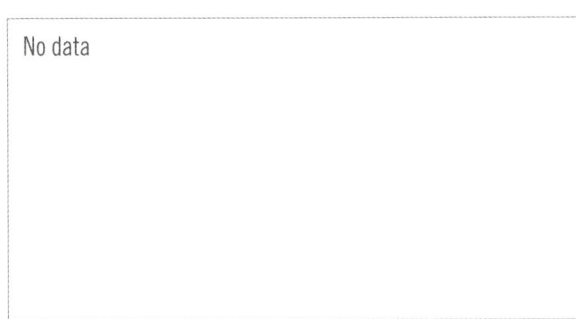

No data

Access to effective treatment: programme data

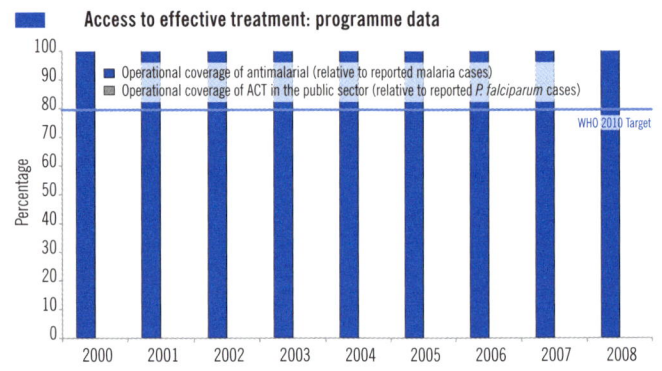

Year	Pregnant women who slept under any net (%)	Pregnant women who slept under an ITN (%)	Children < 5 years with fever (%)	Febrile children < 5 years who sought treatment in HF (%)	Number of households protected by IRS	Number of people protected by IRS	Number of ITNs and/or LLINs	Number of 1st-line treatment courses received	Number of ACT treatment courses received
2000					24 213	125 715		30 800	
2001					25 746	128 730		30 500	
2002					14 334	71 670		24 500	
2003					28 941	144 705		28 500	
2004					50 184	250 920		10 660	
2005					41 370	206 850		17 000	
2006					62 669	313 345		2 600	
2007					21 901	109 505		2 600	
2008					65 475	327 375		980	

IV. FINANCING MALARIA CONTROL

Governmental and external financing

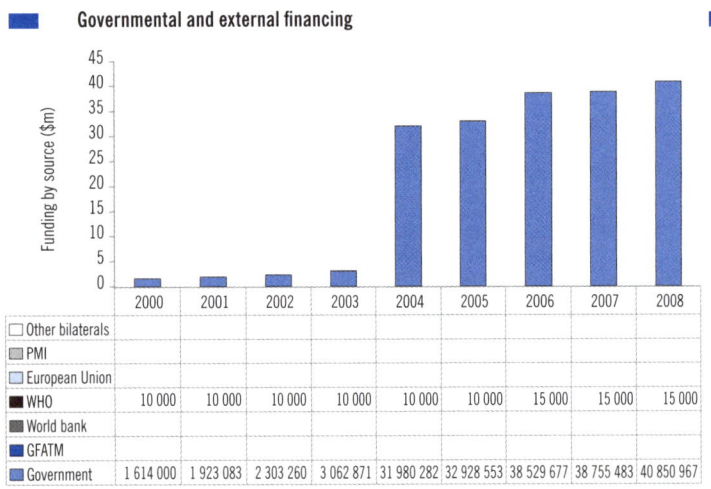

	2000	2001	2002	2003	2004	2005	2006	2007	2008
Other bilaterals									
PMI									
European Union									
WHO	10 000	10 000	10 000	10 000	10 000	10 000	15 000	15 000	15 000
World bank									
GFATM									
Government	1 614 000	1 923 083	2 303 260	3 062 871	31 980 282	32 928 553	38 529 677	38 755 483	40 850 967

Breakdown of expenditure by intervention in 2008

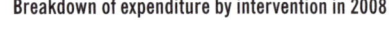
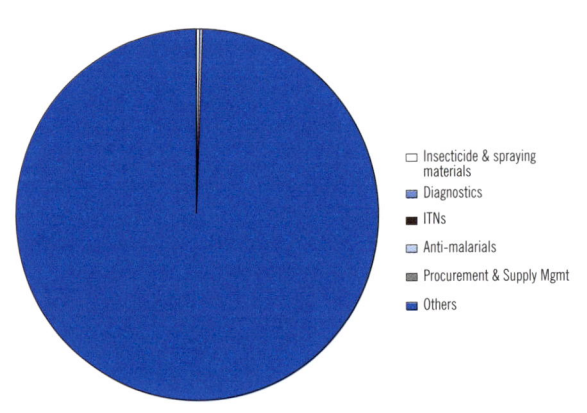

V. SOURCE OF INFORMATION

PROGRAMME DATA		SURVEY AND OTHER DATA	
Reported cases	Surveillance data	Insecticide-treated nets (ITN)	No surveys
Operational coverage of ITNs, IRS and access to medicines	Programme report	Treatment	No surveys
Financial data	Programme report	Use of health services	DHS 2003

UGANDA

Uganda had an estimated 12 million malaria cases in 2006. Transmission occurs all year round in most parts of the country. On average, 10.7 million malaria cases were reported annually during 2004–2008, with no declining trend. About 20% of the suspected cases were parasitologically tested in 2007. The fluctuating numbers of inpatient malaria cases and deaths reported in 2006–2008, due to inconsistent and incomplete surveillance, do not provide a basis for evaluating incidence trends, although the programme reports show a decrease in cases and deaths between 2005 and 2006. The programme delivered nearly 5.9 million LLINs during 2006–2008. Implementation of IRS, which was started in 2006, covered 500 000 households and protected 1 858 149 people at risk in 2008. Nearly 17 million ACT courses were reportedly delivered in 2007 and another 6.4 million in 2008. In the 2006 demographic and health survey, 22% of households owned an ITN, 13% of children slept under an ITN and 3% of febrile children received ACT. Funding for malaria control exceeded US$ 40 million in 2008, supported by the Government (US$ 20 million) and the United States President's Malaria Initiative (US$ 21 million). Although Global Fund grants were significant during 2004–2006, implementation of the latest grant (round 7) has been delayed.

I. EPIDEMIOLOGICAL PROFILE

Population, endemicity and malaria burden

Population (in thousands)	2008	%
All age groups	31 657	
< 5 years	6 182	20
≥ 5 years	25 475	80

Population by malaria endemicity (in thousands)	2008	%
High transmission ≥ 1/1000	28 491	90
Low transmission (0–1/1000)	3 166	10
Malaria-free (0 cases)	0	0
Rural population	27 555	87

Vector and parasite profiles

Major *Anopheles* species	*gambiae, arabiensis, funestus, brochieri, bwambae, coustani, hancocki, hargreavesi, nili, paludis, pharoensis, quadriannulatus*
Plasmodium species	*falciparum, vivax*

Stratification of burden (reported cases, per 1000)

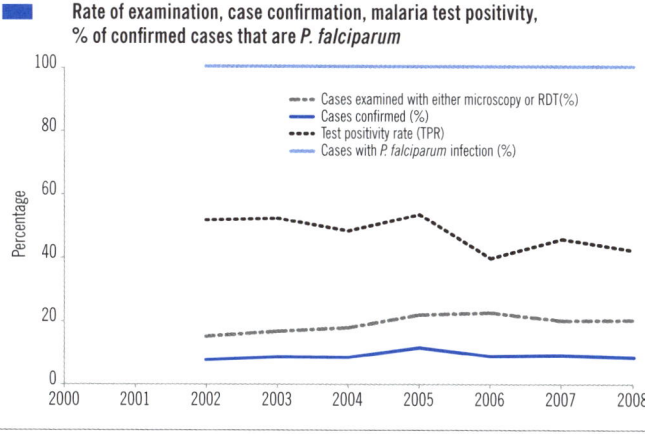

No data / 0 / 0–1 / 1–100 / > 100

Trends in malaria morbidity and mortality

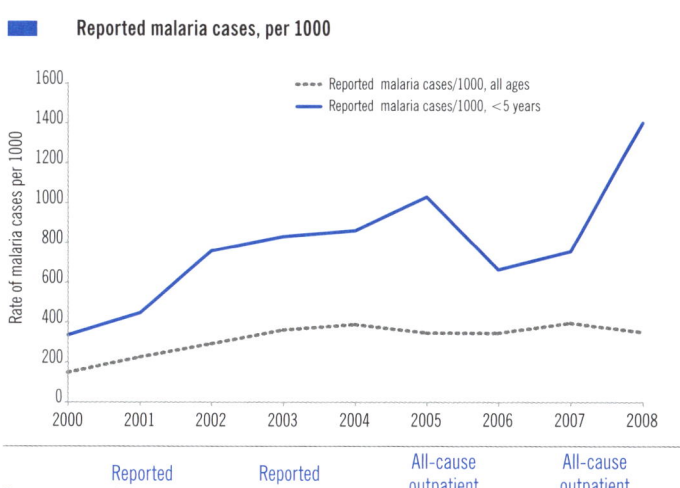

Reported malaria cases, per 1000

- - - Reported malaria cases/1000, all ages
— Reported malaria cases/1000, <5 years

Rate of examination, case confirmation, malaria test positivity, % of confirmed cases that are *P. falciparum*

- - - Cases examined with either microscopy or RDT(%)
— Cases confirmed (%)
···· Test positivity rate (TPR)
— Cases with *P. falciparum* infection (%)

Year	Reported malaria cases, all ages	Reported malaria cases, < 5 years	All-cause outpatient consultations, all ages	All-cause outpatient consultations, < 5 years	Examined	Positive	*P. falciparum*	Reporting completeness of outpatient health facilities (%)	Reporting completeness of districts (%)
2000	3 552 859	1 628 314	10 502 146	4 266 494					
2001	5 624 032	2 233 435	14 525 591	5 384 241					
2002	7 536 748	3 900 000	15 741 520	5 949 360	1 100 374	557 159	546 016		
2003	9 657 332	4 400 000	20 070 390	7 103 940	1 566 474	801 784	785 748		
2004	10 717 076	4 700 000	22 510 595	7 705 537	1 859 780	879 032	861 451		
2005	9 867 174	5 800 000	23 774 349	8 047 500	2 107 011	1 104 310	1 082 224		
2006	10 168 389	3 857 916	25 250 159	9 645 597	2 238 155	867 398	850 050	62	61
2007	12 038 438	4 528 442	30 187 184	13 935 080	2 350 100	1 050 240	1 029 235	77	63
2008	11 029 571	8 656 327	29 237 275	15 071 475	2 173 072	894 505	876 615	29	67

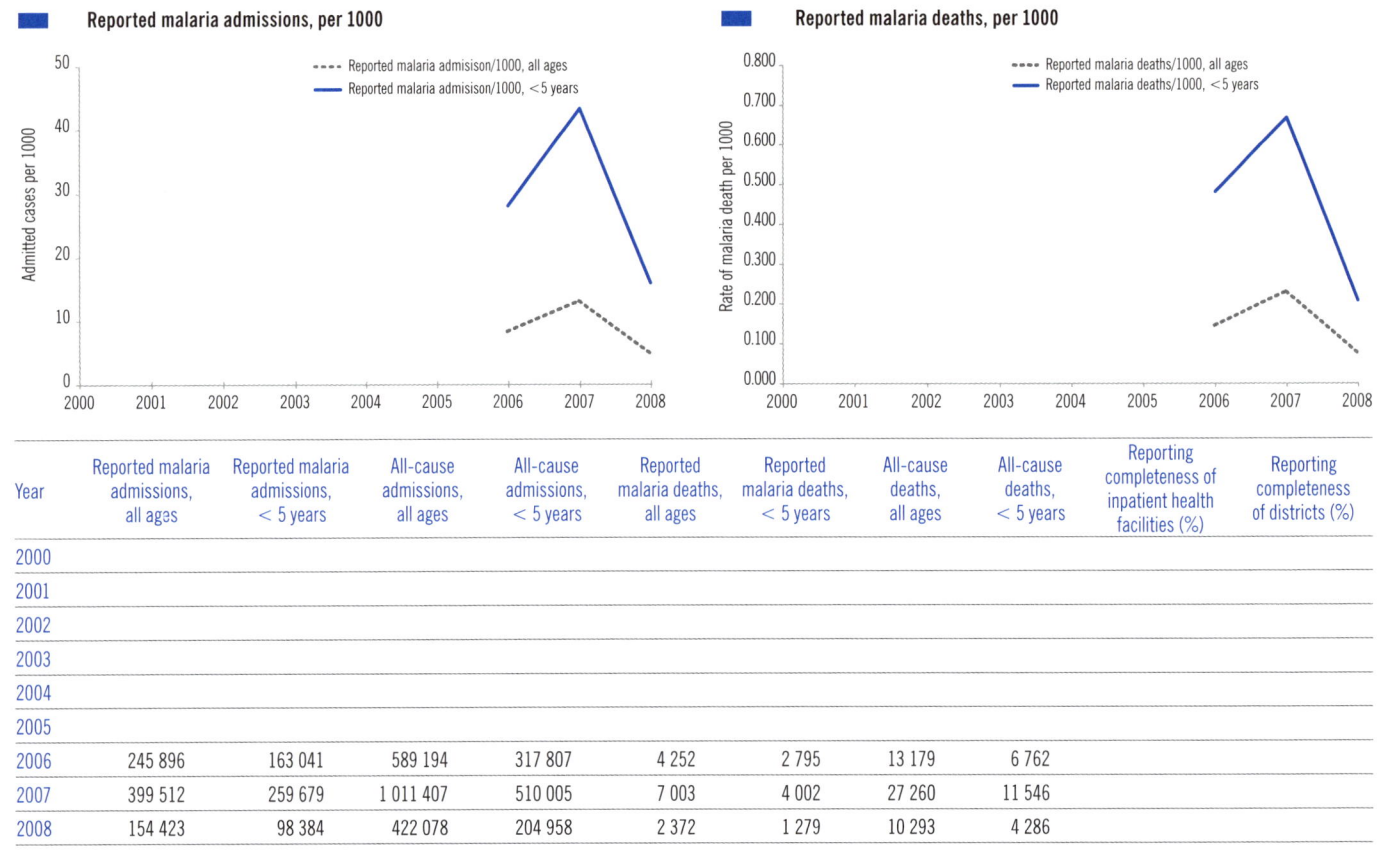

Reported malaria admissions, per 1000

- - - - Reported malaria admission/1000, all ages
——— Reported malaria admission/1000, <5 years

Reported malaria deaths, per 1000

- - - - Reported malaria deaths/1000, all ages
——— Reported malaria deaths/1000, <5 years

Year	Reported malaria admissions, all ages	Reported malaria admissions, < 5 years	All-cause admissions, all ages	All-cause admissions, < 5 years	Reported malaria deaths, all ages	Reported malaria deaths, < 5 years	All-cause deaths, all ages	All-cause deaths, < 5 years	Reporting completeness of inpatient health facilities (%)	Reporting completeness of districts (%)
2000										
2001										
2002										
2003										
2004										
2005										
2006	245 896	163 041	589 194	317 807	4 252	2 795	13 179	6 762		
2007	399 512	259 679	1 011 407	510 005	7 003	4 002	27 260	11 546		
2008	154 423	98 384	422 078	204 958	2 372	1 279	10 293	4 286		

II.   INTERVENTION POLICIES AND STRATEGIES

Intervention	WHO-RECOMMENDED POLICIES / STRATEGIES	Yes or No	Year adopted	OPTIONAL POLICIES / STRATEGIES	Yes or No	Year adoped
Insecticide-treated nets (ITN)	Distribution of ITN/LLINs – Free	Yes	2006	Distribution – Antenatal care	Yes	2004
	Targeting all age groups	Yes	2008	Distribution – EPI routine and campaign	Yes	2004
				Targeting children < 5 years and pregnant women	Yes	2003
				ITN distribution is subsidized	Yes	2004
Indoor residual spraying (IRS)	IRS is a primary vector control intervention	Yes	2006	Insecticide-resistance management implemented	Yes	2007
	DDT is used for IRS (public health) only	Yes	2008	Where IRS is conducted, other options are also implemented, e.g. ITN	Yes	2006
				IRS is used for prevention and control of epidemics	Yes	2001
Intermittent preventive treatment (IPT)	IPT used to prevent malaria during pregnancy	Yes	2000			
Case management	Oral artemisinin monotherapies banned (prohibited from registration or removed from the system)	Yes	2007	Parasitological confirmation for patients ≥ 5 years only	No	–
	Parasitological confirmation for patients of all ages	Yes	1997	Malaria diagnosis is free of charge in the public sector	Yes	2006
	ACT is free of charge for < 5 years old in the public sector	Yes	2006	ACT is free of charge for patients ≥ 5 years in the public sector	Yes	2006
	Diagnosis of malaria of inpatients is based on parasitological confirmation	Yes	1997	ACT is delivered at community level through community agents (beyond the health facilities)	Yes	2006
	Pre-referral treatment with quinine or artemether IM or artesunate suppositories	Yes	2002	Uncomplicated malaria cases are admitted	No	–
	Oversight regulation of case management in the private sectors	No	–			
	RDTs used at community level	No	–			

Antimalarial policy	Type of medicine	Year adopted	Study year	No. of studies	Median	Minimum	Maximum	Percentiles: 25%	75%
				Results of therapeutic efficacy tests					
First-line treatment of *P. falciparum* (unconfirmed)	AL	2004							
First-line treatment of *P. falciparum* (confirmed)	AL	2004							
Treatment failure of *P. falciparum*	QN(7d)	2004							
Treatment of severe malaria	QN(7d)	2004							
Treatment of *P. vivax*	–	–							

III. IMPLEMENTING MALARIA CONTROL

Coverage of ITN: survey data

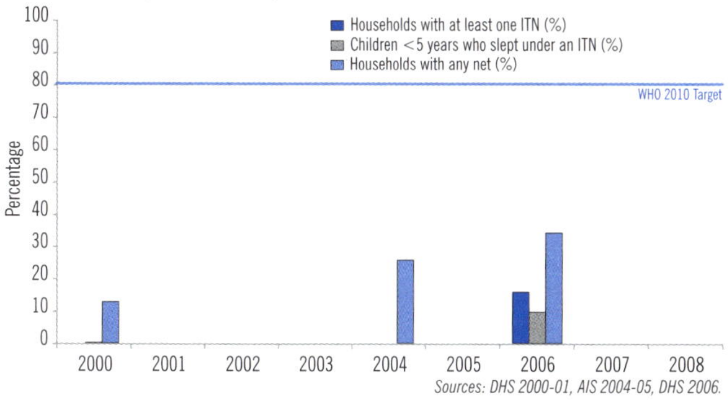

Legend:
- Households with at least one ITN (%)
- Children <5 years who slept under an ITN (%)
- Households with any net (%)

WHO 2010 Target

Sources: DHS 2000-01, AIS 2004-05, DHS 2006.

Coverage of IRS and ITN: programme data

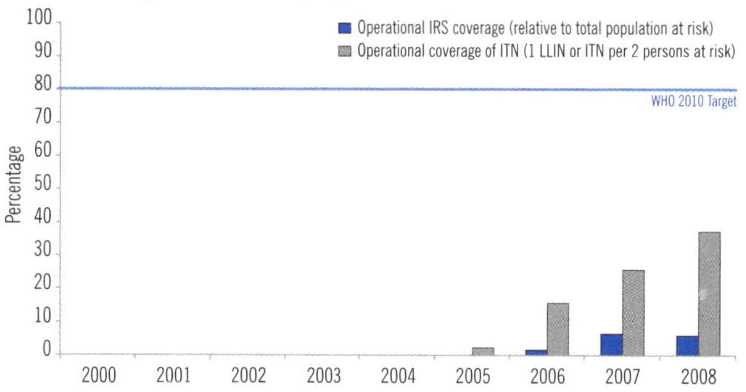

Legend:
- Operational IRS coverage (relative to total population at risk)
- Operational coverage of ITN (1 LLIN or ITN per 2 persons at risk)

WHO 2010 Target

Access by febrile children to effective treatment: survey data

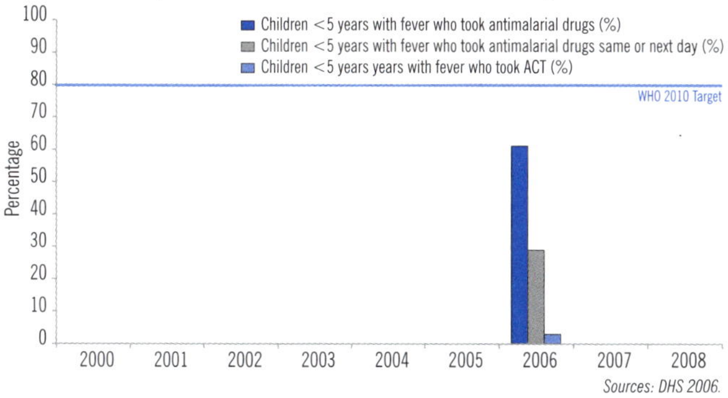

Legend:
- Children <5 years with fever who took antimalarial drugs (%)
- Children <5 years with fever who took antimalarial drugs same or next day (%)
- Children <5 years years with fever who took ACT (%)

WHO 2010 Target

Sources: DHS 2006.

Access to effective treatment: programme data

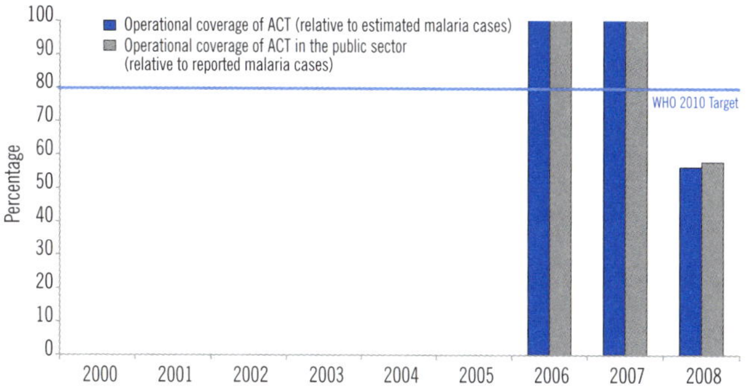

Legend:
- Operational coverage of ACT (relative to estimated malaria cases)
- Operational coverage of ACT in the public sector (relative to reported malaria cases)

WHO 2010 Target

Year	Pregnant women who slept under any net (%)	Pregnant women who slept under an ITN (%)	Children < 5 years with fever (%)	Febrile children < 5 years who sought treatment in HF (%)	Number of households protected by IRS	Number of people protected by IRS	Number of ITNs and/or LLINs	Number of 1st-line treatment courses received	Number of ACT treatment courses received
2000		1	–	–					
2001									
2002									
2003									
2004			–	–					
2005							319 000		
2006	24	10	–	–	103 329	470 000	1 999 449		14 570 670
2007					466 477	1 963 945	1 622 001		16 919 100
2008					499 998	1 858 149	2 273 413		6 389 600

IV. FINANCING MALARIA CONTROL

Governmental and external financing

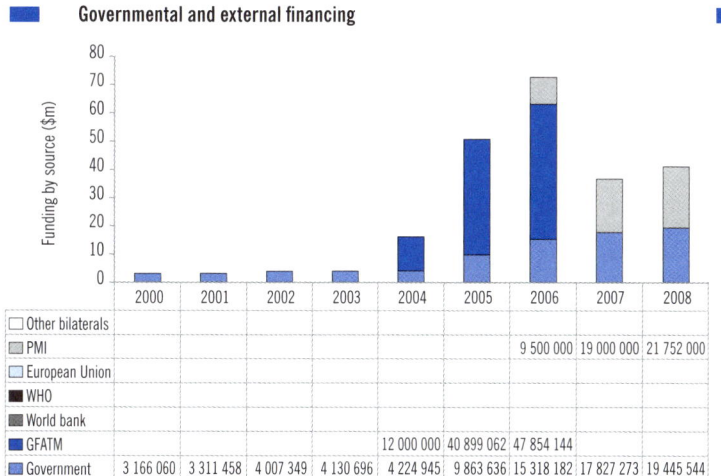

	2000	2001	2002	2003	2004	2005	2006	2007	2008
☐ Other bilaterals									
☐ PMI								9 500 000	19 000 000	21 752 000
☐ European Union									
■ WHO									
■ World bank									
■ GFATM						12 000 000	40 899 062	47 854 144	
☐ Government	3 166 060	3 311 458	4 007 349	4 130 696	4 224 945	9 863 636	15 318 182	17 827 273	19 445 544

Breakdown of expenditure by intervention in 2008

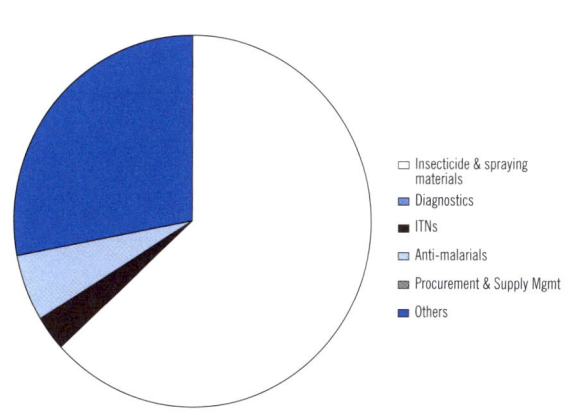

Legend:
- ☐ Insecticide & spraying materials
- ☐ Diagnostics
- ■ ITNs
- ☐ Anti-malarials
- ■ Procurement & Supply Mgmt
- ■ Others

V. SOURCE OF INFORMATION

PROGRAMME DATA		SURVEY AND OTHER DATA	
Reported cases	Surveillance data	Insecticide-treated nets (ITN)	DHS 2000-01, AIS 2004-05, DHS 2006
Operational coverage of ITNs, IRS and access to medicines	Programme report	Treatment	DHS 2006
Financial data	Programme report	Use of health services	DHS 2006

UNITED REPUBLIC OF TANZANIA

The United Republic of Tanzania had an estimated 11 million malaria cases in 2006. Transmission occurs all year round, with seasonal peaks. Most cases are caused by *P. falciparum*, but only a fraction are parasitologically tested. Between 2003 and 2008, 11 million cases and 17 thousand deaths were reported annually. While the nationwide trends are unclear due to limited data from the mainland, the numbers of confirmed malaria cases, inpatient cases and deaths have been significantly reduced in Zanzibar subsequent to the scale-up of LLINs, IRS and ACT. The island delivered 500 000 LLINs during 2006–2008, enough to cover the entire population at risk, implemented IRS covering 213 000 households and protecting the entire 1.1 million population in several rounds, and delivered ACT in all facilities. The data available from the mainland do not show a similar impact. On the mainland, 1.3 million LLINs were distributed during 2006–2008 and 1.8 million conventional ITNs in 2008, adequate to protect less than 10% of the population at risk. IRS was conducted in 2008, covering 100 000 households and protecting 190 000 people at risk. The national malaria control programme delivered 23 million ACT treatment courses in 2007, sufficient to treat all reported cases in the public sector. No information on funding after 2003 was provided by the programme, but it is known that expenditure on malaria control has increased markedly with Global Fund grants providing over US$ 327 million in rounds 1, 4, 7 and 8 and over US$ 20 million annually from the United States President's Malaria Initiative.

I. EPIDEMIOLOGICAL PROFILE

Population, endemicity and malaria burden

Population (in thousands)	2008	%
All age groups	42 484	
< 5 years	7 566	18
≥ 5 years	34 918	82

Population by malaria endemicity (in thousands)	2008	%
High transmission ≥ 1/1000	30 932	73
Low transmission (0–1/1000)	11 552	27
Malaria-free (0 cases)	0	0
Rural population	31 662	75

Vector and parasite profiles

Major *Anopheles* species	*gambiae, arabiensis, funestus, coustani, merus, nili, paludis, pharoensis*
Plasmodium species	*falciparum, vivax*

Stratification of burden (reported cases, per 1000)

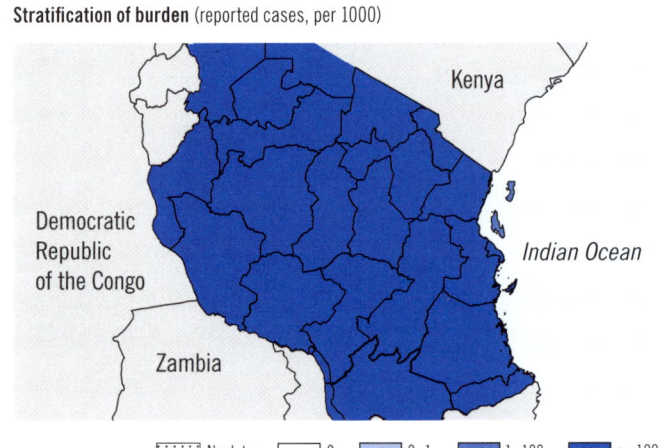

No data | 0 | 0–1 | 1–100 | > 100

Trends in malaria morbidity and mortality

Reported malaria cases, per 1000

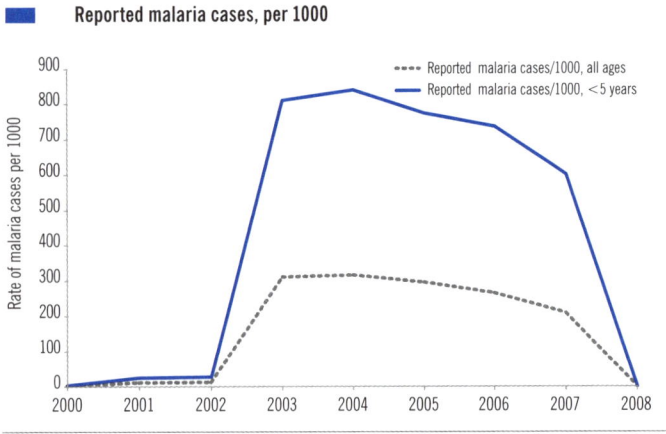

Rate of examination, case confirmation, malaria test positivity, % of confirmed cases that are *P. falciparum*

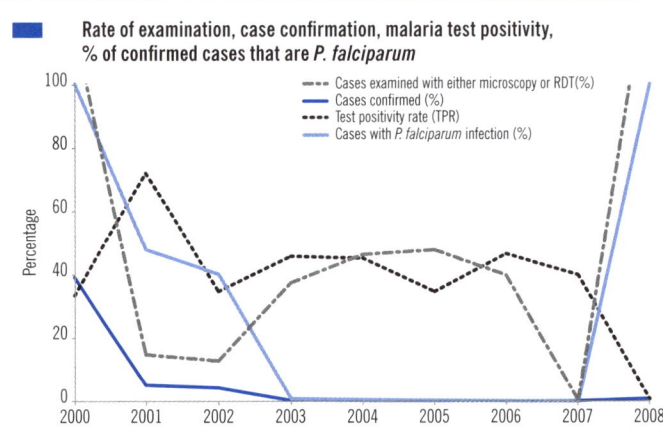

Year	Reported malaria cases, all ages	Reported malaria cases, < 5 years	All-cause outpatient consultations, all ages	All-cause outpatient consultations, < 5 years	Examined	Positive	*P. falciparum*	Reporting completeness of outpatient health facilities (%)	Reporting completeness of districts (%)
2000	45 643	23 350	116 932	54 921	53 533	17 734	17 734		100
2001	369 474	155 189	661 450	317 713	53 804	18 385	18 385		100
2002	413 361	174 899	755 873	368 256	51 968	16 983	16 983		100
2003	11 418 731	5 244 254	28 165 762	12 139 594	4 243 853	15 751	15 705		100
2004	11 930 393	5 605 674	29 595 179	13 093 731	5 489 733	11 981	11 936		100
2005	11 466 713	5 332 548	26 985 965	11 390 100	5 443 908	7 677	7 628		100
2006	10 582 608	5 237 555	24 297 806	11 799 502	4 181 569	1 633	1 585		100
2007	8 571 839	4 410 779	19 109 304	10 055 945	23 511*	293*	293*		100
2008	9 611*	4 689*	110 542*	41 411*	13 183*	67*	67*		100

* Data belongs to Zanzibar only.

Reported malaria admissions, per 1000

- - - - Reported malaria admisison/1000, all ages
——— Reported malaria admisison/1000, <5 years

Reported malaria deaths, per 1000

- - - - Reported malaria deaths/1000, all ages
——— Reported malaria deaths/1000, <5 years

Year	Reported malaria admissions, all ages	Reported malaria admissions, < 5 years	All-cause admissions, all ages	All-cause admissions, < 5 years	Reported malaria deaths, all ages	Reported malaria deaths, < 5 years	All-cause deaths, all ages	All-cause deaths, < 5 years	Reporting completeness of inpatient health facilities (%)	Reporting completeness of districts (%)
2000	9 806	5 407	23 525	10 552	379	252	736	490		
2001	26 029	12 956	70 623	25 944	1 228	1 087	3 241	1 559		
2002	28 062	12 805	70 736	26 296	815	673	2 559	1 249		
2003	195 930	117 174	1 467 822	732 878	15 251	15 121	45 893	21 939		
2004	300 985	178 491	2 242 559	1 204 794	19 859	19 734	60 831	31 245		
2005	737 343	333 465	2 855 465	1 225 897	18 322	18 238	71 687	30 781		
2006	291 913	170 637	2 584 264	1 225 388	20 962	20 913	56 184	21 454		
2007	486 847	1 128*	1 005 042	6 501*	12 593	36*	35 476	187*		
2008	1 878*	861*	19 402*	5 250*	29*	23*	379*	186*		

* Data belongs to Zanzibar only.

II.   INTERVENTION POLICIES AND STRATEGIES

Intervention	WHO-RECOMMENDED POLICIES / STRATEGIES	Yes or No	Year adopted	OPTIONAL POLICIES / STRATEGIES	Yes or No	Year adoped
Insecticide-treated nets (ITN)	Distribution of ITN/LLINs – Free	–	–	Distribution – Antenatal care	Yes	2004
	Targeting all age groups	No	–	Distribution – EPI routine and campaign	Yes	2005
				Targeting children < 5 years and pregnant women	Yes	2004
				ITN distribution is subsidized	–	–
Indoor residual spraying (IRS)	IRS is a primary vector control intervention	No	–	Insecticide-resistance management implemented	No	–
	DDT is used for IRS (public health) only	No	–	Where IRS is conducted, other options are also implemented, e.g. ITN	Yes	2007
				IRS is used for prevention and control of epidemics	Yes	2007
Intermittent preventive treatment (IPT)	IPT used to prevent malaria during pregnancy	Yes	2001			
Case management	Oral artemisinin monotherapies banned (prohibited from registration or removed from the system)	No	–	Parasitological confirmation for patients ≥ 5 years only	–	–
	Parasitological confirmation for patients of all ages	No	–	Malaria diagnosis is free of charge in the public sector	–	–
	ACT is free of charge for < 5 years old in the public sector	Yes	1998	ACT is free of charge for patients ≥ 5 years in the public sector	–	–
	Diagnosis of malaria of inpatients is based on parasitological confirmation	–	–	ACT is delivered at community level through community agents (beyond the health facilities)	–	–
	Pre-referral treatment with quinine or artemether IM or artesunate suppositories	Yes	2001	Uncomplicated malaria cases are admitted	–	–
	Oversight regulation of case management in the private sectors	–	–			
	RDTs used at community level	–	–			

Antimalarial policy	Type of medicine	Year adopted	Study year	Results of therapeutic efficacy tests					
				No. of studies	Median	Minimum	Maximum	Percentiles: 25%	75%
First-line treatment of *P. falciparum* (unconfirmed)	AS + AQ, AL	2004	2002–2005	2	12.1	10.8	13.4	10.8	13.4
First-line treatment of *P. falciparum* (confirmed)	AS + AQ, AL	2004	2002–2007	3	0	0	2.7	0	2.7
Treatment failure of *P. falciparum*	AL, QN(7d)	2004							
Treatment of severe malaria	QN(7d)	2004							
Treatment of *P. vivax*	–	–							

III. IMPLEMENTING MALARIA CONTROL

Coverage of ITN: survey data

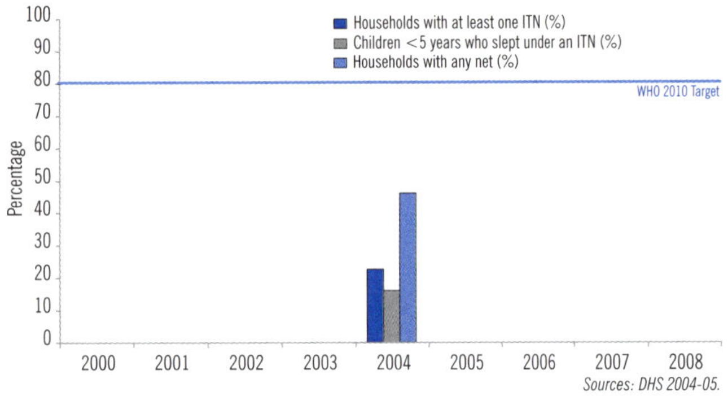

- Households with at least one ITN (%)
- Children <5 years who slept under an ITN (%)
- Households with any net (%)

WHO 2010 Target

Sources: DHS 2004-05.

Coverage of IRS and ITN: programme data

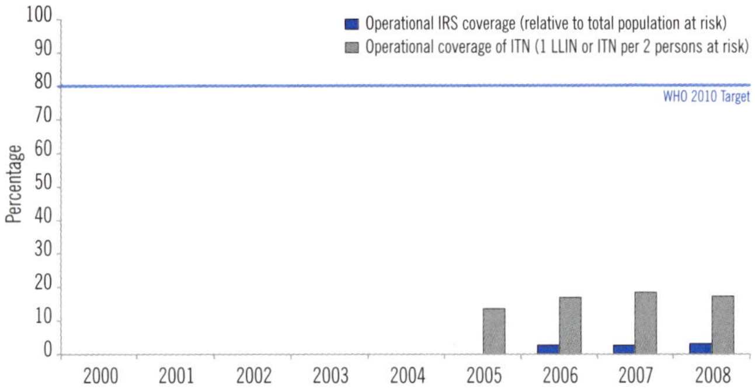

- Operational IRS coverage (relative to total population at risk)
- Operational coverage of ITN (1 LLIN or ITN per 2 persons at risk)

WHO 2010 Target

Access by febrile children to effective treatment: survey data

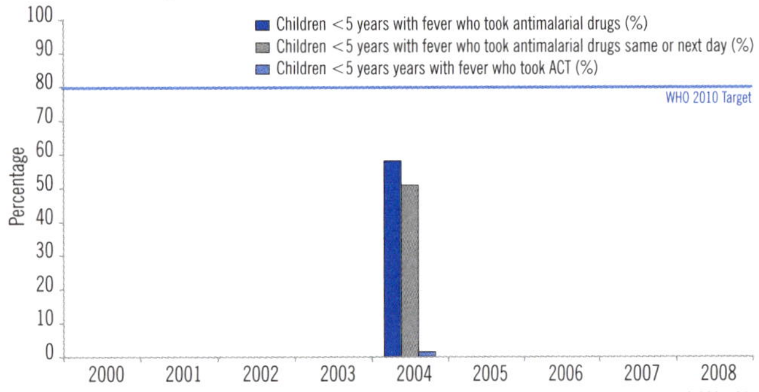

- Children <5 years with fever who took antimalarial drugs (%)
- Children <5 years with fever who took antimalarial drugs same or next day (%)
- Children <5 years years with fever who took ACT (%)

WHO 2010 Target

Sources: DHS 2004-05.

Access to effective treatment: programme data

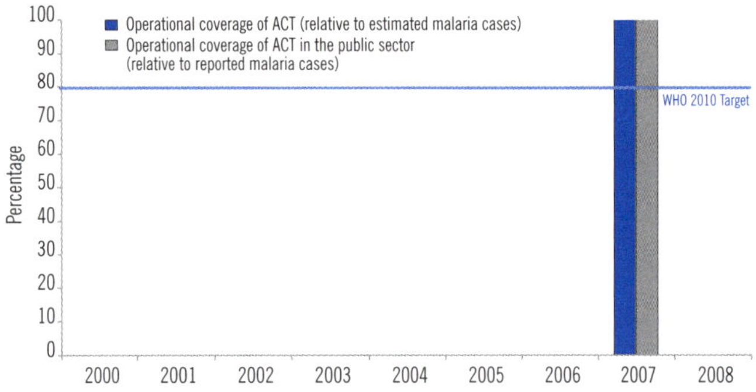

- Operational coverage of ACT (relative to estimated malaria cases)
- Operational coverage of ACT in the public sector (relative to reported malaria cases)

WHO 2010 Target

Year	Pregnant women who slept under any net (%)	Pregnant women who slept under an ITN (%)	Children < 5 years with fever (%)	Febrile children < 5 years who sought treatment in HF (%)	Number of households protected by IRS	Number of people protected by IRS	Number of ITNs and/or LLINs	Number of 1st-line treatment courses received	Number of ACT treatment courses received
2000									
2001									
2002								467 668	28 726	
2003								1 466 181	220 725	
2004		16	–	–			1 792 147	476 712	
2005							2 634 414	363 585	
2006					205 699	1 071 361	3 119 013	227 047	
2007					405 878	1 071 194	2 990 668	23 455 260	23 455 260
2008					295 385	1 308 194	2 271 330		

IV. FINANCING MALARIA CONTROL

Governmental and external financing

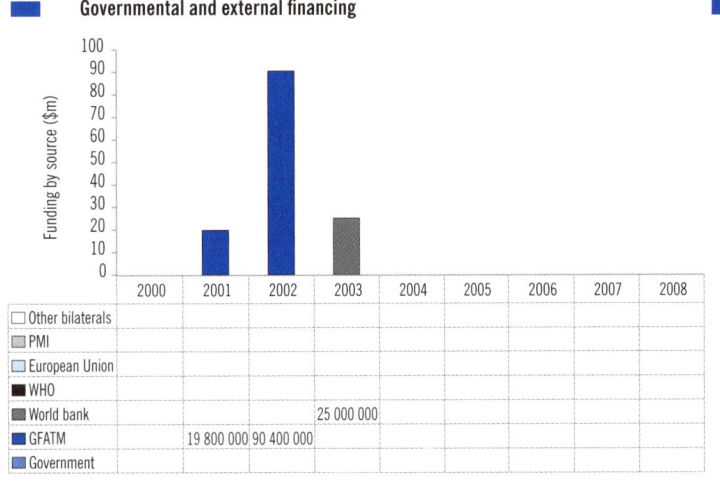

	2000	2001	2002	2003	2004	2005	2006	2007	2008
☐ Other bilaterals									
☐ PMI									
☐ European Union									
■ WHO									
■ World bank			25 000 000						
■ GFATM	19 800 000	90 400 000							
■ Government									

Breakdown of expenditure by intervention in 2008

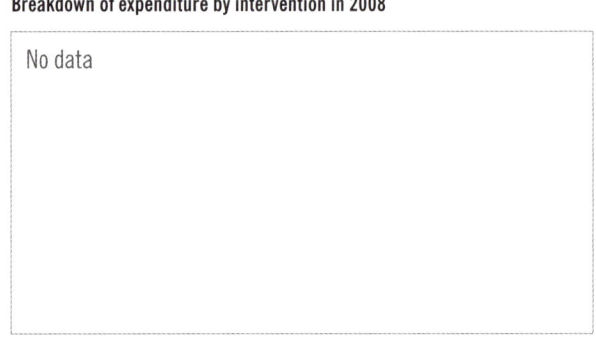

No data

V. SOURCE OF INFORMATION

PROGRAMME DATA		SURVEY AND OTHER DATA	
Reported cases	Surveillance data	Insecticide-treated nets (ITN)	DHS 1999, DHS 2004-05
Operational coverage of ITNs, IRS and access to medicines	Programme report	Treatment	DHS 1999, DHS 2004-05
Financial data	Programme report	Use of health services	DHS 2004

ZAMBIA

Malaria transmission is seasonal, occurring mainly from November to May. Most cases are due to *P. falciparum*, but little confirmation was done in the past. Surveillance data for 2008 showed decreases from the average for 2001–2003 (before interventions) of 55% in the number of inpatient malaria cases and 79% in the number of deaths in children under 5. The decreases for persons of all ages were 52% for inpatient malaria cases, 59% for inpatient deaths and 19% for outpatient cases. The decrease should be interpreted cautiously, however, because data for the third and fourth quarters of 2008 may be incomplete, as the country changed to a new health information system in mid-2008. An analysis by the Ministry of Health and WHO of data for the first and second quarters of each year showed significant decreases in the numbers of inpatient malaria cases and deaths at all ages of 55% and 60%, respectively, in 2008 from the averages for the first and second quarters of 2000–2002. Thus, the apparent impact is likely to be associated with the recent scale-up of interventions. The national malaria control programme delivered nearly 4.8 million LLINs during 2006–2008 (of which 2.1 million were delivered during the 2007 mass campaign), adequate to cover 80% of the population at risk. IRS has recently been expanded, covering 1 149 599 households and protecting 5.7 million (48%) people at risk in 2008. In the 2008 malaria indicator survey, 62% of households owned an ITN and 41% children under 5 slept under one, but only 13% of febrile children received ACT treatment. Funding for malaria has increased significantly, from less than US$ 5 million in 2002 to over US$ 17 million in 2008. The Government's expenditure on malaria is increasing, but major funding also comes from the Global Fund, the United States President's Malaria Initiative, the World Bank, United Nations agencies and nongovernmental organizations.

I.   EPIDEMIOLOGICAL PROFILE

Population, endemicity and malaria burden

Population (in thousands)	2008	%
All age groups	12 620	
< 5 years	2 282	18
≥ 5 years	10 338	82

Population by malaria endemicity (in thousands)	2008	%
High transmission ≥ 1/1000	12 620	100
Low transmission (0–1/1000)	0	0
Malaria-free (0 cases)	0	0
Rural population	8 159	65

Vector and parasite profiles

Major *Anopheles* species	*gambiae, arabiensis, funestus, nili, pharoensis, quadriannulatus*
Plasmodium species	*falciparum, vivax*

Stratification of burden (reported cases, per 1000)

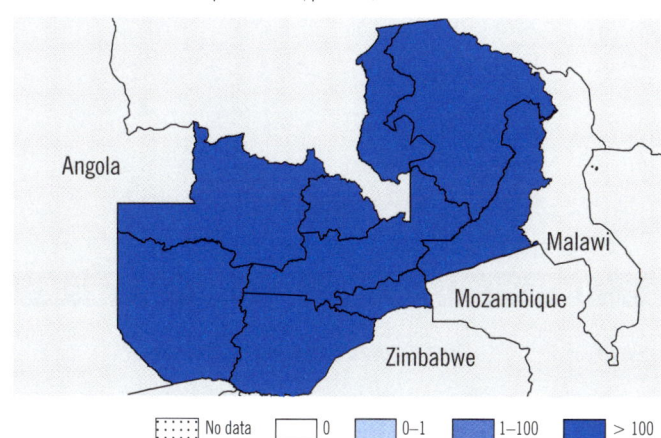

No data | 0 | 0–1 | 1–100 | > 100

Trends in malaria morbidity and mortality

Reported malaria cases, per 1000

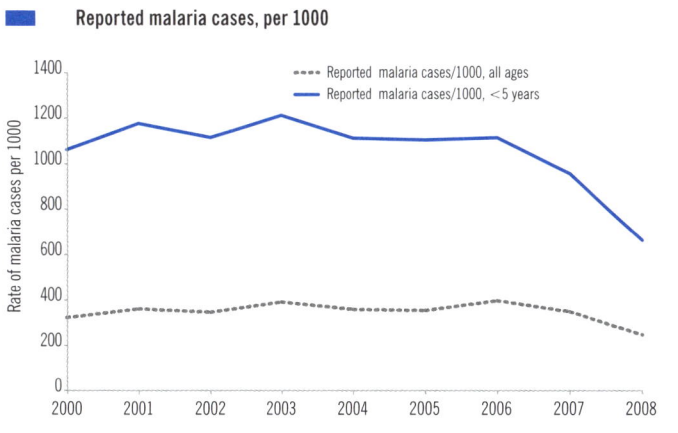

- - - - Reported malaria cases/1000, all ages
——— Reported malaria cases/1000, <5 years

Rate of examination, case confirmation, malaria test positivity, % of confirmed cases that are *P. falciparum*

No data

Year	Reported malaria cases, all ages	Reported malaria cases, < 5 years	All-cause outpatient consultations, all ages	All-cause outpatient consultations, < 5 years	Examined	Positive	*P. falciparum*	Reporting completeness of outpatient health facilities (%)	Reporting completeness of districts (%)
2000	3 337 796	2 016 333	9 230 639	4 856 786					
2001	3 838 402	2 295 738	10 133 545	5 334 699					
2002	3 760 335	2 230 107	10 347 966	5 299 233					
2003	4 346 172	2 480 157	11 970 827	5 972 557					
2004	4 078 234	2 324 580	11 252 589	5 534 795					
2005	4 121 356	2 360 307	11 567 755	5 680 460					
2006	4 731 338	2 434 135	13 283 617	5 872 543					
2007	4 248 295	2 133 915	13 277 766	5 559 399					
2008	3 080 301	1 508 448	11 565 345	4 675 281					

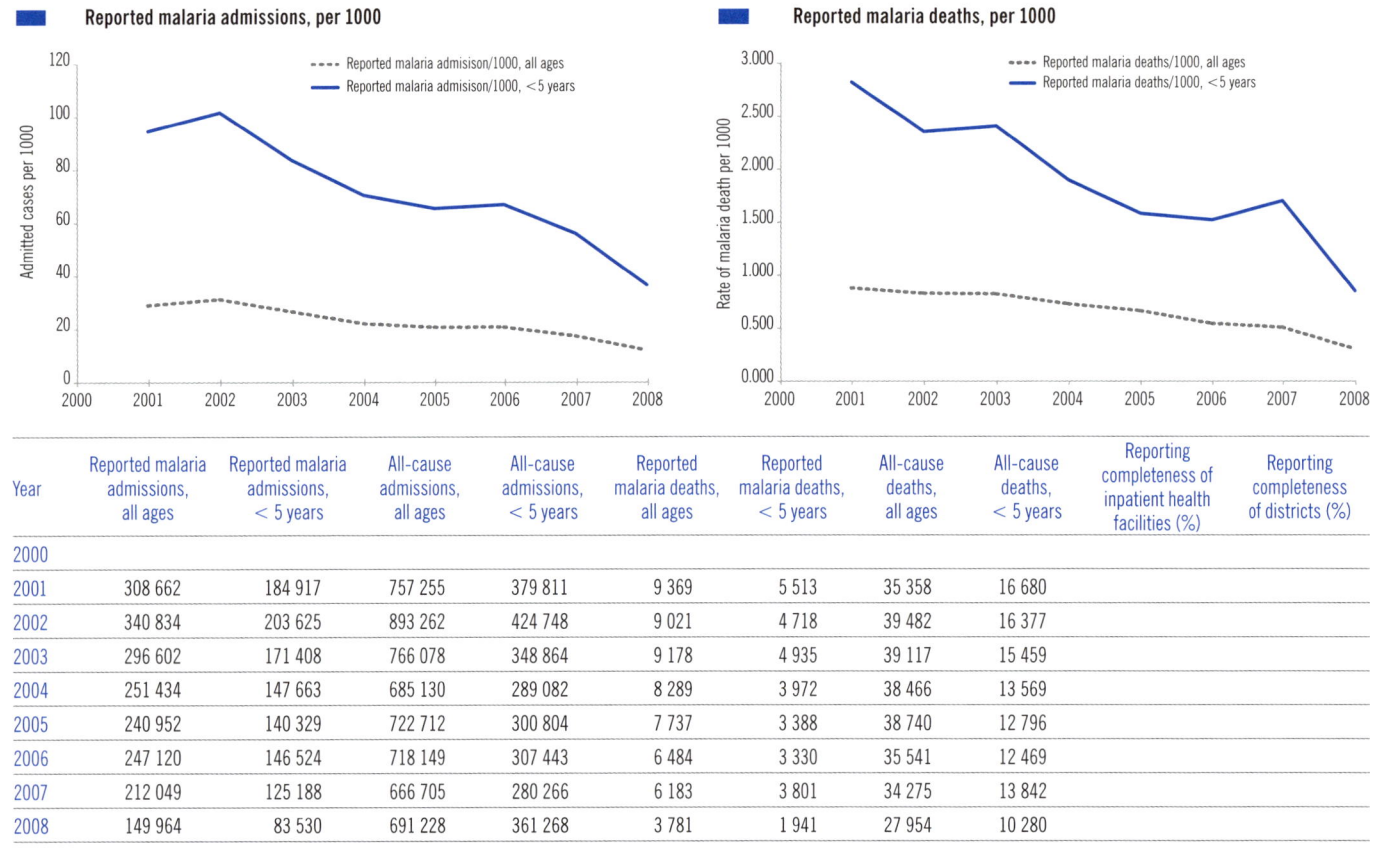

Reported malaria admissions, per 1000

- ---- Reported malaria admission/1000, all ages
- —— Reported malaria admission/1000, <5 years

Reported malaria deaths, per 1000

- ---- Reported malaria deaths/1000, all ages
- —— Reported malaria deaths/1000, <5 years

Year	Reported malaria admissions, all ages	Reported malaria admissions, < 5 years	All-cause admissions, all ages	All-cause admissions, < 5 years	Reported malaria deaths, all ages	Reported malaria deaths, < 5 years	All-cause deaths, all ages	All-cause deaths, < 5 years	Reporting completeness of inpatient health facilities (%)	Reporting completeness of districts (%)
2000										
2001	308 662	184 917	757 255	379 811	9 369	5 513	35 358	16 680		
2002	340 834	203 625	893 262	424 748	9 021	4 718	39 482	16 377		
2003	296 602	171 408	766 078	348 864	9 178	4 935	39 117	15 459		
2004	251 434	147 663	685 130	289 082	8 289	3 972	38 466	13 569		
2005	240 952	140 329	722 712	300 804	7 737	3 388	38 740	12 796		
2006	247 120	146 524	718 149	307 443	6 484	3 330	35 541	12 469		
2007	212 049	125 188	666 705	280 266	6 183	3 801	34 275	13 842		
2008	149 964	83 530	691 228	361 268	3 781	1 941	27 954	10 280		

II.   INTERVENTION POLICIES AND STRATEGIES

Intervention	WHO-RECOMMENDED POLICIES / STRATEGIES	Yes or No	Year adopted	OPTIONAL POLICIES / STRATEGIES	Yes or No	Year adoped
Insecticide-treated nets (ITN)	Distribution of ITN/LLINs – Free	Yes	2005	Distribution – Antenatal care	Yes	2001
	Targeting all age groups	Yes	1998	Distribution – EPI routine and campaign	Yes	2003
				Targeting children < 5 years and pregnant women	Yes	2000
				ITN distribution is subsidized	Yes	2001
Indoor residual spraying (IRS)	IRS is a primary vector control intervention	Yes	2000	Insecticide-resistance management implemented	Yes	2000
	DDT is used for IRS (public health) only	Yes	2001	Where IRS is conducted, other options are also implemented, e.g. ITN	Yes	2001
				IRS is used for prevention and control of epidemics	Yes	2001
Intermittent preventive treatment (IPT)	IPT used to prevent malaria during pregnancy	Yes	2001			
Case management	Oral artemisinin monotherapies banned (prohibited from registration or removed from the system)	Yes	2003	Parasitological confirmation for patients ≥ 5 years only	Yes	2001
	Parasitological confirmation for patients of all ages	Yes	2001	Malaria diagnosis is free of charge in the public sector	Yes	2000
	ACT is free of charge for < 5 years old in the public sector	Yes	2003	ACT is free of charge for patients ≥ 5 years in the public sector	Yes	2003
	Diagnosis of malaria of inpatients is based on parasitological confirmation	Yes	2003	ACT is delivered at community level through community agents (beyond the health facilities)	Yes	2007
	Pre-referral treatment with quinine or artemether IM or artesunate suppositories	Yes	1998	Uncomplicated malaria cases are admitted	Yes	2000
	Oversight regulation of case management in the private sectors	No	–			
	RDTs used at community level	Yes	2007			

				Results of therapeutic efficacy tests						
Antimalarial policy	Type of medicine	Year adopted	Study year	No. of studies	Median	Minimum	Maximum	Percentiles:	25%	75%
First-line treatment of *P. falciparum* (unconfirmed)	AL	2002	2004–2005	10	0	0	0		0	0
First-line treatment of *P. falciparum* (confirmed)	AL	2002								
Treatment failure of *P. falciparum*	QN(7d)	2002								
Treatment of severe malaria	QN(7d)	2002								
Treatment of *P. vivax*	–	–								

III. IMPLEMENTING MALARIA CONTROL

Coverage of ITN: survey data

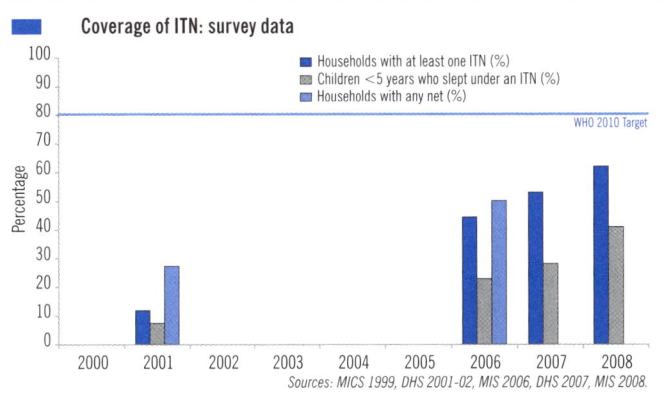

Legend:
- Households with at least one ITN (%)
- Children <5 years who slept under an ITN (%)
- Households with any net (%)

WHO 2010 Target

Sources: MICS 1999, DHS 2001-02, MIS 2006, DHS 2007, MIS 2008.

Coverage of IRS and ITN: programme data

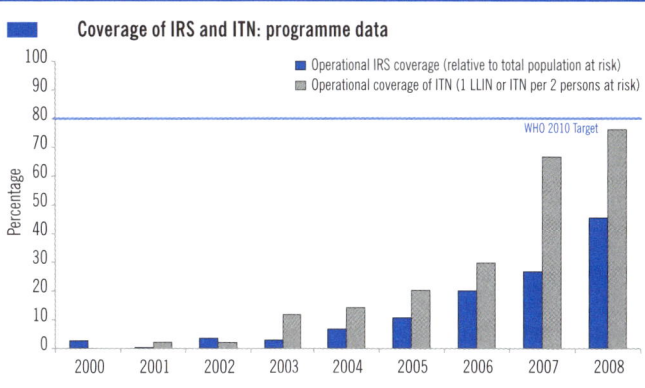

Legend:
- Operational IRS coverage (relative to total population at risk)
- Operational coverage of ITN (1 LLIN or ITN per 2 persons at risk)

WHO 2010 Target

Access by febrile children to effective treatment: survey data

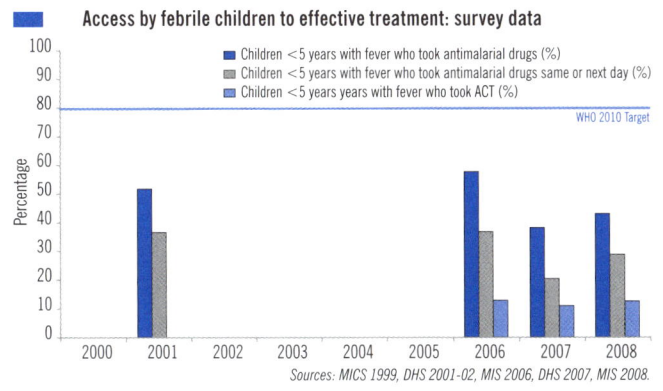

Legend:
- Children <5 years with fever who took antimalarial drugs (%)
- Children <5 years with fever who took antimalarial drugs same or next day (%)
- Children <5 years years with fever who took ACT (%)

WHO 2010 Target

Sources: MICS 1999, DHS 2001-02, MIS 2006, DHS 2007, MIS 2008.

Access to effective treatment: programme data

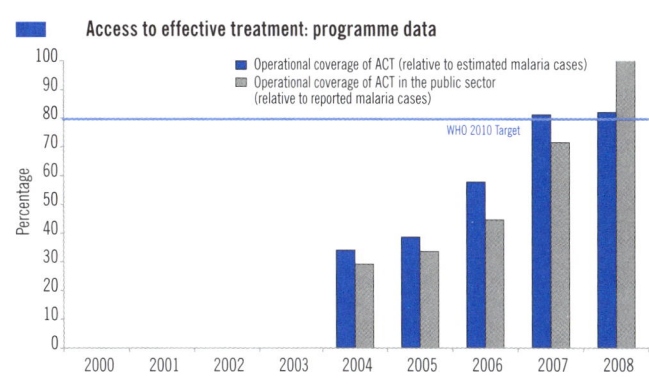

Legend:
- Operational coverage of ACT (relative to estimated malaria cases)
- Operational coverage of ACT in the public sector (relative to reported malaria cases)

WHO 2010 Target

Year	Pregnant women who slept under any net (%)	Pregnant women who slept under an ITN (%)	Children < 5 years with fever (%)	Febrile children < 5 years who sought treatment in HF (%)	Number of households protected by IRS	Number of people protected by IRS	Number of ITNs and/or LLINs	Number of 1st-line treatment courses received	Number of ACT treatment courses received
2000						279 321			
2001	17	9	–	–		37 890	115 891		
2002						391 926	112 020		
2003						324 137	557 071		
2004						772 644	176 082	1 184 698	1 184 698
2005						1 251 701	516 999	1 379 955	1 379 955
2006		24	–	–		2 408 080	1 162 578	2 111 348	2 111 348
2007			–	–		3 288 475	2 458 183	3 036 982	3 036 982
2008			–	–		5 747 995	1 188 443	3 142 405	3 142 405

IV. FINANCING MALARIA CONTROL

Governmental and external financing

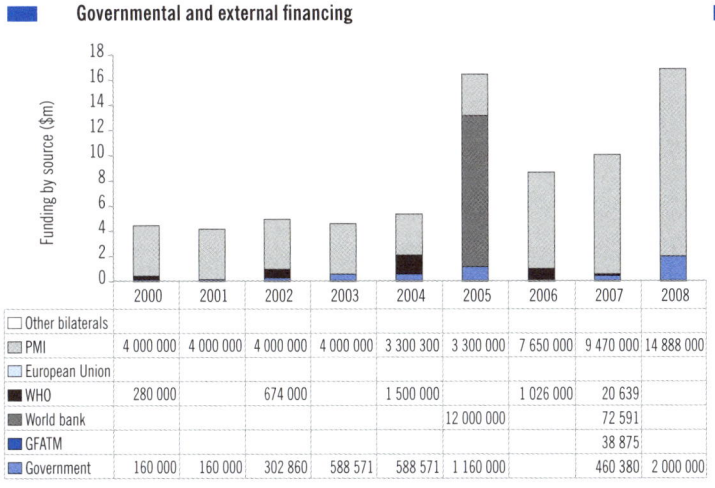

	2000	2001	2002	2003	2004	2005	2006	2007	2008
Other bilaterals									
PMI	4 000 000	4 000 000	4 000 000	4 000 000	3 300 300	3 300 000	7 650 000	9 470 000	14 888 000
European Union									
WHO	280 000		674 000		1 500 000		1 026 000	20 639	
World bank						12 000 000		72 591	
GFATM								38 875	
Government	160 000	160 000	302 860	588 571	588 571	1 160 000		460 380	2 000 000

Breakdown of expenditure by intervention in 2008

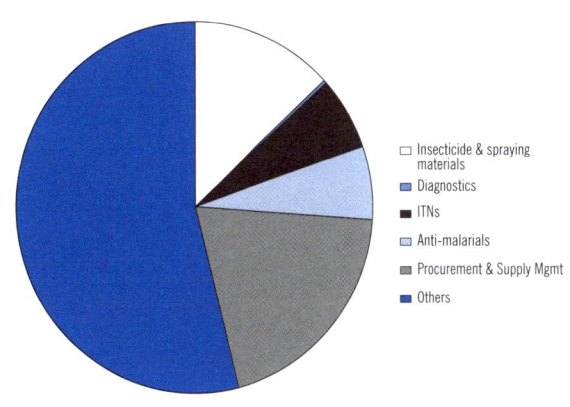

Legend:
- Insecticide & spraying materials
- Diagnostics
- ITNs
- Anti-malarials
- Procurement & Supply Mgmt
- Others

V. SOURCE OF INFORMATION

PROGRAMME DATA		SURVEY AND OTHER DATA	
Reported cases	Surveillance data	Insecticide-treated nets (ITN)	MICS 1999, DHS 2001-02, MIS 2006, DHS 2007, MIS 2008
Operational coverage of ITNs, IRS and access to medicines	Programme report	Treatment	MICS 1999, DHS 2001-02, MIS 2006, DHS 2007, MIS 2008
Financial data	Programme report	Use of health services	DHS 2001

ANNEXES

Annex 1. Methods for preparing the country profiles

This annex describes the methods used for preparing country profiles but which also apply to other sections.

A.1   Epidemiological profile

Population

The total population of each country is taken from the World population prospects, 2008 revision *(1)*. The population of children < 5 years of age is also given, as this age group is particularly susceptible to malaria infection and disease.

Population by malaria endemicity

The country population is subdivided into three levels of malaria endemicity, as reported by the national malaria control programme:

1. Areas of high transmission, where the reported incidence of malaria due to all species was 1 or more per 1000 population per year in 2008

2. Areas of low transmission, where the reported malaria case incidence from all species was < 1 per 1000 population per year in 2008 but greater than 0. Transmission in these areas is generally highly seasonal, with or without epidemic peaks.

3. Malaria-free areas, where there is no continuing, local, mosquito-borne malaria transmission, and all reported malaria cases are imported *(2)*. An area is designated malaria-free when no cases have occurred for several years. Areas may be malaria-free due to environmental factors or as a result of effective control efforts. In practice, malaria-free areas can be accurately designated by national programmes only after taking into account the local epidemiological situation and the results of entomological and biomarker investigations. If a national malaria control programme did not provide the number of people living in high- and low-risk areas, the numbers were inferred from subnational case incidence data provided by the programme.

Population at risk

The total population living in areas where malaria is endemic (low and high transmission), excluding the population living in malaria-free areas. The population at risk is often used as the denominator in calculating operational coverage of malaria interventions, and hence in assessing current and future needs, taking into account the population already covered.

Maps of malaria, country profiles

Epidemiological maps for each country are based on the malaria cases reported in 2008 at the first or lower administrative levels.

Four levels of endemicity are depicted:

- ≥ 100 cases per 1000 population per year;
- ≥ 1 cases per 1000 population per year and < 100 cases;
- < 1 case per 1000 population per year but > zero; and
- 0 recorded cases.

The first two categories correspond to the high-transmission category described above. It should be noted that case incidence rates for 2008 do not necessarily reflect the endemicity of areas in previous years. If subnational data on population or malaria cases were lacking, an administrative unit was labelled "no data" on the map. In some cases, the subnational data provided by a malaria control programme did not correspond to a mapping area known to WHO. This may be the result of modifications to administrative boundaries or the use of names not verifiable by WHO.

Vector and parasite profile

The species of mosquito responsible for malaria transmission in a county and the species of *Plasmodium* involved are listed according to information provided by WHO regional offices.

Reported malaria cases

Reported malaria cases = probable + confirmed.

Probable malaria cases = suspected cases not tested, but reported as malaria

In high transmission countries of the WHO African Region, where there is no adequate parasitological testing, probable cases are usually equal to suspected malaria cases.

Slide examination, case confirmation, Plasmodium *spp.*

A table in the epidemiolical profile gives the reported number of slides examined, the number positive and the number with a *P. falciparum* infection (including mixed *P. falciparum* and *P. vivax*). The graph shows four indicators:

- *percentage of cases examined microscopically:* number of cases examined under a microscope or with a RDT in every 100 suspected malaria cases. It indicates the extent to which a programme can provide diagnostic services to patients attending health facilities.

- *percentage of cases confirmed:* number of confirmed malaria cases per 100 reported (probable and confirmed) malaria cases. This indicates the extent to which a country programme depends on confirmation of malaria cases for diagnosis, treatment and epidemiological assessment.

- *malaria test positivity rate:* number of parasitologically positive cases per 100 cases examined (by RDT or microscopically). This measures the prevalence of malaria parasites among people who seek care and are examined in health facilities.

- *percentage of cases with P. falciparum infection:* number of *P. falciparum* cases per 100 microscopically confirmed malaria cases.

A.2 Intervention policies and targets

This section of the profile shows the policies and strategies adopted by each country for malaria prevention, diagnosis and treatment. Policies may vary according to the epidemiological setting, socioeconomic factors and the capacity of the national malaria programme or country health system. Adoption of policies does not necessarily imply immediate implementation, nor does it indicate full, continuous implementation nationwide. Policies and strategies are divided into those recommended by WHO and those that are optional. WHO-recommended policies and strategies include (see also Chapter 2):

- provision of free or highly-subsidized long-lasting insecticide-impregnated nets to persons in all age groups at risk for malaria (3);

- use of IRS, including with DDT (4);

- use of intermittent preventive treatment in highly endemic countries with comparatively low levels of resistance to sulfadoxine-pyrimethamine (5);

- parasitological confirmation for persons in all age groups;

- banning of oral artemisinin monotherapies; and

- provision of ACT, free or highly subsidized in the public sector, for malaria cases infected with P. falciparum (6).

Optional policies or strategies are those adopted by countries after taking local epidemiological and other circumstances into account. "Yes" implies that the policy or strategy is adopted regardless of the scale of implementation; "No" implies that the policy is not adopted; and "Not applicable" implies that the policy is irrelevant to the country situation. The year of adoption of a policy is that in which it was approved by a national malaria control programme. It does not take into account any change that may have occurred after the reports were received.

A.3 Implementing malaria control

Coverage with ITNs, from survey data

The percentage of households that own at least one mosquito net and the percentage of children under 5 years who slept under a net are taken from nationally representative household surveys, such as multiple indicator cluster surveys, demographic health surveys and malaria indicator surveys. Other available national surveys were also included. The results of subnational surveys undertaken to support local project implementation are difficult to interpret nationwide and hence are not presented in the profiles, although they can be useful for assessing progress locally. It should be noted that most multiple indicator cluster and demographic health surveys are conducted during the dry season, for logistical reasons, and the estimates may not reflect use during peak malaria transmission (when ITN use may be higher).

Coverage with IRS and ITNs from programme data

Because many countries do not have recent national survey data, the numbers of mosquito nets distributed and houses sprayed were derived from the national malaria control programme and used to estimate operational coverage with ITNs and IRS. "Administrative" or operational coverage with ITN was calculated as the number of ITNs

distributed, divided by the population at risk (sum of populations living in low- and high-transmission areas) divided by 2 (a ratio of one ITN for every two persons, following WHO recommendations) and multiplied by 100 (2). As, on average, long-lasting insecticidal nets are considered to have a useful lifespan of 3 years, the cumulative total of mosquito nets distributed over the past 3 years is taken as the numerator for any particular year. Other ITNs are considered to have an average lifespan of 1 year; some nets will be effective for longer if re-treated with insecticide. Therefore, the numerator for long-lasting insecticidal nets and ITNs is the sum of the cumulative long-lasting insecticidal nets of the latest 3 years and the number of ITNs during the latest year. Re-treatment is not taken into account in this report and is in any case becoming less frequent with the advent of the long-lasting insecticidal nets. Such operational estimates contain no information about the geographical distribution of ITNs or their distribution within households. ITNs may be clustered in certain subpopulations, thus depriving others at risk, and the number of ITNs delivered to a household may exceed or fall short of the recommended ratio of one net per two people.

Operational coverage with IRS is calculated as the number of people living in a household where IRS has been conducted during the preceding 12 months, divided by the population at risk (the sum of populations living in low- and high-transmission areas) multiplied by 100. Respondents were asked to convert, where necessary, records of the number of built structures sprayed to number of households, where the average household consists of more than one structure. The number of people protected by IRS, provided by national malaria control programmes, was taken as the numerator. Programme data are the most important source of information for estimating coverage, as household surveys do not generally include questions on IRS. In addition, IRS is often focalized, carried out on a limited geographical scale, for which nationally representative household surveys may not provide an adequate sample size for coverage to be measured accurately. The percentage of people protected by IRS is a measure of the extent to which IRS is implemented or the extent to which the population at risk benefits from IRS nationwide. The data show neither the quality of spraying nor the geographical distribution of IRS coverage in a country, which is typically focal.

Access by febrile children to effective treatment, from survey data

Estimates of the percentage of children under 5 years of age with fever who were treated with antimalarial medicines, together with the type of antimalarial medicine, were obtained from nationally representative household surveys such as multiple indicator cluster, demographic health and malaria indicator surveys. These estimates should be interpreted with the following provisos:

- Not all cases of fever are malaria, particularly in low-transmission areas, so 100% of febrile children cannot be expected to receive an antimalarial agent, particularly if they seek formal health care and laboratory diagnosis excludes malaria.

- Most multiple indicator cluster and demographic health surveys are conducted during the dry season, and the data may not reflect the year-round incidence of malarial disease or the provision of antimalarial treatment during the period of peak incidence.

- As it may be difficult to exclude some non-malarious areas from the analysis, the rates of antimalarial treatment relative to the estimated need may appear unduly low.

- Respondents to household surveys may not recall accurately the type of medicine given to children. The graph in the profile shows the use of any antimalarial agent and use of ACT. Access to ACT may also appear unduly low in countries where chloroquine is used to treat *P. vivax*, especially where *P. vivax* causes a high proportion of malaria cases. As ACT was introduced comparatively recently, surveys commonly report only on the use of any antimalarial agent.

- In the absence of diagnosis, care-givers and patients may consider other diseases as the cause of the fever and hence provide other medicines, such as paracetamol or antibiotics.

Access to effective treatment, from programme data

Access to effective treatment is estimated as the number of ACT treatment courses delivered by a national malaria control programme per 100 cases requiring treatment in a year. The number requiring treatment in a year depends not only on the incidence of malaria but also on the rate of case confirmation. In countries in which all cases are confirmed, the number requiring treatment will be the number of confirmed cases. In countries where cases are not confirmed, it will be the number of reported malaria cases.

A.4 Financing malaria control

Government and external financing

National malaria control programme budgets and expenditures may be used to assess the extent to which the programmes can maintain or scale up access to malaria prevention, diagnosis and treatment. The data shown are those reported by the programme. The first graph shows financial contributions by source or name of agency by year. The government contribution is usually the declared government expenditure for the year. When government expenditure was not reported by the programme, the government budget was used. External contributions are contributions allocated to the programme by external agencies, which may or may not be disbursed. Additional information about contributions from specific donors, as reported by the donors themselves, is given in Annex 5.

Breakdown of expenditure by intervention

The pie chart shows the proportion of all malaria funding, spent on different activities: ITNs, IRS, diagnosis, treatment and other programme-related expenses. All countries were requested to convert their local currencies into 2008 US$. The quantities have not been adjusted for purchasing power parity. When annual plans are completed as anticipated, the amounts shown should be about the same as the total amount received by the programme. Some divergence may occur, however, due to unexpectedly slow or fast disbursement of donor contributions or implementation or to changes in plans, prices and other factors. There may also be differences in the completeness of data, and the expenditures on activities listed may not include all items of expenditure. Despite the various uncertainties associated with these data, the graphs highlight major changes in programme funding and expenditure.

A.5 Sources of information

The sources of data are shown at the end of each profile. The WHO Global Malaria Programme has created a database containing the information used in compiling this Report. The data, together with profiles for all 109 malaria endemic countries, are available from www.who. int/topics/malaria/en/.

References

1. *World population prospects*. New York, United Nations, United Nations Population Division, 2008.

2. *Malaria elimination: a field manual for low and moderate endemic countries*. Geneva, World Health Organization, 2007.

3. *WHO position statement on ITNs*. Geneva, World Health Organization, Global Malaria Programme, Global Malaria Programme, 2007.

4. *Use of indoor residual spraying for scaling up global malaria control and elimination*. Geneva, World Health Organization, 2006 (WHO/HTM/MAL/2006.1112).

5. *A strategic framework for malaria prevention and control during pregnancy in the African Region*. Brazzaville WHO Regional Office for Africa, 2004 (AFRO/MAL/04/01).

6. *Guidelines for the treatment of malaria*. Geneva, World Health Organization, Global Malaria Programme, 2006 (WHO/HTM/MAL/2006.1108).

Annex 2 – Reported malaria cases and deaths, 2008

WHO region / Country/area	Population	Inpatient malaria cases	Malaria attributed deaths	Outpatient malaria cases	Malaria case definition	Mic. slides/RDTs taken	Mic. slides/RDTs positive	P. falciparum	P. vivax	Cases at community level
Africa										
Algeria	34,373,429	-	-	196	Probable and confirmed	11,964	196	185	10	-
Angola	18,020,665	106,345	9,465	2,151,072	Probable and confirmed	2,659,344	1,377,992	-	-	-
Benin	8,662,088	-	-	-	Suspected	-	-	-	-	-
Botswana	1,921,123	-	12	1,201	Probable and confirmed	1,201	1,201	-	-	-
Burkina Faso	15,233,882	356,989	7,834	3,688,338	Suspected	138,414	36,514	-	-	-
Burundi	8,074,253	16,788	226	876,741	Suspected	1,492,068	876,741	-	-	-
Cameroon	19,088,388	270,038	7,673	-	Suspected	-	-	-	-	142,121
Cape Verde	498,672	-	2	35	Probable and confirmed	6,033	35	35	0	-
Central African Republic	4,339,261	13,116	456	-	Suspected	-	-	-	-	-
Chad	10,913,667	3,757	1,018	472,460	Suspected	64,171	57,644	24,015	23,742	-
Comoros	660,723	-	47	-	Suspected	-	-	-	-	-
Congo	3,615,152	-	-	-	Suspected	-	-	-	-	-
Côte d'Ivoire	20,591,300	41,189	1,249	-	Suspected	-	-	-	-	-
Democratic Republic of the Congo	64,703,615	299,158	18,928	4,518,616	Suspected	2,314,880	1,462,300	1,196	27	4,710
Equatorial Guinea	659,200	7,571	-	77,456	Suspected	59,759	50,758	-	-	-
Eritrea	4,926,873	3,494	19	4,702	Probable and confirmed	42,482	4,702	1,269	2,028	55,619
Ethiopia	80,713,435	25,739	1,169	2,532,645	Probable and confirmed	986,323	458,561	274,657	173,300	-
Gabon	1,448,156	15,459	156	187,714	Suspected	151,137	40,701	40,701	-	-
Gambia	1,660,200	17,575	403	10,910	Suspected	-	10,910	-	-	-
Ghana	23,350,928	272,802	3,889	3,200,149	Suspected	827,436	827,438	-	-	-
Guinea	9,833,056	47,474	441	33,405	Suspected	-	33,405	33,405	-	-
Guinea-Bissau	1,575,447	-	487	128,758	Suspected	31,083	11,299	-	-	-
Kenya	38,765,310	-	-	6,078,783	Suspected	874,866	839,904	839,904	-	-
Liberia	3,793,394	46,887	345	606,952	Suspected	606,952	606,952	-	-	-
Madagascar	19,110,939	5,367	276	142,658	Suspected	299,000	89,138	-	-	-
Malawi	14,846,184	181,248	7,748	-	Suspected	-	-	-	-	-
Mali	12,705,737	151,910	1,227	-	Suspected	-	-	-	-	-
Mauritania	3,215,039	10,263	-	302	Suspected	1,555	302	-	-	-
Mauritius	1,279,800	-	-	-	-	-	-	-	-	-
Mozambique	22,382,535	120,259	4,424	-	Suspected	-	-	-	-	-
Namibia	2,129,855	4,907	171	4,907	Probable and confirmed	-	4,907	-	-	185,827
Niger	14,704,319	-	2,691	413,252	Suspected	1,466,095	413,252	-	-	-
Nigeria	151,212,257	538,487	8,677	143,079	Suspected	-	143,079	-	-	20,156
Rwanda	9,720,691	20,018	563	228,015	Probable and confirmed	1,640,106	228,015	-	-	-
Sao Tome and Principe	160,176	1,049	16	1,647	Probable and confirmed	38,583	1,572	-	-	-
Senegal	12,211,179	23,719	722	398,881	Suspected	505,045	202,466	33,062	-	73,340
Sierra Leone	5,559,852	3,554	871	154,459	Suspected	235,800	154,459	-	-	21,907
South Africa	49,667,629	-	43	-	Probable and confirmed	-	-	-	-	-
Swaziland	1,167,836	178	5	58	Probable and confirmed	0	58	58	0	-
Togo	6,458,607	20,014	2,663	898,112	Suspected	273,471	273,471	151,960	-	119,557
Uganda	31,656,865	154,423	2,372	9,751,004	Suspected	2,173,072	894,505	876,615	-	125,670
United Republic of Tanzania	42,483,926	1,878	29	67	Suspected	13,183	67	67	-	-
Zambia	12,620,220	149,964	3,781	493,805	Probable and confirmed	602,941	92,900	-	-	-
Zimbabwe	12,462,881	-	-	-	-	-	-	-	-	-

Annex 2 – Reported malaria cases and deaths, 2008 (continued)

WHO region	Country/area	Population	Inpatient malaria cases	Malaria attributed deaths	Outpatient malaria cases	Malaria case definition	Mic. slides/ RDTs taken	Mic. slides/ RDTs positive	P. falciparum	P. vivax	Cases at community level
Americas	Argentina	39,882,981	-	-	130	Probable and confirmed	1,104	130	0	130	-
	Bahamas	337,668	-	-	12	Probable and confirmed	35	12	-	-	-
	Belize	300,644	-	-	-	Probable and confirmed	-	-	-	-	-
	Bolivia (Plurinational State of)	9,694,113	-	-	9,894	Probable and confirmed	159,826	9,748	782	8,912	-
	Brazil	191,971,509	4,039	51	315,642	Probable and confirmed	2,721,017	315,642	46,289	266,299	-
	Colombia	45,012,093	223	22	80,559	Probable and confirmed	465,381	80,559	21,475	56,838	-
	Costa Rica	4,519,126	-	-	966	Probable and confirmed	17,304	966	0	966	-
	Dominican Republic	9,952,711	-	9	1,262	Probable and confirmed	153,093	1,262	1,839	1	-
	Ecuador	13,481,427	-	-	-	Probable and confirmed	-	-	-	-	-
	El Salvador	6,133,911	-	-	33	Probable and confirmed	97,872	33	0	32	-
	French Guiana	-	-	-	514	Probable and confirmed	11,994	514	1,077	920	-
	Guatemala	13,686,129	289	-	3,264	Probable and confirmed	120,464	3,264	40	7,148	-
	Guyana	763,437	-	1	11,815	Probable and confirmed	137,247	11,815	5,252	5,920	-
	Haiti	9,876,401	-	-	36,774	Probable and confirmed	168,950	36,774	36,768	6	-
	Honduras	7,318,788	-	-	8,225	Probable and confirmed	119,378	8,225	570	7,615	-
	Jamaica	2,707,664	-	-	86	Probable and confirmed	30,796	86	-	-	-
	Mexico	108,555,486	-	-	2,357	Probable and confirmed	1,246,780	2,357	0	2,357	-
	Nicaragua	5,667,325	-	-	764	Probable and confirmed	533,173	764	61	703	-
	Panama	3,398,820	22	-	744	Probable and confirmed	200,574	744	4	740	-
	Paraguay	6,237,857	-	-	1,341	Probable and confirmed	92,339	1,341	-	-	-
	Peru	28,836,700	-	-	-	Probable and confirmed	-	-	-	-	-
	Suriname	515,123	50	-	2,086	Probable and confirmed	28,137	2,086	802	639	-
	Venezuela (Bolivarian Republic of)	28,120,630	-	-	32,037	Probable and confirmed	414,137	32,037	5,021	26,437	-
Eastern Mediterranean	Afghanistan	27,208,326	4,434	46	467,123	Probable and confirmed	549,494	82,564	4,360	78,204	159,509
	Djibouti	849,251	41	-	3,569	Probable and confirmed	2,896	119	119	-	-
	Egypt	81,527,170	-	2	76	Probable and confirmed	-	76	76	-	-
	Iran (Islamic Republic of)	73,311,800	89	3	5,955	Probable and confirmed	218,273	5,955	938	10,337	-
	Iraq	30,096,252	1	0	6	Probable and confirmed	1,105,054	6	2	4	-
	Morocco	31,605,616	-	1	118	Probable and confirmed	-	118	118	-	-
	Oman	2,785,359	-	2	94	Probable and confirmed	-	94	94	-	-
	Pakistan	176,952,123	-	-	2,558,998	Probable and confirmed	2,054,533	59,284	24,550	79,868	-
	Saudi Arabia	25,200,516	-	1	1,491	Probable and confirmed	1,114,841	1,491	833	658	-
	Somalia	8,926,327	-	-	24,136	Probable and confirmed	73,985	23,905	23,427	-	-
	Sudan*	41,347,723	111,934	1,125	3,073,996	Probable and confirmed	127,512	457,362	-	-	-
	Syrian Arab Republic	21,226,921	-	1	46	Probable and confirmed	-	46	46	-	-
	Yemen	-	-	-	-		-	-	-	-	-

Annex 2 – Reported malaria cases and deaths, 2008 (continued)

WHO region	Country/area	Population	Inpatient malaria cases	Malaria attributed deaths	Outpatient malaria cases	Malaria case definition	Mic. slides/ RDTs taken	Mic. slides/ RDTs positive	P. falciparum	P. vivax	Cases at community level
Europe	Armenia	3,077,084	0	-	1	Probable and confirmed	471	1	1	0	-
	Azerbaijan	8,730,533	0	0	73	Probable and confirmed	183,949	73	73	72	0
	Georgia	4,307,011	0	-	6	Probable and confirmed	6	6	6	7	-
	Kyrgyzstan	5,413,644	18	0	18	Probable and confirmed	40,833	18	0	18	-
	Russian Federation	141,394,300	-	-	-	Probable and confirmed	-	-	-	-	-
	Tajikistan	6,836,084	-	-	318	Probable and confirmed	158,068	318	2	316	-
	Turkey	73,914,259	23	3	136	Probable and confirmed	55,856	136	23	191	-
	Turkmenistan	5,043,615	1	-	1	Probable and confirmed	75,524	1	-	1	-
	Uzbekistan	27,191,284	27	0	27	Probable and confirmed	883,807	27	27	27	-
South-East Asia	Bangladesh	160,000,129	3,042	154	168,662	Probable and confirmed	442,506	84,690	70,331	14,409	-
	Bhutan	686,787	240	4	329	Probable and confirmed	47,268	329	136	148	-
	Democratic People's Republic of Korea	23,818,755	-	-	-	Probable and confirmed	-	-	-	-	-
	Democratic Republic of Timor-Leste	1,098,385	-	31	143,594	Probable and confirmed	92,870	45,973	45,973	11,295	-
	India	1,181,411,912	-	1,061	1,532,467	Probable and confirmed	95,368,303	1,532,467	771,670	747,971	-
	Indonesia	227,345,081	-	669	1,206,261	Probable and confirmed	1,243,744	343,048	163,222	175,237	-
	Myanmar	49,563,015	47,553	1,088	566,204	Probable and confirmed	948,937	411,494	447,993	3,096	-
	Nepal	28,809,526	79	-	106,100	Probable and confirmed	153,331	3,888	629	623	-
	Sri Lanka	20,060,639	-	0	670	Probable and confirmed	1,047,104	670	46	-	-
	Thailand	67,386,383	2,689	101	26,150	Probable and confirmed	1,910,982	26,150	12,108	13,886	26,150
Western Pacific	Cambodia	14,562,007	4,513	209	42,124	Probable and confirmed	130,995	42,124	15,095	4,625	24,439
	China	1,344,919,642	-	23	16,650	Probable and confirmed	4,316,976	16,650	1,222	15,323	-
	Lao People's Democratic Republic	6,205,337	1,110	13	18,566	Probable and confirmed	262,973	17,648	4,697	247	-
	Malaysia	27,014,343	3,617	29	5,598	Probable and confirmed	588,489	5,598	2,268	3,820	-
	Papua New Guinea	6,576,821	23,508	628	1,450,609	Probable and confirmed	246,641	84,452	60,000	16,806	-
	Philippines	90,348,440	343	-	23,655	Probable and confirmed	287,189	23,655	11,807	4,806	-
	Republic of Korea	48,152,296	482	0	1,052	Probable and confirmed	1,052	1,052	-	-	-
	Solomon Islands	510,671	731	21	102,140	Probable and confirmed	279,972	40,535	29,492	11,173	-
	Vanuatu	233,866	257	1	3,477	Probable and confirmed	30,267	3,477	1,579	1,850	-
	Viet Nam	87,095,913	8,758	25	11,355	Probable and confirmed	1,369,452	11,355	8,901	2,348	-

Notes:

Mayotte is one of the 108 countries/areas with malarious areas but is not included in the annexes.

Mauritius is one of the countries listed but it has had no ongoing local transmission for over a decade.

*Data for Sudan only represents 15 northern states.

Annex 3.A – Reported malaria cases, 1990–2008

WHO region	Country/area	1990	1991	1992	1993	1994	1995	1996	1997	1998	1999	2000	2001	2002	2003	2004	2005	2006	2007	2008
Africa	Algeria	152	229	106	84	206	107	221	197		701	541	435	307	427	163	299	117	288	196
	Angola	243,673	1,143,701	782,988	722,981	667,376	156,603	623,396	893,232	1,169,028	1,471,993	2,080,348	1,249,761	1,862,662	3,246,258	2,489,170	889,572	1,029,198	1,295,535	1,377,992
	Benin	92,870	118,796	290,868	403,327	546,827	579,300	80,004	670,857	650,025	709,348		717,290	782,818	819,256	853,034	803,462	861,847		
	Botswana	10,750	14,364	4,995	55,331	29,591	17,599		101,887	59,696	72,640	8,056	4,716	1,588	1,830	3,453	530	2,548	464	1,201
	Burkina Faso	496,513	448,917	420,186	502,275	472,355	501,020	582,658	672,752	721,480	867,866					18,256	21,335	44,265	44,246	36,514
	Burundi		787,796	664,413	478,693	189,066	932,794	974,226	670,857	831,481	1,936,584	308,095	312,015	327,138	353,459	363,395	327,464	649,756	860,606	876,741
	Cameroon	869,048	568,938	773,539	828,429		784,321	931,311	787,796	664,413							277,413	634,507	313,083	1,650,749
	Cape Verde	69	80	38	44	21	127	77	20	41	29	144	107	18	68	45	68	80	18	35
	Central African Republic	174,436	125,038	89,930	82,072	82,057	100,962	95,259	99,718	105,664	127,964	89,614	140,742	194,976	162,344	187,910	131,856	114,403	119,477	152,260
	Chad	212,554	246,410	229,444	234,869	278,225	293,564	278,048	343,186	395,205	392,815	40,078	38,287	20,049	39,383	28,328	31,668	45,155	58,288	57,644
	Comoros				12,012	13,860	15,707	15,509	9,491	3,844	9,793			43,933	45,195	12,874	31,668	20,559		
	Congo	32,428	32,391	21,121	15,504	35,957	28,008	14,000	9,793	17,122							6,086	157,757		
	Côte d'Ivoire	511,916	466,895	553,875	421,043		755,812	1,109,011	983,089	141,353	1,508,042		1,193,288	1,109,751	1,136,810	1,275,138	1,280,914	1,253,408	1,277,670	1,343,654
	Democratic Republic of the Congo	25,552	22,598	25,100	17,867	14,827	12,530	129,908	141,353	255,150	147,062	897	1,531	1,735	2,438	2,684	2,971	2,050	759,059	1,462,300
	Equatorial Guinea															4,119	9,073	6,541	9,195	50,758
	Eritrea						81,183					50,810	9,716	6,078	10,346			33,458		4,702
	Ethiopia	57,450	80,247	206,262	305,616	358,469	412,609	478,411	509,804	604,960	647,919		392,377	427,795	463,797	578,904	538,942	447,780	451,816	458,561
	Gabon	222,538	215,414	188,035	100,629	70,928	54,849	74,310	57,450	80,247	127,899	50,810	53,167	62,976	58,212	70,075	70,644	33,458	45,186	40,701
	Gambia						325,555	266,189	299,824	135,909	620,767		481,590	620,767	540,165	395,043	329,426	427,598	439,798	10,910
	Ghana	1,438,713	1,372,771	1,446,947	1,697,109	1,672,709	1,928,316	2,189,860	2,227,762	1,745,214	2,895,079	3,349,528	3,044,844	3,140,893	3,552,896	475,441	655,093	472,255	476,484	827,438
	Guinea	21,762	17,718	56,073	158,748	607,560	600,317	772,731	802,210	817,949	807,895	4,800	6,238	16,561	107,925	103,069	50,452	41,228	28,646	33,405
	Guinea-Bissau	81,835	64,123				197,386	6,457	10,632	2,113	80,718	246,316	202,379				14,659	15,120	14,284	11,299
	Kenya							3,777,022	826,151	777,754	1,141,474	4,216,531	3,262,931				9,181,224	8,926,058	9,610,691	839,904
	Liberia							239,998									44,875	761,415	492,272	606,952
	Madagascar	3,870,904				196,358		12,794	73	52		6,946	8,538	5,272	6,909	7,638	6,753	5,689	43,674	89,138
	Malawi	248,904	282,256	280,562	4,686,201	4,736,974		6,183,290	2,761,269	2,985,659	4,193,145	3,646,212	3,823,796	2,784,001	3,358,960	2,871,098	3,688,389	4,204,468	4,442,197	4,986,779
	Mali	26,903	42,112	45,687	43,892	156,080	181,204	168,131	189,571	253,513	530,197	546,634	612,896	723,077	809,428	969,214	962,706	1,022,592	1,291,853	
	Mauritania												243,942	224,614	318,120	224,840	223,472	1,061		302
	Mauritius	54	48	66	54	65	46	82	65	73	52									
	Mozambique				380,530	401,519	275,442	345,177	390,601	353,110	429,571			194,024					6,155,082	4,831,491
	Namibia											31,975	41,636	23,984	20,295	36,043	23,339	27,690	4,242	4,907
	Niger	1,116,992	909,656	1,219,348	981,943	1,175,004	1,133,926	1,149,435	1,148,542	948,823	1,145,112	1,340,142		888,345	56,460	76,030	56,043	3,956	138,902	413,252
	Nigeria	1,282,012	1,331,494	1,373,247	733,203	371,550	1,391,931	1,145,759	1,331,494	1,279,581	906,552		150	2,122,663	2,608,479	3,310,022	3,532,108	3,982,372	2,969,950	143,079
	Rwanda				13,285	450,071	628,773	7,192	209,312	249,744	409,670	2,476,608	423,493	506,028	553,150	589,315	683,769	573,686	382,686	228,015
	Sao Tome and Principe						51,938	47,074	47,757	46,026	37,026		42,086	50,586	42,656	46,486	18,139	5,146	2,080	1,572
	Senegal					450,071	628,773					44,959	14,261	15,261	28,272	23,171	38,746	49,366	95,169	202,466
	Sierra Leone	6,822	4,693	2,872	13,285	10,289	8,750	7,192	23,121	26,445	51,444	460,881	2,206	3,702	3,945	2,206	4,808	4,932	653,987	154,459
	South Africa							38,875	23,754	4,410	30,420	64,624	26,506	15,649	13,459	13,399	7,755	12,098	6,327	7,796
	Swaziland											0	1,395	670	342	574	279	155	84	58
	Togo	810,509	780,825	634,166	561,328	328,488		352,334	366,672	368,472	412,619	498,826	557,159	583,872	490,256	516,942	437,662	566,450	221,110	273,471
	Uganda			2,446,659	1,470,662	2,191,277	1,431,068	2,317,840		2,845,811	3,070,800	3,552,859	5,624,032	557,159	801,784	879,032	1,104,310	867,398	1,050,240	894,505
	United Republic of Tanzania	10,715,736	8,715,736	7,681,524	8,777,340	7,976,590	2,438,040	4,969,273	1,131,655	30,504,654	423,967	17,734	18,385	16,983	15,751	11,981	7,677	1,633	293	67
	Zambia	1,933,696	2,340,994	2,953,692	3,514,000	3,514,000	2,742,118	3,215,866		3,399,630	3,385,616	3,337,796	3,838,402	3,760,335	4,346,172	4,078,234	4,121,356	4,731,338	4,248,295	3,080,301
	Zimbabwe	662,613	581,168	420,137	877,734	324,188	761,791	1,696,192	1,849,383	1,719,960	1,804,479					16,990	18,954	19,702	30,521	92,900
Americas	Argentina	1,660	803	643	758	948	1,065	2,048	592	339	222	458	219	97	138	123	248	188	387	130
	Bahamas											2	4	1	3	2	1	49	6	12
	Belize	3,033	3,317	5,341	8,586	9,957	9,413	6,605	4,014	2,614	1,850									
	Bolivia (Plurinational State of)	19,680	19,031	24,486	27,475	34,749	46,911	64,012	51,478	73,913	50,037	31,468	15,765	14,276	20,343	14,910	20,142	18,995	14,610	9,748
	Brazil	560,396	614,431	609,860	466,190	564,406	565,727	455,194	392,976	471,892	609,594	613,241	388,303	348,259	408,765	464,901	606,067	549,469	458,041	315,642
	Colombia	99,489	184,156	184,023	129,377	127,218	187,082	135,923	180,898	185,455	66,845	144,432	231,233	204,916	180,956	142,241	121,629	120,096	128,462	80,559
	Costa Rica	1,151	3,273	6,951	5,033	4,445	4,515	5,480	4,898	5,148	3,998	1,879	1,363	1,021	718	1,289	3,541	2,903	1,223	966
	Dominican Republic	356	377	698	987	1,670	1,808	1,414	816	2,006	3,589	461	431	455	743	1,321	1,990	1,789	1,620	1,262
	Ecuador	71,670	59,400	41,089	46,859	30,006	18,128	11,882	16,365	43,696	87,620									
	El Salvador	9,269	5,933	4,539	3,887	2,803	3,362	5,888	2,719	1,182	1,230	745	360	117	83	111	65	48	48	33
	French Guiana	5,909	3,573	4,072	3,974	4,241	4,711	4,724	3,195	3,462	5,307	3,708	3,823	3,661	3,839	6,075	3,414	4,074	2,797	3,264
	Guatemala	41,711	57,829	57,560	41,868	22,057	20,268	24,178	32,099	47,689	45,098	53,311	3,735	3,309	3,072	3,418	3,017	4,304	1,864	514
	Guyana	22,681	42,204	39,702	33,172	39,566	59,311	18,877	32,103	41,200	27,283	24,018	27,122	21,895	27,627	28,866	38,984	21,064	11,657	11,815
	Haiti	4,806	25,511	13,457	853	23,140				34,449	1,196	16,897	9,837	9,837	9,837	10,802	21,778	32,739	29,825	36,774

Annex 3.A – Reported malaria cases, 1990–2008 (continued)

WHO region	Country/area	1990	1991	1992	1993	1994	1995	1996	1997	1998	1999	2000	2001	2002	2003	2004	2005	2006	2007	2008
Americas	Honduras	53,095	73,352	70,838	44,513	52,110	59,446	74,487	65,863	42,979	46,740	35,125	24,149	17,223	14,123	17,293	16,007	11,561	10,270	8,225
	Jamaica											97	65	53	113	652	379	382	199	86
	Mexico	44,513	26,565	16,170	15,793	12,864	7,329	6,293	4,805	25,023	13,450	7,390	4,996	4,624	3,819	3,406	2,967	2,514	2,361	2,357
	Nicaragua	35,785	27,653	26,866	44,037	41,490	69,444	75,606	42,819	33,903	38,676	23,878	10,482	7,695	6,717	6,897	6,642	3,114	1,356	764
	Panama	381	1,115	727	481	684	730	476	505	1,039	936	1,036	928	2,244	4,500	5,095	3,667	1,663	1,281	744
	Paraguay	2,912	2,983	1,289	436	583	898	637	567	2,091	9,947	6,853	2,710	2,778	1,392	694	376	823	1,341	1,341
	Peru	28,882	33,705	54,922	95,222	122,039	192,629	208,132	183,740	247,004	166,579	68,321	79,473	85,742	85,742	93,581	86,272	64,871	56,538	.
	Suriname	1,608	1,490	1,404	.	4,704	6,606	16,649	11,323	12,412	13,939	11,361	16,003	12,837	10,982	8,378	9,131	3,289	1,104	2,086
	Venezuela (Bolivarian Republic of)	46,910	43,454	21,416	12,539	13,727	16,371	18,858	22,400	21,862	19,086	29,736	20,006	29,491	31,719	46,655	45,049	37,062	41,749	32,037
Eastern Mediterranean	Afghanistan	317,479	297,605	.	.	88,302	.	303,955	202,767	288,070	.	.	.	414,631	360,940	242,022	116,444	86,129	92,202	82,564
	Djibouti	3,237	7,338	7,468	4,166	6,140	5,982	6,105	4,314	5,920	6,140	4,667	4,312	5,021	5,036	122	413	1,796	210	119
	Egypt	150	48	32	34	1,054	644	50	22	26	122	17	11	10	45	43	23	29	30	80
	Iran (Islamic Republic of)	77,470	96,340	76,971	64,581	51,089	67,532	56,362	38,684	32,951	23,110	19,716	19,303	15,558	23,562	13,821	18,966	15,909	6,947	5,955
	Iraq	3,924	1,764	5,752	49,863	98,243	98,705	49,840	13,959	9,684	4,143	1,860	1,265	952	347	155	47	24	3	6
	Morocco	1,674	988	810	396	412	394	204	250	242	120	59	59	107	73	56	100	83	75	142
	Oman	65,440	38,548	29,654	33,746	14,430	3,602	2,530	2,052	2,186	1,802	694	635	590	740	615	544	443	705	965
	Pakistan	79,689	66,586	99,015	92,634	108,586	111,836	98,035	77,480	73,516	91,774	82,526	125,292	107,666	125,152	101,640	97,049	100,956	92,971	59,284
	Saudi Arabia	15,666	9,962	19,623	18,380	10,032	18,751	21,007	20,631	40,796	13,166	.	3,074	2,612	1,724	1,232	1,059	1,278	2,864	1,491
	Somalia	.	.	.	3,049	.	.	.	.	.	9,055	.	10,364	15,732	7,571	11,436	12,516	16,430	16,058	23,905
	Sudan*	7,508,704	6,947,787	9,326,944	9,867,778	8,562,205	6,347,143	4,595,092	4,065,460	5,062,000	4,215,308	368,557	203,491	280,550	933,267	537,899	628,417	595,683	560,428	457,362
	Syrian Arab Republic	214	108	912	1,932	1,166	1,252	690	260	120	86	42	79	27	24	13	28	34	37	51
	Yemen																			
Europe	Armenia	0	0	0	0	196	502	347	841	1,156	616	141	79	52	29	45	7	0	1	1
	Azerbaijan	24	113	27	23	667	2,840	13,135	9,911	5,175	2,315	1,526	1,058	506	482	386	242	143	110	73
	Georgia	1	2	1	0	6	7	7	13	16	51	173	439	472	315	256	155	60	23	6
	Kyrgyzstan	1	1	2	0	6	3	26	13	11	5	12	28	2,744	468	93	226	320	96	18
	Russian Federation	216	169	160	209	335	425	611	831	1,081	792									
	Tajikistan	175	294	404	619	2,411	6,103	16,561	29,794	19,351	13,493	19,064	11,387	6,160	5,428	3,588	2,309	1,344	635	318
	Turkey	8,680	12,218	18,676	47,210	84,345	82,096	60,884	35,456	36,842	20,963	9,465	7,710	7,814	8,025	4,278	1,627	605	250	136
	Turkmenistan	1	17	11	3	9	10	14	14	137	49	24	8	18	51	4	1	.	0	1
	Uzbekistan	28	12	25	36	21	27	51	52	74	85	126	77	74	74	66	102	76	89	27
South-East Asia	Bangladesh	53,875	63,578	115,660	125,402	166,564	152,729	100,864	68,594	60,023	63,723	54,223	54,216	62,269	54,654	58,894	48,121	32,857	59,857	84,690
	Bhutan	9,497	22,126	28,900	28,116	39,852	23,188	15,696	9,029	7,693	12,237	5,935	5,982	6,511	3,806	2,670	1,825	1,868	793	329
	Democratic People's Republic of Korea									1,085	7,980	.	115,615	88,852	16,538	15,827	6,728	6,913		
	Democratic Republic of Timor-Leste									10,332		15,212	83,049	26,651	33,411	39,164	43,093	37,896	46,869	45,973
	India	2,018,783	2,117,460	2,125,826	2,207,431	2,511,453	2,988,231	3,035,588	2,660,057	2,222,748	2,284,713	2,031,790	2,085,484	1,841,227	1,869,403	1,915,363	1,816,569	1,785,109	1,508,927	1,532,467
	Indonesia	171,908	132,412	103,277	136,367	145,920	123,226	179,878	161,285	160,282	.	.	267,592	273,793	223,074	268,852	437,323	347,597		343,048
	Myanmar	989,042	939,257	789,672	702,239	701,043	656,547	664,507	568,262	548,066	121,031	120,029	170,502	173,096	177,530	152,070	165,737	216,470	332,056	411,494
	Nepal	22,856	29,135	23,234	16,380	9,442	9,718	6,628	8,957	8,498	9,699	7,981	6,396	12,750	9,506	4,895	5,050	4,969	4,220	3,888
	Sri Lanka	287,384	400,263	399,349	327,020	273,434	142,294	184,319	218,550	211,691	210,039	.	66,522	41,411	10,510	3,720	1,640	591	198	670
	Thailand	273,880	198,383	168,370	115,220	102,119	82,743	87,622	97,540	131,055	125,379	.	63,528	44,555	37,355	26,690	29,782	30,294	33,178	26,150
Western Pacific	Cambodia	123,796	102,930	91,000	99,200	85,012	76,923	74,883	88,029	58,874	64,679	62,442	53,601	46,902	71,265	59,745	49,436	78,696	42,518	42,124
	China	117,359	101,600	74,000	59,000	62,000	47,118	33,382	26,800	27,090	26,797	.	21,237	25,520	28,491	27,197	21,936	35,383	29,304	16,650
	Lao People's Democratic Republic	22,044	41,048	38,500	41,787	52,601	52,021	77,894	72,190	39,031	28,050	40,106	27,076	21,420	18,894	16,183	13,615	18,382	19,037	17,648
	Malaysia	50,500	39,189	36,853	39,890	58,958	59,208	51,921	26,649	13,491	11,106	8,257	8,384	6,792	4,271	4,217	4,250	4,094	4,064	5,598
	Papua New Guinea	104,900	86,500	86,500	66,797	65,000	99,000	71,013	38,105	20,900	18,564	79,839	94,484	75,748	72,620	91,055	92,957	93,938	86,912	84,452
	Philippines	86,200	86,400	95,778	64,944	61,959	56,852	40,545	42,005	50,709	37,061	36,596	34,787	37,005	48,441	50,850	46,342	35,405	36,235	23,655
	Republic of Korea	0	0	0	1	20	107	396	1,724	3,992	3,621	4,183	2,556	1,799	1,171	864	1,369	2,051	2,227	1,052
	Solomon Islands	116,500	141,400	153,359	126,123	131,687	118,521	84,795	68,125	72,808	63,169	68,107	76,493	74,936	92,227	90,297	76,390	75,337	65,404	40,535
	Vanuatu	28,805	19,466	13,330	10,469	3,771	8,318	5,654	6,099	6,181	5,152	6,220	7,656	14,342	15,245	13,579	8,339	8,055	5,471	3,477
	Viet Nam	123,796	187,994	225,928	156,069	140,120	100,116	84,625	65,859	72,091	75,102	74,316	68,699	47,807	38,790	24,909	19,496	22,637	16,389	11,355

Notes:

Cases reported before 2000 can be probable and confirmed or only confirmed cases depending on the country.

Cases reported can be autochthonous malaria cases only or may inlcude imported cases.

Mauritius is one of the countries listed but it has had no ongoing local transmission for over a decade.

*Data for Sudan, after 1999, only represents 15 northern states.

Annex 3.B – Reported malaria deaths, 1990–2008

WHO region	Country/area	1990	1991	1992	1993	1994	1995	1996	1997	1998	1999	2000	2001	2002	2003	2004	2005	2006	2007	2008
Africa	Algeria									2	6	2	1							
	Angola										25,572	9,510	9,473	14,434	38,598	12,459	13,768	10,220	9,812	9,465
	Benin										544		468	707	560	944	322	1,226	1,195	
	Botswana								141	23	49		29	23	18	19	11	40	6	12
	Burkina Faso									2,624	2,808		4,233	4,032	4,860	4,205	5,224	8,083	6,472	7,834
	Burundi											691	417	483	425	689	776	434	167	226
	Cameroon																836	930	1,811	7,673
	Cape Verde												0	2	4	4	2	7	2	2
	Central African Republic									374	484	439	535		417	859	668	865	578	456
	Chad											712	957	98	1,021	13	558	837	617	1,018
	Comoros										50					28	92	56		47
	Côte d'Ivoire									1,337	974								797	1,249
	Democratic Republic of the Congo											3,856	416	2,152	989	13,613	15,322	8,295	14,637	18,928
	Eritrea									404	169		133	86	79	24	49	47	42	19
	Ethiopia												1,681	1,607	2,138	3,327	1,086	1,357	991	1,169
	Gabon											2,016	1,693	1,141	692	466	353	238	216	156
	Gambia												275	259	192	153	426	150	424	403
	Ghana									2,798	2,826	6,108	1,717	2,376	2,103	1,575	2,037	3,125	4,622	3,889
	Guinea									13	13	626	517	440	586	528	490			441
	Guinea-Bissau												635	780	1,137	565	565	507	370	487
	Kenya	57,649								665	1,545	48,767	48,286	47,697	51,842	25,403	44,328	40,079		
	Liberia																41	877	310	345
	Madagascar								35,982		640	591	742	575	817	715	699	441	428	276
	Malawi										4,747		3,355	5,775	4,767	3,457	5,070	7,132	8,541	7,748
	Mali										583	748	562	826	1,309	1,012	1,285	1,914	1,782	1,227
	Mauritania									279	525							67		
	Mozambique									896	1,189								5,816	4,424
	Namibia						250		547	404	531	424	1,728	1,504	1,106	1,185	1,325	571	181	171
	Niger	2,284	1,947						1,018	1,823	2,165		2,366	2,769	2,248	1,333	2,060	1,150	1,420	2,691
	Nigeria					1,686	3,268	4,773	4,603	6,197	4,123	1,244	4,317	4,092	5,343	6,032	6,494	6,586	10,289	8,677
	Rwanda									2,736	1,881		4,275	3,167	2,679	2,362	2,581	2,486	1,772	563
	Sao Tome and Principe									154		254	248	321	193	169	85	26	3	16
	Senegal								1,205	1,029	1,235	1,275	1,515	1,226	1,602	1,524	1,587	1,678	1,935	722
	Sierra Leone												328	461	157	126	50	90	324	871
	South Africa	35	19		45	12		163	104	198	406		81	96	142	88	63	87	37	43
	Swaziland						44			109	149		62	46	30	28	17	27	14	5
	Togo									475	766		1,394	1,661	1,130	1,183	1,024	819	1,236	2,663
	Uganda																	4,252	7,003	2,372
	United Republic of Tanzania											379	1,228	815	15,251	19,859	18,322	20,962	12,593	29
	Zambia	4,863	4,998	3,315	4,689	5,775					8,580		9,369	9,021	9,178	8,289	7,737	6,484	6,183	3,781
	Zimbabwe								1,192	1,248	1,139			1,844	1,044	1,809	1,916	802	285	
Americas	Argentina									23			0	0	0	0	0	0		
	Bolivia (Plurinational State of)													8	4	0	0	0		
	Brazil												142	93	103	100	122	105	94	51
	Colombia												58	40	24	25	28	53		22
	Dominican Republic									14		6	17	11	12	16	16	10	14	9
	Ecuador									16			0	0	0	0	0	0		
	El Salvador									9			0	0						
	Guatemala																			
	Guyana									34			32			16	44	40		
	Haiti									25							58	64		
	Honduras												0	0	0	0	2	0		
	Mexico															0	0			

Annex 3.B — Reported malaria deaths, 1990–2008 (continued)

WHO region	Country/area	1990	1991	1992	1993	1994	1995	1996	1997	1998	1999	2000	2001	2002	2003	2004	2005	2006	2007	2008
Americas	Nicaragua	–	–	–	–	–	–	–	–	–	–	–	2	8	7	1	6	1	–	–
	Panama	–	–	–	–	–	–	–	–	–	–	–	–	4	6	6	–	–	1	–
	Suriname	–	–	–	–	–	–	–	–	–	–	24	23	16	18	7	2	–	1	–
	Venezuela (Bolivarian Republic of)	–	–	–	–	–	–	–	–	–	–	–	–	–	–	–	–	–	–	–
Eastern Mediterranean	Afghanistan	–	–	–	–	22	–	–	–	–	–	–	–	–	–	–	–	–	25	46
	Djibouti	–	–	–	–	–	–	–	–	–	–	–	–	–	–	–	–	29	1	–
	Egypt	–	–	–	–	0	–	–	–	–	–	–	–	–	–	–	–	–	–	–
	Iran (Islamic Republic of)	–	–	–	–	–	–	–	22	–	3	–	2	2	5	1	1	1	0	3
	Iraq	–	–	–	–	0	–	–	–	–	–	–	0	0	0	0	0	0	0	0
	Morocco	–	–	–	–	–	–	–	0	–	–	–	–	–	–	0	0	0	–	–
	Saudi Arabia	–	–	–	–	–	–	–	6	–	–	–	0	0	0	0	0	0	2	1
	Somalia	–	–	–	–	–	–	–	–	28	–	–	8	8	54	79	15	58	33	21
	Sudan*	–	–	–	–	932	–	1,944	1,825	1,958	2,622	2,162	2,252	2,125	2,479	1,814	1,703	1,686	1,254	1,125
	Yemen	–	–	–	–	–	–	–	–	–	–	–	–	–	–	–	–	73	–	–
Europe	Armenia	–	–	–	–	–	–	–	–	0	0	0	0	0	0	0	0	0	0	0
	Azerbaijan	–	0	–	–	–	–	0	–	0	0	0	0	0	0	0	0	0	0	0
	Georgia	–	–	0	0	0	0	0	0	–	0	–	0	0	0	0	0	0	0	0
	Kyrgyzstan	0	0	0	0	0	0	0	4	0	0	0	0	0	–	0	0	0	0	0
	Russian Federation	1	1	–	1	3	2	3	7	0	3	–	–	–	–	–	–	–	1	3
	Tajikistan	–	–	–	–	–	–	–	7	0	–	–	–	–	–	–	–	–	–	–
	Turkey	0	0	0	0	0	0	0	0	0	0	–	–	–	–	–	–	–	–	–
	Turkmenistan	0	0	0	0	0	0	0	0	0	–	–	–	–	–	–	–	–	–	–
	Uzbekistan	0	1	0	1	0	0	0	0	–	0	0	0	0	0	0	0	0	1	0
South-East Asia	Bangladesh	–	–	–	–	–	1,393	794	469	528	552	478	490	588	577	535	501	307	228	154
	Bhutan	–	–	–	–	–	–	25	14	17	–	–	–	–	14	7	5	7	2	4
	Democratic Republic of Timor-Leste	–	–	–	–	–	–	–	–	–	–	–	–	–	–	61	88	58	60	31
	India	–	–	–	–	–	–	2,803	879	666	–	892	1,015	973	1,006	949	963	1,708	1,311	1,061
	Indonesia	–	–	–	–	–	–	148	199	45	–	–	–	–	–	–	–	494	–	669
	Myanmar	–	–	–	–	–	–	3,424	2,943	3,182	3,648	2,756	2,814	2,634	2,476	1,982	1,707	1,647	1,265	1,088
	Nepal	–	–	–	–	0	0	15	2	7	–	–	1	3	5	7	10	42	3	–
	Sri Lanka	–	–	–	–	–	–	26	61	115	–	77	52	30	4	1	0	–	1	0
	Thailand	1,287	–	–	–	–	–	826	764	688	740	–	848	722	650	460	142	226	97	101
Western Pacific	Cambodia	1,020	–	1,408	1,100	1,009	614	745	811	621	891	608	476	457	492	382	296	396	241	209
	China	35	1,163	52	19	43	34	30	46	24	67	–	28	42	52	31	48	38	18	23
	Lao People's Democratic Republic	372	457	438	418	609	620	608	606	427	338	350	244	195	187	105	77	21	14	13
	Malaysia	43	–	25	23	28	35	40	25	27	21	35	46	39	21	35	33	21	18	29
	Papua New Guinea	457	–	500	448	281	415	514	390	651	567	699	619	678	559	644	731	668	559	628
	Philippines	913	924	864	811	784	643	536	514	561	755	–	–	–	–	–	–	–	–	–
	Republic of Korea	0	0	0	0	0	0	0	0	0	0	–	–	–	–	–	–	0	–	0
	Solomon Islands	33	46	33	40	49	51	30	27	33	23	–	55	59	71	34	38	12	15	21
	Vanuatu	32	32	26	13	8	4	0	0	–	0	2	4	12	14	3	2	1	2	1
	Viet Nam	3,340	4,646	2,632	1,026	604	348	203	152	183	190	142	78	44	50	24	18	38	20	25

Notes:

Deaths reported before 2000 can be probable and confirmed or only confirmed deaths depending on the country.

*Data for Sudan, after 1999, only represents 15 northern states.

Annex 4.A – Recommended policies and strategies for malaria control, 2009

| WHO region/subregion | Country/area | Insecticide-treated nets | | Indoor residual spraying | | ACT policy adopted | Oral artemisinin monotherapies banned | Parasitological confirmation for all age groups | ACT is free of charge for under 5 years old in the public sector | Treatment | | | | Malaria in pregnancy |
		Distribution - Free	Targeting - All age groups	IRS is the primary vector control intervention	DDT is used for IRS (public health only)					Diagnosis of malaria inpatients is based on laboratory testing	Pre-referral treatment with quinine or artemether IM or artesunate suppositories	Oversight regulation of case management in the private sectors	RDTs used at community level	IPT Strategy used to prevent malaria during pregnancy
Africa	Algeria	N	Y	Y	N	NA	Y	Y	N	Y	N	N	N	N
	Angola	N	Y	Y	N	Y	Y	Y	Y	N	N	N	N	Y
	Benin	N	Y	Y	N	Y	Y	Y	Y	N	N	Y	N	Y
	Botswana	Y	Y	Y	N	Y	N	Y	Y	Y	N	Y	N	N
	Burkina Faso	Y	N	N	N	Y	N	N	Y	Y	N	N	N	Y
	Burundi	N	N	N	N	Y	Y	N	N	N	N	N	N	Y
	Cameroon	N	N	N	N	Y	N	Y	N	Y	N	Y	N	Y
	Cape Verde	Y	Y	N	N	Y	N	Y	N	Y	N	N	N	N (N)
	Central African Republic	N	N	N	N	Y	Y	N	N	Y	Y	Y	N	Y
	Chad	N	N	N	N	Y	Y	Y	N	N	N	-	N	Y
	Comoros	N	N	N	N	Y	Y	Y	N	Y	-	Y	-	Y
	Congo	-	-	-	N	Y	N	N	N	-	N	Y	N	Y
	Côte d'Ivoire	N	N	N	N	Y	Y	Y	N	Y	N	Y	N	Y
	Democratic Republic of the Congo	Y	Y	Y	Y	Y	N	Y	Y	Y	Y	Y	N	Y
	Equatorial Guinea	Y	Y	N	Y	Y	Y	Y	Y	Y	Y	N	-	Y
	Eritrea	Y	N	Y	Y	Y	N	Y	Y	Y	N	N	N	N
	Ethiopia	Y	Y	Y	Y	Y	Y	N	Y	N	Y	Y	Y	N
	Gabon	Y	N	N	N	Y	Y	Y	Y	N	N	Y	N	Y
	Gambia	N	N	N	Y	Y	N	Y	Y	Y	N	Y	N	Y
	Ghana	Y	Y	Y	N	Y	N	N	Y	Y	N	Y	N	Y
	Guinea	N	N	N	N	Y	Y	Y	Y	Y	N	Y	N	Y
	Guinea-Bissau	N	N	N	N	Y	N	Y	Y	N	N	Y	N	Y
	Kenya	N	-	N	-	Y	Y	N	Y	N	N	Y	-	Y
	Liberia	Y	-	-	N	Y	-	N	N	-	N	-	-	Y
	Madagascar	Y	Y	Y	N	Y	Y	Y	Y	Y	N	Y	N	Y
	Malawi	Y	N	Y	N	Y	Y	N	Y	N	N	-	-	Y
	Mali	N	Y	Y	N	Y	Y	Y	Y	Y	Y	Y	N	Y
	Mauritania	Y	-	-	-	NA	N	-	-	-	N	-	-	-
	Mauritius	-	-	-	-	NA	Y	Y	N	-	N	Y	N	-
	Mozambique	N	Y	Y	Y	Y	Y	N	N	N	Y	Y	N	Y
	Namibia	N	Y	Y	Y	Y	Y	Y	N	N	N	Y	N	Y
	Niger	Y	Y	N	N	Y	N	N	Y	Y	Y	Y	N	Y
	Nigeria	Y	Y	N	N	Y	Y	Y	Y	Y	Y	Y	N	Y
	Rwanda	N	Y	Y	N	Y	N	Y	Y	Y	Y	N	N	N
	Sao Tome and Principe	Y	N	Y	N	Y	Y	Y	Y	Y	Y	Y	N	Y
	Senegal	Y	Y	Y	N	Y	Y	N	Y	N	N	N	N	Y
	Sierra Leone	N	N	N	N	Y	-	N	Y	N	N	-	N	Y
	South Africa	-	Y	Y	Y	Y	Y	Y	N	Y	Y	Y	N	Y
	Swaziland	N	Y	Y	Y	Y	Y	Y	Y	Y	Y	Y	N	Y
	Togo	N	N	N	N	Y	N	N	Y	Y	Y	Y	N	Y
	Uganda	N	Y	Y	N	Y	Y	Y	Y	N	Y	Y	N	Y
	United Republic of Tanzania	N	Y	Y	N	Y	Y	N	Y	N	Y	Y	N	Y
	Zambia	Y	Y	Y	Y	Y	Y	Y	Y	N	N	Y	N	Y
	Zimbabwe	Y	Y	Y	Y	Y	Y	Y	Y	N	Y	-	-	N
Americas	Argentina	-	Y	Y	N	NA	N	N	N	N	N	-	N	N
	Belize	-	-	Y	N	NA	-	N	N	N	N	-	N	N
	Bolivia (Plurinational State of)	Y	Y	N	N	Y	Y	Y	N	N	Y	Y	N	Z
	Brazil	Y	Y	N	N	Y	Y	Y	Y	Y	Y	Y	N	Z
	Colombia	N	N	N	N	NA	N	N	N	N	N	N	N	N
	Costa Rica	Y	N	Y	N	NA	-	N	N	N	Z	-	N	N
	Dominican Republic	N	N	N	N	Y	Z	Y	Z	Y	Y	Y	N	N
	Ecuador	Y	-	-	N	Y	-	Y	N	N	N	-	-	N
	El Salvador	Y	Y	Y	N	NA	-	N	N	N	N	N	N	N
	French Guiana	Y	-	-	N	NA	Z	Y	N	N	Y	N	N	N
	Guatemala	Y	N	N	N	Y	N	Y	Y	N	N	N	N	N
	Guyana	Y	Y	N	N	Y	Y	Y	Y	Y	N	N	N	N
	Haiti	Y	N	N	N	NA	N	N	Y	Y	N	N	N	Y
	Honduras	-	Y	Y	N	NA	-	N	-	-	-	-	-	-

Annex 4.A – Recommended policies and strategies for malaria control, 2009

WHO region/subregion · Country/area	Insecticide-treated nets: Distribution - Free	Insecticide-treated nets: Targeting - All age groups	Indoor residual spraying: IRS is the primary vector control intervention	Indoor residual spraying: DDT is used for IRS (public health only)	Treatment: ACT policy adopted	Treatment: Oral artemisinin monotherapies banned	Treatment: Parasitological confirmation for all age groups	Treatment: ACT is free of charge for under 5 years old in the public sector	Treatment: Diagnosis of malaria inpatients is based on laboratory testing	Treatment: Pre-referral treatment with quinine or artemether IM or artesunate suppositories	Treatment: Oversight regulation of case management in the private sectors	Treatment: RDTs used at community level	Malaria in pregnancy: IPT Strategy used to prevent malaria during pregnancy
Africa													
Algeria	N	N	Y	N	NA	N	Y	NA	Y	Y	N	N	N
Angola	Y	N	Y	N	Y	Y	Y	Y	Y	Y	N	N	Y
Benin	Y	N	Y	N	Y	Y	N	Y	Y	Y	Y	N	Y
Botswana	N	Y	Y	Y	Y	Y	Y	N	Y	Y	Y	N	Y
Burkina Faso	Y	Y	N	N	Y	Y	Y	N	Y	Y	Y	N	Y
Burundi	Y	N	N	N	Y	Y	N	N	Y	Y	N	N	N
Cameroon	Y	N	N	N	N	Y	Y	N	Y	Y	Y	N	Y
Cape Verde	Y	Y	N	N	Y	Y	Y	Y	Y	Y	Y	N	Y
Central African Republic	Y	N	N	N	Y	Y	Y	Y	N	Y	-	-	Y
Chad	Y	N	N	N	Y	Y	Y	N	N	N	Y	N	Y
Comoros	Y	-	N	N	Y	Y	Y	N	-	-	-	-	Y
Congo	Y	N	N	N	Y	Y	Y	N	N	N	N	N	Y
Côte d'Ivoire	Y	N	N	N	Y	Y	Y	N	Y	Y	Y	N	Y
Democratic Republic of the Congo	Y	Y	N	N	Y	Y	Y	N	Y	Y	Y	Y	Y
Equatorial Guinea	Y	Y	Y	Y	Y	Y	Y	Y	-	Y	N	N	Y
Eritrea	Y	Y	N	Y	Y	Y	Y	N	Y	Y	Y	Y	N
Ethiopia	Y	Y	N	N	Y	Y	Y	Y	Y	Y	Y	Y	Y
Gabon	Y	Y	N	N	Y	Y	Y	N	Y	Y	Y	N	Y
Gambia	Y	Y	N	N	Y	Y	Y	N	Y	Y	Y	N	Y
Ghana	N	N	N	N	Y	Y	Y	N	Y	Y	Y	N	Y
Guinea	Y	N	N	N	Y	Y	Y	N	Y	Y	Y	N	Y
Guinea-Bissau	Y	Y	N	N	Y	Y	Y	N	Y	Y	N	N	Y
Kenya	Y	N	Y	N	Y	Y	Y	N	Y	Y	Y	N	Y
Liberia	Y	Y	N	N	Y	Y	Y	Y	Y	Y	N	N	Y
Madagascar	Y	Y	Y	Y	Y	Y	Y	N	-	-	-	N	Y
Malawi	Y	N	N	N	Y	Y	Y	N	Y	Y	N	N	Y
Mali	Y	Y	N	N	Y	Y	Y	N	Y	Y	N	Y	Y
Mauritania	N	N	-	-	-	-	-	-	-	-	-	-	-
Mauritius	Y	-	-	-	NA	-	-	-	-	-	-	-	-
Mozambique	Y	N	Y	Y	Y	N	Y	Y	Y	Y	N	N	Y
Namibia	Y	N	Y	Y	Y	Y	Y	N	Y	Y	Y	N	Y
Niger	Y	Y	N	N	Y	Y	Y	N	Y	Y	N	N	Y
Nigeria	Y	Y	N	N	Y	Y	Y	N	Y	Y	Y	Y	Y
Rwanda	Y	Y	Y	N	Y	Y	Y	Y	Y	Y	-	N	Y
Sao Tome and Principe	Y	Y	Y	Y	Y	Y	Y	Y	Y	Y	Y	N	Y
Senegal	Y	Y	Y	N	Y	Y	Y	N	Y	Y	Y	N	Y
Sierra Leone	Y	Y	N	N	Y	Y	Y	Y	Y	Y	N	N	Y
South Africa	-	-	Y	Y	Y	Y	Y	N	Y	Y	Y	-	-
Swaziland	-	-	Y	Y	Y	Y	Y	N	Y	Y	N	N	-
Togo	N	N	N	N	Y	N	N	N	N	N	N	N	Y
Uganda	Y	Y	Y	N	Y	Y	Y	Y	Y	Y	N	N	Y
United Republic of Tanzania	-	N	Y	Y	Y	Y	Y	Y	Y	Y	Y	Y	Y
Zambia	Y	N	Y	Y	Y	Y	Y	N	Y	Y	Y	Y	Y
Zimbabwe	Y	Y	Y	Y	Y	Y	Y	N	Y	Y	Y	Y	Y
Americas													
Argentina	N	N	Y	N	NA	N	Y	N	Y	N	N	-	N
Belize	-	-	Y	N	NA	-	Y	-	Y	Y	-	-	-
Bolivia (Plurinational State of)	Y	Y	Y	N	Y	Y	Y	Y	Y	Y	Y	Y	-
Brazil	Y	Y	Y	N	Y	Y	Y	Y	Y	Y	Y	Y	-
Colombia	N	N	N	N	NA	N	Y	N	Y	Y	Z	Y	-
Costa Rica	Y	Y	N	N	Y	-	Y	Y	Y	Y	-	Y	-
Dominican Republic	N	N	N	N	N	N	Y	Y	Y	N	N	N	-
Ecuador	-	Y	-	-	NA	-	Y	-	Y	-	-	N	-
El Salvador	Y	Y	N	N	NA	N	Y	-	Y	Y	Z	Y	-
French Guiana	-	-	Y	N	NA	-	Y	-	Y	Y	N	Y	-
Guatemala	Y	Y	N	N	NA	Y	Y	N	Y	Y	N	N	-
Guyana	N	Y	N	Y	NA	Y	Y	N	Y	Y	N	Y	-
Haiti	N	-	Y	N	NA	Y	Y	N	Y	Y	N	N	-
Honduras	-	-	Y	N	NA	-	-	-	-	-	-	-	-

| WHO region/subregion | Country/area | Insecticide-treated nets | | Indoor residual spraying | | ACT policy adopted | Treatment | | | | | | | Malaria in pregnancy |
		Distribution - Free	Targeting - All age groups	IRS is the primary vector control intervention	DDT is used for IRS (public health only)		Oral artemisinin monotherapies banned	Parasitological confirmation for all age groups	ACT is free of charge for under 5 years old in the public sector	Diagnosis of malaria inpatients is based on laboratory testing	Pre-referral treatment with quinine or artemether IM or artesunate suppositories	Oversight regulation of case management in the private sectors	RDTs used at community level	IPT Strategy used to prevent malaria during pregnancy
Americas	Jamaica	-	-	-	-	NA	-	-	-	-	-	-	-	-
	Mexico	Y	Y	Y	N	NA	Y	Y	N	-	-	-	-	-
	Nicaragua	N	Y	N	N	NA	Y	Y	N	-	N	N	-	-
	Panama	Y	N	Y	N	N	-	Y	-	-	-	-	-	-
	Paraguay	Y	N	Y	N	N	-	Y	-	-	-	-	-	-
	Peru	-	Y	-	N	Y	Y	Y	N	Y	Y	N	-	-
	Suriname	Y	Y	N	N	Y	Y	Y	Y	-	Y	-	Y	N
	Venezuela (Bolivarian Republic of)	Y	Y	Y	N	Y	Y	Y	Y	Y	Y	Y	-	-
Eastern Mediterranean	Afghanistan	Y	Y	N	N	Y	Y	Y	Y	Y	Y	-	N	N
	Djibouti	Y	N	N	N	Y	Y	N	Y	-	N	-	-	Y
	Egypt	-	-	-	-	Y	Y	-	Y	-	-	-	-	-
	Iran (Islamic Republic of)	Y	Y	Y	N	Y	Y	Y	Y	Y	Y	Y	N	N
	Iraq	Y	Y	Y	N	Y	Y	Y	Y	Y	N	Y	Y	N
	Morocco	-	-	-	-	NA	-	-	-	-	-	-	-	-
	Oman	-	-	-	-	Y	Y	-	Y	-	-	-	-	-
	Pakistan	Y	N	N	N	Y	Y	N	Y	Y	Y	N	N	N
	Saudi Arabia	Y	N	N	N	Y	Y	Y	Y	Y	Y	Y	Y	N
	Somalia	Y	Y	N	N	Y	Y	N	Y	Y	Y	N	Y	Y
	Sudan	Y	Y	Y	N	Y	Y	Y	Y	Y	Y	-	-	Y
	Syrian Arab Republic	-	-	-	-	NA	-	-	-	-	-	-	-	-
	Yemen	Y	N	Y	N	Y	Y	Y	Y	Y	Y	N	N	N
Europe	Armenia	N	N	Y	N	NA	N	Y	N	Y	N	-	N	N
	Azerbaijan	N	N	Y	N	NA	N	Y	N	Y	N	Y	N	N
	Georgia	Y	N	Y	N	NA	N	Y	N	Y	N	N	N	N
	Kyrgyzstan	Y	Y	Y	N	-	N	Y	N	Y	Y	N	N	N
	Russian Federation	Y	-	-	-	NA	-	-	-	-	-	-	-	-
	Tajikistan	Y	Y	Y	N	Y	N	Y	Y	Y	N	-	N	N
	Turkey	N	N	N	N	NA	N	Y	Y	Y	N	Y	N	N
	Turkmenistan	N	N	Y	N	NA	N	Y	Y	Y	N	Y	N	N
	Uzbekistan	Y	Y	Y	N	-	Y	Y	Y	Y	N	-	N	-
South-East Asia	Bangladesh	Y	Y	N	N	Y	Y	Y	Y	Y	Y	N	Y	N
	Bhutan	Y	Y	Y	N	Y	Y	Y	Y	Y	Y	N	Y	N
	Democratic People's Republic of Korea	N	Y	N	N	NA	N	N	Y	Y	N	N	N	N
	Democratic Republic of Timor-Leste	Y	Y	N	Y	Y	Y	Y	Y	-	Y	-	N	-
	India	Y	N	Y	Y	Y	N	Y	Y	Y	Y	Y	Y	N
	Indonesia	Y	Y	N	N	Y	Y	Y	Y	N	Y	Y	Y	N
	Myanmar	Y	Y	N	N	Y	N	Y	Y	Y	Y	-	Y	N
	Nepal	Y	Y	Y	N	Y	Y	Y	Y	Y	Y	N	Y	N
	Sri Lanka	Y	Y	Y	N	Y	Y	Y	Y	-	N	Y	Y	N
	Thailand	Y	Y	Y	N	Y	Y	Y	Y	Y	Y	-	Y	-
Western Pacific	Cambodia	Y	Y	N	N	Y	Y	Y	Y	Y	Y	Y	Y	N
	China	Y	Y	N	N	Y	Y	Y	Y	Y	N	Y	N	N
	Lao People's Democratic Republic	N	Y	N	N	Y	Y	Y	Y	Y	Y	Y	Y	N
	Malaysia	Y	Y	Y	N	Y	N	Y	N	Y	Y	N	N	N
	Papua New Guinea	Y	Y	N	Y	Y	N	Y	Y	Y	Y	N	Y	Y
	Philippines	Y	Y	Y	N	Y	Y	Y	Y	Y	Y	N	Y	N
	Republic of Korea	N	N	N	N	NA	N	Y	N	Y	N	-	-	-
	Solomon Islands	Y	Y	Y	N	Y	Y	N	Y	Y	Y	-	N	N
	Vanuatu	Y	Y	N	N	Y	N	N	Y	Y	Y	N	N	N
	Viet Nam	Y	Y	Y	N	Y	Y	Y	Y	Y	Y	Y	Y	N

(Y) = Actually implemented.

(N) = Not implemented.

(-) = Question not answered or not applicable.

*The policies for Sudan only represents the northern states.

Annex 4.A – Recommended policies and strategies for malaria control, 2009 (continued)

WHO region/subregion	Country/area	Insecticide-treated nets: Distribution - Free	Insecticide-treated nets: Targeting - All age groups	Indoor residual spraying: IRS is the primary vector control intervention	Indoor residual spraying: DDT is used for IRS (public health only)	ACT policy adopted	Oral artemisinin monotherapies banned	Parasitological confirmation for all age groups	ACT is free of charge for under 5 years old in the public sector	Diagnosis of malaria inpatients is based on laboratory testing	Pre-referral treatment with quinine or artemether IM or artesunate suppositories	Oversight regulation of case management in the private sectors	RDTs used at community level	IPT Strategy used to prevent malaria during pregnancy
	Jamaica	Y	-	-	-	NA	-	-	-	-	-	-	-	-
	Mexico	Y	Y	Y	N	NA	-	-	-	-	-	-	-	-
	Nicaragua	N	N	N	N	NA	N	N	N	-	-	-	-	-
	Panama	N	Y	N	N	N	-	N	-	-	N	-	-	-
	Paraguay	N	Y	Y	N	N	-	N	-	-	-	-	-	-
	Peru	Y	-	-	N	Y	N	N	-	N	-	N	N	N
	Suriname	Y	Y	N	N	Y	N	Y	Y	N	-	-	-	-
	Venezuela (Bolivarian Republic of)	Y	Y	Y	N	Y	Y	Y	Y	Y	Y	N	N	N
Eastern Mediterranean	Afghanistan	Y	Y	N	N	Y	Y	Y	Y	Y	N	N	Y	Y
	Djibouti	N	N	N	N	Y	Y	Y	N	Y	N	N	-	-
	Egypt	-	-	-	-	Y	-	N	-	-	-	-	-	-
	Iran (Islamic Republic of)	Y	Y	Y	N	Y	Y	Y	Y	Y	N	N	N	N
	Iraq	Y	Y	Y	N	Y	Y	Y	Y	Y	Y	N	N	N
	Morocco	-	-	-	-	Y	-	-	N	-	-	-	-	-
	Oman	-	-	-	-	NA	-	-	-	-	-	-	-	-
	Pakistan	N	Y	Y	N	Y	Y	Y	Y	N	N	N	N	N
	Saudi Arabia	N	N	N	N	Y	Y	Y	Y	Y	Y	N	N	N
	Somalia	Y	Y	N	N	NA	Y	Y	Y	Y	Y	Y	Y	Y
	Sudan*	Y	N	N	N	Y	Y	N	Y	Y	N	-	N	Y
	Syrian Arab Republic	-	-	-	-	NA	-	-	-	-	-	-	-	-
	Yemen	N	Y	Y	N	Y	Y	Y	Y	N	N	N	N	N
Europe	Armenia	N	Y	Y	N	NA	N	Y	N	N	N	N	N	N
	Azerbaijan	N	Y	Y	N	NA	N	Y	N	Y	N	N	N	N
	Georgia	N	Y	Y	N	NA	N	Y	N	N	N	N	N	N
	Kyrgyzstan	Y	Y	-	Y	-	N	-	N	N	-	-	N	N
	Russian Federation	-	-	-	-	-	-	-	-	-	-	-	-	-
	Tajikistan	Y	Y	Y	N	Y	Y	Y	N	Y	N	N	N	N
	Turkey	N	Y	N	N	NA	Y	Y	N	Y	N	N	N	N
	Turkmenistan	N	Y	Y	N	NA	N	Y	N	Y	N	N	N	N
	Uzbekistan	Y	Y	Y	N	-	N	Y	N	N	N	N	N	-
South-East Asia	Bangladesh	Y	N	N	N	Y	Y	Y	N	N	Y	N	N	N
	Bhutan	Y	Y	Y	N	Y	Y	Y	Y	N	Y	N	N	N
	Democratic People's Republic of Korea	Y	Y	N	-	NA	N	N	Y	-	N	-	N	-
	Democratic Republic of Timor-Leste	Y	N	N	N	Y	Y	Y	Y	Y	-	N	-	N
	India	Y	Y	Y	Y	Y	Y	N	Y	Y	Y	N	N	N
	Indonesia	Y	Y	N	N	Y	Y	Y	Y	N	Y	N	N	N
	Myanmar	Y	Y	Y	N	Y	Y	N	Y	Y	Y	N	N	N
	Nepal	Y	Y	Y	N	Y	Y	Y	Y	Y	Y	N	N	N
	Sri Lanka	Y	Y	Y	N	Y	Y	Y	Y	N	Y	-	N	N
	Thailand	Y	Y	Y	N	Y	Y	Y	Y	Y	Y	N	N	-
Western Pacific	Cambodia	Y	N	N	N	Y	Y	Y	Y	Y	N	-	N	N
	China	Y	N	N	N	Y	Y	Y	Y	N	Y	N	N	N
	Lao People's Democratic Republic	Y	Y	N	N	Y	Y	Y	Y	Y	N	N	N	N
	Malaysia	Y	Y	Y	N	Y	N	Y	Y	N	N	N	N	N
	Papua New Guinea	Y	Y	Y	Y	Y	Y	Y	Y	Y	N	Y	N	Y
	Philippines	Y	Y	N	N	Y	Y	Y	Y	Y	Y	Y	N	N
	Republic of Korea	N	N	N	N	NA	N	N	N	N	N	N	N	N
	Solomon Islands	Y	N	N	N	Y	Y	Y	Y	N	N	N	N	N
	Vanuatu	Y	N	N	N	Y	N	Y	Y	N	N	-	-	-
	Viet Nam	Y	Y	Y	N	Y	Y	Y	Y	Y	Y	N	N	N

(Y) = Actually implemented.

(N) = Not implemented.

(-) = Question not answered or not applicable.

Mauritius is one of the countries listed but it has had no ongoing local transmission for over a decade.

*The policies for Sudan only represents the northern states.

Annex 4.B – Antimalarial drug policy, 2009

WHO region	Country/area	P. falciparum				P. vivax
		Uncomplicated unconfirmed	Uncomplicated confirmed	Severe	Prevention during pregnancy	Treatment
Africa	Algeria	-	-	-	-	CQ
	Angola	AL	AL	QN(7d)	SP(IPT)	-
	Benin	AL	AL	QN(7d)	SP(IPT)	-
	Botswana	AL	AL	QN(7d)	CQ+PG	-
	Burkina Faso	AS+AQ;AL	AS+AQ;AL	QN(7d)	SP(IPT)	-
	Burundi	AS+AQ	AS+AQ	QN(7d)	-	-
	Cameroon	AS+AQ	AS+AQ	QN(7d)	SP(IPT)	-
	Cape Verde	AL	AL	QN(7d)	CQ	-
	Central African Republic	AL	AL	QN(7d)	SP(IPT)	-
	Chad	AS+AQ;AL	AS+AQ;AL	QN(7d)	SP(IPT)	-
	Comoros	AL	AL	QN(7d)	SP(IPT)	-
	Congo	AS+AQ	AS+AQ	QN(7d)	SP(IPT)	-
	Côte d'Ivoire	AS+AQ	AS+AQ	QN(7d)	SP(IPT)	-
	Democratic Republic of the Congo	AS+AQ	AS+AQ	QN(7d)	SP(IPT)	-
	Equatorial Guinea	AS+AQ	AS+AQ	QN(7d)	-	CQ+PQ
	Eritrea	CQ+SP	AS+AQ	QN(7d)	-	CQ
	Ethiopia	AL	AL	QN(7d)	SP(IPT)	-
	Gabon	AS+AQ	AS+AQ	QN(7d)	SP(IPT)	-
	Gambia	AL	AL	QN(7d)	SP(IPT)	-
	Ghana	AS+AQ;AL	AS+AQ;AL	QN(7d)	SP(IPT)	-
	Guinea	AS+AQ	AS+AQ	QN(7d)	SP(IPT)	-
	Guinea-Bissau	AL	AL	QN(7d)	SP(IPT)	-
	Kenya	AL	AL	QN(7d)	SP(IPT)	-
	Liberia	AS+AQ	AS+AQ	QN(7d)	SP(IPT)	-
	Madagascar	AS+AQ	AS+AQ	QN(7d)	SP(IPT)	-
	Malawi	AL	AL	QN(7d)	SP(IPT)	-
	Mali	AL	AL	QN(7d)	SP(IPT)	-
	Mauritania	AS+AQ	AS+AQ	QN(7d)	-	CQ
	Mauritius	-	-	-	-	-
	Mozambique	AL	AL	QN(7d)	SP(IPT)	-
	Namibia	AL	AL	QN(7d)	SP(IPT)	-
	Niger	AL	AL	QN(7d)	SP(IPT)	-
	Nigeria	AL;AS+AQ	AL;AS+AQ	QN(7d)	SP(IPT)	-
	Rwanda	AL	AL	QN(7d)	SP(IPT)	-
	Sao Tome and Principe	AS+AQ	AS+AQ	QN(7d)	SP(IPT)	-
	Senegal	AS+AQ	AS+AQ;AL	QN(7d)	SP(IPT)	-
	Sierra Leone	AS+AQ	AS+AQ	QN(7d)	SP(IPT)	-
	South Africa	AL	AL	QN(7d)	CQ+PG	-
	Swaziland	-	-	QN(7d)	CQ+PG	-
	Togo	AL;AS+AQ	AL;AS+AQ	QN(7d)	SP(IPT)	-
	Uganda	AL	AL	QN(7d)	SP(IPT)	-
	United Republic of Tanzania	AL;AS+AQ	AL;AS+AQ	QN(7d)	SP(IPT)	-
	Zambia	AL	AL	QN(7d)	SP(IPT)	-
	Zimbabwe	AL	AL	QN(7d)	SP(IPT)	-

Annex 4.B – Antimalarial drug policy, 2009 (continued)

WHO region	Country/area	P. falciparum Uncomplicated unconfirmed	Uncomplicated confirmed	Severe	Prevention during pregnancy	P. vivax Treatment
Americas	Argentina	-	-	-	-	CQ+PQ
	Belize	-	-	-	-	CQ+PQ
	Bolivia	-	AS+MQ	-	-	CQ+PQ
	Brazil	-	AL	AS; AM; QN	-	CQ+PQ(7d)
	Colombia	-	AL; AS+MQ	QN(7d)	-	CQ+PQ
	Costa Rica	-	-	-	-	CQ+PQ
	Dominican Republic	-	CQ+PQ(3d)	-	-	-
	Ecuador	-	AS+SP; AL	-	-	CQ+PQ
	El Salvador	-	-	-	-	CQ+PQ
	French Guiana	-	QN+T	-	-	CQ+PQ
	Guatemala	-	-	-	-	CQ+PQ
	Guyana	-	AL	-	-	CQ+PQ
	Haiti	-	CQ+PQ	-	-	-
	Honduras	-	-	-	-	CQ+PQ
	Mexico	-	-	-	-	CQ+PQ
	Nicaragua	-	CQ+PQ(7d)	QN+CL	-	CQ+PQ(7d)
	Panama	-	-	-	-	CQ+PQ
	Paraguay	-	CQ+PQ	-	-	CQ+PQ
	Peru	-	AS+MQ; AS+SP	-	-	CQ+PQ
	Suriname	-	AL	-	-	CQ+PQ
	Venezuela (Bolivarian Republic of)	-	AS+MQ	-	-	CQ+PQ
Eastern Mediterranean	Afghanistan	CQ+SP	AS+SP	QN(7d); AS+SP	-	CQ
	Djibouti	AS+SP	AS+SP	QN	-	CQ+PQ(14d)
	Egypt	-	AL	QN(7d)	-	CQ+PQ(14d)
	Iran (Islamic Republic of)	-	AS+SP	QN; AS	-	CQ+PQ(14d)
	Iraq	-	AL	QN(7d)	-	CQ+PQ(14d)
	Morocco	-	AL	QN(7d)	-	CQ+PQ(14d)
	Oman	-	AL+PQ	QN(7d); AS	-	CQ+PQ(14d)
	Pakistan	AS+SP	AS+SP	QN; AM	-	CQ+PQ(5d)
	Saudi Arabia	-	AS+SP	QN(7d)	-	CQ+PQ(14d)
	Somalia	AS+SP	AS+SP	QN	SP(IPT)	-
	Sudan*	AS+SP; AS+AQ	AS+SP; AS+AQ	QN; AM; AS+SP	SP(IPT)	CQ+PQ(14d)
	Syrian Arab Republic	-	SP	QN(7d)	-	CQ+PQ(14d)
	Yemen	AS+SP	AS+SP	QN(7d)	-	CQ+PQ(14d)

Annex 4.B – Antimalarial drug policy, 2009 (continued)

WHO region	Country/area	P. falciparum				P. vivax
		Uncomplicated unconfirmed	Uncomplicated confirmed	Severe	Prevention during pregnancy	Treatment
Europe	Armenia	-	-	-	-	CQ+PQ(14d)
	Azerbaijan	-	-	-	-	CQ+PQ(14d)
	Georgia	-	-	-	-	CQ+PQ(14d)
	Tajikistan	-	AS+SP;AL	QN(7d)	-	CQ+PQ(14d)
	Turkey	-	-	-	-	CQ+PQ(14d)
	Turkmenistan	-	-	-	-	CQ+PQ(14d)
South-East Asia	Bangladesh	CQ+PQ	AL	QN; AM	-	CQ+PQ(14d)
	Bhutan	-	AL	QN; AM	-	CQ+PQ(14d)
	Democratic People's Republic of Korea	-	-	-	-	CQ+PQ(14d)
	Democratic Republic of Timor-Leste	CQ+PQ	AL	QN; AM	-	CQ+PQ(14d)
	India	CQ+PQ	AS+SP	QN; AM	-	CQ+PQ(14d)
	Indonesia	CQ+PQ	AS+AQ+PQ;DHA-PPQ	QN; AM	-	CQ+PQ(14d)
	Myanmar	CQ	AS+MQ;AL;DHA-PPQ	QN; AS	-	CQ+PQ(14d)
	Nepal	CQ+PQ	AL	QN	-	CQ+PQ(14d)
	Sri Lanka	-	AL	QN(7d)	-	CQ+PQ(14d)
	Thailand	-	AS+MQ	QN; AS	-	CQ+PQ(14d)
Western Pacific	Cambodia	AS+MQ	AS+MQ	AM+MQ	-	CQ
	China	-	PPQ;ART+NQ;ART+PPQ;AS+AQ	AM; AS; AM; PYR	-	CQ+PQ(8d)
	Lao People's Democratic Republic	CQ	AL	AS+AL	CQ(weekly); SP(IPT)	CQ+PQ(14d)
	Malaysia	-	AS+MQ;AL	QN+T	-	CQ+PQ(14d)
	Papua New Guinea	AL	AL	AS; AM	SP(IPT); CQ	CQ+PQ(14d)
	Philippines	AL	AL+PQ	QN+T	CQ(weekly); SP(IPT)	CQ+PQ(14d)
	Republic of Korea	-	-	-	-	AL+PQ(1d)
	Solomon Islands	-	AL	AS	CQ	AL+PQ(14d)
	Vanuatu	AL	AL	QN(7d)	CQ(weekly)	AL+PQ(14d)
	Viet Nam	-	DHA-PPQ	AS; QN	CQ(weekly)	CQ+PQ(14d)

AL=Artemether-lumefantrine
AM=Artemether
AQ=Amodiaquine
ART=Artemisinin
AS=Artesunate
CL=Clindamycine
CQ=Chloroquine

D=Doxycycline
DHA=Dihydroartemisinin
MQ=Mefloquine
NQ=Naphroquine
PG=Proguanil
PPQ=Piperaquine
PQ=Primaquine

PYR=Pyronaridine
QN=Quinine
SP=Sulfadoxine-pyrimethamine
T=Tetracycline

*The drug policy for Sudan represents only the northern states.

Mauritius is one of the countries listed but it has had no ongoing local transmission for over a decade.

Annex 5 – Operational coverage of insecticide-treated nets, indoor residual spraying and antimalarial treatment, 2007–2008

WHO region	Country/area	Year	No. of ITN + LLIN sold or delivered	No. of LLIN sold or delivered	No. of ITN sold or delivered	% ITN coverage	No. of houses sprayed	No. of people protected by IRS	% IRS coverage	Any 1st-line treatment courses delivered (including ACT)	ACT treatment courses delivered	% Any antimalarial coverage total	% ACT coverage total	% Any antimalarial coverage public	% ACT coverage public
Africa	Algeria	2007	-	-	-	-	-	-	-	297	-	-	-	-	-
	Algeria	2008	-	-	-	-	-	-	-	152	-	-	-	-	-
	Angola	2007	1,495,165	1,495,165	-	26.5	110,826	612,776	3.5	2,031,760	2,031,760	20.2	20.2	33.2	33.2
	Angola	2008	1,471,200	1,471,200	-	42.1	133,687	736,231	4.1	2,363,970	2,363,970	23.1	23.1	38	38
	Benin	2007	2,000,000	2,000,000	-	48.8	-	-	-	-	-	-	-	-	-
	Benin	2008	20,000	20,000	-	47.8	-	-	-	-	-	-	-	-	-
	Botswana	2007	-	-	-	0.3	-	342,536	37.9	16,983	16,983	56.7	56.7	588.3	588.3
	Botswana	2008	-	-	-	0.3	-	344,989	37.6	17,886	17,886	59	59	612.3	612.3
	Burkina Faso	2007	24,000	13,000	11,000	2.0	-	-	-	4,981,270	811,507	21.8	3.5	67.7	11
	Burkina Faso	2008	724,548	724,547	1	11.3	-	-	-	2,408,905	2,408,905	10.3	10.3	32.1	32.1
	Burundi	2007	1,203,763	1,203,763	-	58.6	-	-	-	2,263,515	2,263,515	31.9	31.9	68.1	68.1
	Burundi	2008	895,355	895,355	-	85.3	24,007	-	-	2,006,361	2,006,361	28	28	59.6	59.6
	Cameroon	2007	244,425	-	244,425	2.8	-	-	-	2,566,785	2,566,785	17.5	17.5	49.6	49.6
	Cameroon	2008	802,105	802,105	-	8.6	-	-	-	1,814,725	1,814,725	12.1	12.1	34.3	34.3
	Cape Verde	2007	-	-	-	-	200	1,000	0.8	-	-	-	-	-	-
	Cape Verde	2008	-	-	-	-	500	2,500	1.9	-	-	-	-	-	-
	Central African Republic	2007	498,050	498,050	0	29.1	-	-	-	1,192,266	1,192,266	22	22	58.9	58.9
	Central African Republic	2008	846,966	846,966	0	67.6	-	-	-	1,242,306	1,242,306	22.4	22.4	60.1	60.1
	Chad	2007	83,000	-	-	1.6	-	-	-	-	-	-	-	-	-
	Chad	2008	126,000	-	-	2.3	-	-	-	-	-	-	-	-	-
	Comoros	2007	95,000	95,000	95,000	29.4	-	-	-	104,640	83,020	17.3	-	44.3	-
	Comoros	2008	20,000	20,000	-	6.1	-	-	-	295,590	295,590	47.9	-	122.5	-
	Congo	2007	-	-	-	-	-	-	-	-	-	-	-	-	-
	Congo	2008	-	-	-	-	-	-	-	-	-	-	-	-	-
	Côte d'Ivoire	2007	169,832	-	169,832	5.0	-	-	-	721,314	476,203	3.3	2.2	12.6	8.3
	Côte d'Ivoire	2008	1,034,486	-	1,034,486	13.3	-	-	-	-	-	-	-	-	-
	Democratic Republic of the Congo	2007	2,385,684	2,385,684	-	17.1	-	-	-	1,348,304	1,348,304	1.8	2169.5	5.6	6810.4
	Democratic Republic of the Congo	2008	5,788,513	5,788,513	-	34.5	22,000	82,975	0.1	1,723,655	1,723,655	2.3	2769.8	7.1	8695.1
	Equatorial Guinea	2007	152,992	152,992	-	47.6	-	216,200	33.7	-	-	-	-	-	-
	Equatorial Guinea	2008	65,913	65,913	65,913	66.4	-	371,136	56.3	58,241	47,933	10.1	8.3	21.7	17.8
	Eritrea	2007	159,360	159,360	159,360	10.0	86,153	305,978	6.4	-	37,429	-	161.9	-	1183.5
	Eritrea	2008	134,399	134,399	134,399	15.2	75,019	251,641	5.1	-	22,662	-	99.2	-	725.3
	Ethiopia	2007	7,178,443	7,178,443	7,178,443	60.8	2,523,902	5,303,213	9.9	5,450,400	4,032,640	-	18.9	94.2	143
	Ethiopia	2008	3,316,696	3,316,696	3,316,696	71.3	5,641,275	28,206,375	51.4	8,000,000	8,000,000	12.5	37	-	280.3
	Gabon	2007	352,994	2,874	350,120	50.1	-	-	-	1,260,759	952,000	110.6	101.9	261.5	241
	Gabon	2008	10,640	1,640	9,000	2.3	-	-	-	190,259	0	16.8	-	39.6	-
	Gambia	2007	224,979	77,163	147,816	31.9	-	-	-	1,188,325	1,188,325	-	-	-	-
	Gambia	2008	428,083	290,393	137,690	64.8	-	-	-	-	-	98.2	98.2	146.6	146.6
	Ghana	2007	4,281,460	1,934,460	2,347,000	57.3	154,000	240,000	1.0	2,018,967	1,852,967	9.9	9.1	24.1	22.1
	Ghana	2008	2,357,717	257,717	2,100,000	56.2	68,252	601,973	2.6	9,616,195	9,783,983	46.7	47.5	113.2	115.2
	Guinea	2007	312,500	312,500	-	9.0	-	-	-	-	-	-	-	-	-
	Guinea	2008	246,000	246,000	246,000	13.8	-	-	-	29,347	29,347	-	0.4	-	1.3
	Guinea-Bissau	2007	91,700	91,700	-	35.6	-	-	-	-	-	-	-	-	-
	Guinea-Bissau	2008	2,064	2,064	-	35.1	-	-	-	110,627	110,627	5.8	5.8	9.9	9.9
	Kenya	2007	1,996,875	1,591,492	405,383	58.5	390,058	3,459,207	12.1	-	-	-	-	-	-
	Kenya	2008	2,786,742	2,437,621	349,121	73.2	307,207	3,061,966	10.4	-	-	-	-	-	-
	Liberia	2007	342,639	342,639	-	43.5	-	-	-	675,225	675,225	27.9	27.9	71.3	71.3
	Liberia	2008	714,500	714,500	-	61.2	21,904	160,000	4.2	595,000	595,000	24.1	24.1	61.7	61.7
	Madagascar	2007	3,359,244	-	-	36.1	248,269	1,241,344	6.7	-	558,000	-	12.8	-	47.7
	Madagascar	2008	907,739	-	-	9.5	1,312,811	6,564,056	34.3	1,167,480	1,167,480	-	26.6	-	99.4
	Malawi	2007	673,238	255,266	417,972	11.0	-	-	-	-	-	-	-	-	-
	Malawi	2008	2,354,094	858,026	1,496,068	36.8	-	-	-	-	-	-	-	-	-
	Mali	2007	2,982,346	-	-	49.5	87,198	405,936	3.3	-	1,162,048	-	-	-	-
	Mali	2008	682,461	-	-	12.2	-	-	-	-	2,842,500	-	-	-	-
	Mauritania	2007	20,850	-	20,850	4.5	-	-	-	-	-	-	-	-	-
	Mauritania	2008	-	-	-	6.3	-	-	-	-	-	-	-	-	-

Annex 5 – Operational coverage of insecticide-treated nets, indoor residual spraying and antimalarial treatment, 2007–2008 (continued)

WHO region	Country/area	Year	No. of ITN + LLIN sold or delivered	No. of LLIN sold or delivered	No. of ITN sold or delivered	% ITN coverage	No. of houses sprayed	No. of people protected by IRS	% IRS coverage	Any 1st-line treatment courses delivered (including ACT)	ACT treatment courses delivered	% Any antimalarial coverage total	% ACT coverage total	% Any antimalarial coverage public	% ACT coverage public
Africa	*Mauritius*	2007													
		2008													
	Mozambique	2007	1,586,534	1,586,534	-	17.4	1,682,369	6,465,517	29.6	6,155,082	6,155,082	27.2	27.2	49.2	49.2
		2008	2,086,367	2,086,367	-	35.6	1,945,389	6,545,395	29.2	4,831,491	4,831,491	20.9	20.9	37.9	37.9
	Namibia	2007	58,500	30,000	28,500	27.4	658,635	487,372	34.8	4,433	4,433	3.5	3.5	6.5	6.5
		2008	397,282	312,382	84,900	78.5	205,748	233,440	16.4	5,193	5,193	4.1	4.1	7.6	7.6
	Niger	2007	710,000	710,000	-	47.7				1,162,636	1,162,636	11.3	14	39.6	48.7
		2008	700,000	700,000	-	45.8				2,033,971	1,593,782	19.7	15.4	68.8	53.9
	Nigeria	2007	3,225,594	1,003,573	2,222,021	9.5	600	3,000	0.0	13,019,950	13,000,000	8.2	8.2	33.3	33.3
		2008	6,700,000	6,700,000	-	15.2				12,000,000	12,000,000	7.5	7.5	30.2	30.2
	Rwanda	2007	1,162,275	1,162,275	-	66.0	152,072	705,035	7.5						
		2008	17,926			64.6	189,756	885,957	9.1						
	Sao Tome and Principe	2007	573,799	573,799	-	728.0	22,857	117,428	74.5	5,451	5,451	14.9	14.9	47.7	47.7
		2008	787,385	787,385	-	1699.6				3,679	3,679	9.9	9.9	31.6	31.6
	Senegal	2007	1,572,261	1,572,261	-	6.7		678,971	5.7	990,141	990,141	21.8	162.3	51.8	386.7
		2008	2,273,413	2,273,413	-	32.3		635,666	5.2	320,335	320,335	6.9	51.6	16.5	123
	Sierra Leone	2007	319,199	319,199	-	59.8				240,404		2.7		6.4	
		2008	541,265	541,265	-	77.8				828,857		9.1		21.4	
	South Africa	2007						4	0.0						
		2008						4	0.0						
	Swaziland	2007	29,236	29,236	-	21.6	102,541	93	0.0		0				
		2008	20,000	20,000	-	30.7	94,766	94	0.0		0				
	Togo	2007	43,946	43,946	0	3.5				555,204	555,204	7.9	17.7	26.9	60.6
		2008	1,261,706	1,261,706	0	42.5				800,000	800,000	11.1	24.9	37.9	85.2
	Uganda	2007	1,622,001	1,622,001	-	23.6	466,477	1,963,945	6.4		16,919,100	87.8	87.8		308.4
		2008	2,273,413	2,273,413	-	37.2	499,998	1,858,149	5.9		6,389,600	32.3	32.3		113.6
	United Republic of Tanzania	2007	2,990,668	322,516	2,668,152	17.2	405,878	1,071,194	2.6	23,455,260	23,455,260	102.5	150	194.2	284
		2008	2,783,740	927,461	1,856,279	17.2	295,385	1,308,194	3.1						
	Zambia	2007	2,458,183	2,458,183	-	58.8		3,288,475	26.7	3,036,982	3,036,982				
		2008	1,188,443	1,188,443	-	76.2		5,747,995	45.5	3,142,405	3,142,405				
	Zimbabwe	2007	517,835	517,835	-	8.3	303,143	1,659,393	13.3						
		2008				8.3	156,658	929,660	7.5						
Americas	Argentina	2007					6,580	26,320	1.1	355		91.7	91.7	142.9	142.9
		2008					5,628	22,512	0.9	106		81.5	81.5	127	127
	Bahamas	2007													
		2008													
	Belize	2007													
		2008													
	Bolivia (Plurinational State of)	2007	14,000	14,000	-	1.7		50,000	0.8	14,610	1,622	100		287	
		2008	5,000	5,000	-	1.9		125,000	2.0	9,894	782	100		287	
	Brazil	2007	10,000	10,000	0	0.1				459,513	45,918	100.3	77	917.3	703.9
		2008								347,086	45,717	110	111.2	1005.4	1017
	Colombia	2007	87,394	87,394	-	1.3		143,640	1.0	155,132	33,240	120.8	105.6	672.3	587.7
		2008	194,363	105,759	88,604	3.8		211,294	1.4	79,230	46,350	98.4	234.7	547.5	1306.8
	Costa Rica	2007						0		12,230	12,230	1000		10328.3	
		2008					627			9,660	9,660	1000		10328.3	
	Dominican Republic	2007						11,008	0.2	2,711	2,711	167.3		9552.7	
		2008	6,000	6,000	0	0.2		17,092	0.2	1,840	2	145.8	0.1	8322.9	6.4
	Ecuador	2007													
		2008													
	El Salvador	2007													
		2008													
	French Guiana	2007													
		2008													
	Guatemala	2007	427,277	427,277	-	21.3									
		2008	427,277	427,277	-	31.1					1,817,097		9085485		102193472.6

Annex 5 – Operational coverage of insecticide-treated nets, indoor residual spraying and antimalarial treatment, 2007–2008 (continued)

WHO region	Country/area	Year	No. of ITN + LLIN sold or delivered	No. of LLIN sold or delivered	No. of ITN sold or delivered	% ITN coverage	No. of houses sprayed	No. of people protected by IRS	% IRS coverage	Any 1st-line treatment courses delivered (including ACT)	ACT treatment courses delivered	% Any antimalarial coverage total	% ACT coverage total	% Any antimalarial coverage public	% ACT coverage public
Americas	Guyana	2007	2,784	2,784	-	9.1	-	-	-	11,657	4,351	100	84	763.7	641.3
		2008	4,287	4,287	-	10.3	-	-	-	11,815	5,252	100	100	763.7	763.7
	Haiti	2007	89,049	89,049	-	1.8	-	-	-	-	-	-	-	-	-
		2008	125,713	125,713	-	4.3	-	-	-	-	-	-	-	-	-
	Honduras	2007	-	-	-	0.1	-	-	-	-	-	-	-	-	-
		2008	-	-	-	0.1	-	-	-	-	-	-	-	-	-
	Jamaica	2007	-	-	-	-	-	-	-	-	-	-	-	-	-
		2008	-	-	-	-	-	-	-	-	-	-	-	-	-
	Mexico	2007	-	-	-	-	-	-	-	-	-	-	-	-	-
		2008	-	-	-	-	-	-	-	-	-	-	-	-	-
	Nicaragua	2007	-	-	-	-	-	-	-	-	-	-	-	-	-
		2008	-	-	-	-	-	-	-	-	-	-	-	-	-
	Panama	2007	-	-	-	-	-	-	-	-	-	-	-	-	-
		2008	6,649	-	6,649	0.4	-	11,975	0.4	-	-	-	-	-	-
	Paraguay	2007	-	-	-	-	-	-	-	-	-	-	-	-	-
		2008	-	-	-	-	-	-	-	-	-	-	-	-	-
	Peru	2007	-	-	-	-	-	-	-	-	-	-	-	-	-
		2008	-	-	-	-	-	-	-	-	-	-	-	-	-
	Suriname	2007	7,742	-	-	28.3	-	-	-	-	-	-	-	-	-
		2008	14,372	-	-	52.1	-	-	-	-	-	-	-	-	-
	Venezuela (Bolivarian Republic of)	2007	6,000	-	-	0.2	-	-	-	-	-	-	-	-	-
		2008	-	-	-	-	2,827,542	10,116,563	131.2	1,814,681	-	5664.3	-	85020.6	-
Eastern Mediterranean	Afghanistan	2007	345,245	345,245	-	2.9	-	-	-	-	-	-	-	-	-
		2008	916,723	916,723	-	9.6	-	-	-	-	-	-	-	-	-
	Djibouti	2007	-	-	-	5.3	-	-	-	-	-	-	-	-	-
		2008	45,000	45,000	-	15.8	-	-	-	-	7,102	-	28.8	-	247.5
	Egypt	2007	-	-	-	-	-	-	-	-	-	-	-	-	-
		2008	-	-	-	-	-	-	-	-	-	-	-	-	-
	Iran (Islamic Republic of)	2007	40,000	40,000	-	0.7	-	-	-	-	-	-	-	-	-
		2008	50,000	50,000	-	0.9	-	-	-	-	-	-	-	-	-
	Iraq	2007	-	-	-	2.5	-	-	-	30	0	1000	-	3124.8	-
		2008	240,000	240,000	-	5.6	-	-	-	64	24	1066.7	1200	3333.1	3749.8
	Morocco	2007	-	0	0	-	-	-	-	2,864	-	100	-	301.3	-
		2008	250,000	250,000	-	3.6	-	-	-	1,491	-	100	-	301.3	-
	Oman	2007	-	-	-	-	-	-	-	-	-	-	-	-	-
		2008	-	-	-	-	-	-	-	-	-	-	-	-	-
	Pakistan	2007	90,000	-	-	0.4	-	-	-	4,513,876	-	178.9	-	1068.7	-
		2008	41,400	41,400	-	0.3	602,314	4,938,975	3.0	6,762,058	-	264.2	-	1578.9	-
	Saudi Arabia	2007	-	0	-	-	-	-	-	-	-	100	-	100	-
		2008	-	-	0	-	-	-	-	-	-	100	-	100	-
	Somalia	2007	456,000	-	-	10.4	120	720	0.0	-	-	-	-	-	-
		2008	162,187	162,187	-	3.6	231	1,386	0.0	141,379	141,379	585.8	597.7	6563	6697
	Sudan*	2007	1,910,000	830,000	1,080,000	13.3	641,123	3,846,738	9.5	3,337,103	2,677,199	109.8	-	353.6	-
		2008	1,806,540	1,756,540	50,000	16.5	456,337	2,281,687	5.5	3,073,996	3,073,996	100	-	322.1	-
	Syrian Arab Republic	2007	-	-	-	-	-	-	-	-	-	-	-	-	-
		2008	-	-	-	-	-	-	-	-	-	-	-	-	-
	Yemen	2007	450,000	450,000	0	5.8	125,849	-	-	34,500	0	51	-	563.4	-
		2008	700,000	700,000	0	11.8	208,326	-	-	26,163	0	59.4	-	656	-
Europe	Armenia	2007	-	0	-	-	652	2,608	-	2	0	200	-	-	-
		2008	-	0	-	-	476	2,120	-	1	0	100	-	-	-
	Azerbaijan	2007	-	0	0	-	36,813	150,933	3.8	110	0	100	-	121.1	-
		2008	-	0	0	-	31,522	127,665	3.2	73	0	100	-	121.1	-
	Georgia	2007	-	-	-	-	4,260	-	-	25	0	108.7	-	129.9	-
		2008	-	-	-	-	4,260	-	-	8	0	133.3	-	159.4	-
	Kyrgyzstan	2007	20,000	0	20,000	1.0	24,800	123,000	3.0	96	0	100	-	101.7	-
		2008	68,000	0	68,000	3.2	51,610	313,003	7.4	18	0	100	-	101.7	-

WHO region	Country/area	Year	No. of ITN + LLIN sold or delivered	No. of LLIN sold or delivered	No. of ITN sold or delivered	% ITN coverage	No. of houses sprayed	No. of people protected by IRS	% IRS coverage	Any 1st-line treatment courses delivered (including ACT)	ACT treatment courses delivered	% Any antimalarial coverage total	% ACT coverage total	% Any antimalarial coverage public	% ACT coverage public
Europe	Russian Federation	2007	-	-	-	-	-	-	-	-	-	-	-	-	-
		2008	-	-	-	-	-	-	-	-	-	-	-	-	-
	Tajikistan	2007	26,438	26,438	-	1.6	183,464	552,912	10.8	635	7	100	206.1	115.1	237.2
		2008	19,494	19,494	-	2.3	624,000	632,622	12.2	318	2	100	117.6	115.1	135.4
	Turkey	2007	-	-	-	-	21,901	109,505	1.8	2,600	-	1040	-	1386.1	-
		2008	-	-	-	-	65,475	327,375	5.3	980	-	720.6	-	960.4	-
	Turkmenistan	2007	-	0	0	-	-	-	-	0	0	-	-	-	-
		2008	-	0	0	-	-	-	-	1	0	100	-	-	-
	Uzbekistan	2007	3,000	3,000	0	0.3	21,699	130,192	6.6	89	0	100	-	119.5	-
		2008	10,000	10,000	0	1.3	22,396	134,376	6.7	27	0	100	-	119.5	-
South-East Asia	Bangladesh	2007	-	-	-	0.0	-	-	-	241,398	114,990	97.2	64.7	2551.9	1700.5
		2008	1,863,940	1,200,000	663,940	3.2	-	-	-	164,394	110,280	97.5	91.5	2559.8	2402.1
	Bhutan	2007	4,561	4,561	-	40.3	39,763	185,905	37.2	793	379	100	115.6	17657.4	20415
		2008	10,000	10,000	-	43.7	19,914	97,494	19.2	329	181	100	133.1	17657.4	23499.9
	Democratic People's Republic of Korea	2007	-	-	-	0.3	500,000	5,205	0.0	-	-	-	-	-	-
		2008	-	-	-	0.3	-	-	-	-	-	-	-	-	-
	Democratic Republic of Timor-Leste	2007	95,914	95,914	-	22.1	-	-	-	213,402	34,174	99.1	22.2	1370.5	307
		2008	79,226	79,226	-	35.9	-	-	-	143,594	34,406	100	33.5	1383.3	463.6
	India	2007	7,000,000	0	7,000,000	4.8	-	70,853,795	24.3	1,508,927	550,000	100	78.6	4150.3	3263.9
		2008	7,240,000	0	7,240,000	4.9	-	53,773,347	18.2	1,532,497	622,000	100	87.6	4150.4	3634.4
	Indonesia	2007	250,000	-	250,000	4.0	40,000	-	-	-	-	-	-	-	-
		2008	-	-	-	3.5	1,383	-	-	338,629	327,440	28.1	57.1	81.1	164.8
	Myanmar	2007	298,579	127,384	171,195	2.2	3,098	10,479	0.0	-	226,397	-	46.4	-	1168.7
		2008	693,858	112,865	580,993	5.1	2,902	11,284	0.0	-	187,102	-	42.7	-	1075.4
	Nepal	2007	154,300	154,300	-	2.3	-	-	-	68,097	25,488	100	250.4	427.8	1071.3
		2008	380,899	380,899	-	5.5	56,263	904,540	3.8	106,100	33,816	100	213.2	427.8	912.2
	Sri Lanka	2007	-	0	0	3.1	92,609	358,104	5.6	198	198	100	1422.5	476.3	6774.8
		2008	253,000	253,000	0	11.0	189,090	727,431	11.3	670	640	100	226.8	476.3	89319.6
	Thailand	2007	66,212	-	66,212	0.0	152,899	493,224	1.2	33,178	33,178	100	226.8	39386.8	89319.6
		2008	-	-	-	0.4	201,730	650,742	1.6	26,150	26,150	100	226.8	39386.8	89319.6
Western Pacific	Cambodia	2007	456,581	120,598	335,983	12.0	0	0	0.0	91,839	150,819	216	989.9	1138.1	5215.8
		2008	742,748	214,973	527,775	22.2	0	0	0.0	110,001	81,090	261.1	537.2	1376	2830.6
	China	2007	815,174	168,533	646,641	1.2	389	-	-	321,520	66,952	1097.2	3113	28839.7	81825.6
		2008	1,209,127	581,992	627,135	2.0	382	-	-	241,127	12,200	1448.2	998.4	38066.3	26242.1
	Lao People's Democratic Republic	2007	422,900	134,000	288,900	13.9	-	-	-	164,160	164,160	806.1	3697.3	5476.2	25116.8
		2008	395,275	73,000	322,275	17.1	-	-	-	287,160	287,160	1546.7	7094	10507	48191
	Malaysia	2007	176,462	1,000	175,462	7.5	-	301,733	6.4	5,456	-	134.3	-	24607.8	-
		2008	204,455	503	203,952	8.5	-	362,460	7.5	7,390	-	132	-	24197.1	-
	Papua New Guinea	2007	53,500	53,500	-	16.0	-	24,699	0.4	-	-	-	-	-	-
		2008	438,441	438,441	-	29.0	-	-	-	-	-	-	-	-	-
	Philippines	2007	620,010	-	-	2.9	-	853,099	2.0	-	110,000	-	10.7	-	27.1
		2008	444,390	-	-	2.0	-	15,570,992	35.9	-	-	-	-	-	-
	Republic of Korea	2007	-	-	-	-	-	-	-	-	-	-	-	-	-
		2008	-	-	-	-	-	-	-	-	-	-	-	-	-
	Solomon Islands	2007	70,000	70,000	-	49.7	34,875	154,854	31.3	-	-	-	-	-	-
		2008	61,805	61,805	-	72.8	30,292	143,443	28.2	-	-	-	-	-	-
	Vanuatu	2007	29,154	29,154	0	45.8	-	-	-	230,691	-	4216.6	-	16047.3	-
		2008	47,241	47,241	0	85.3	-	-	-	208,213	-	5988.3	-	22789.9	-
	Viet Nam	2007	600,000	-	600,000	1.4	-	1,767,840	2.1	1,300,000	112,500	7932.1	928	157429.1	18417.4
		2008	300,000	-	300,000	0.7	-	1,659,873	1.9	811,000	109,725	7142.2	1306.3	141751.6	25926.7

Mauritius is one of the countries listed but it has had no ongoing local transmission for over a decade.

*Data for Sudan only represents 15 northern states.

Annex 6.A – Household surveys of mosquito nets ownership and usage, 2006–2008

WHO region/subregion	Country/area	Year	Source	Subgroup	% of HH with ≥1 any net	% of HH with ≥1 ever treated net	% of HH with ≥1 ITN	% of children <5 years who slept under any net	% of children <5 years who slept under ever treated net	% of children <5 years who slept under an ITN	% of pregnant women who slept under any net	% of pregnant women who slept under ever treated net	% of pregnant women who slept under an ITN
Africa	Angola	2006	MIS 2006-07	Total	33	-	28	21	-	18	-	-	22
		2006	MIS 2006-07	Urban	34	-	29	19	-	17	-	-	15
		2006	MIS 2006-07	Rural	31	-	26	22	-	19	-	-	26
		2007	MIS 2007	Total	-	-	28	-	-	17	-	-	-
		2007	MIS 2007	Rural	-	-	-	-	-	-	-	-	-
		2008	MICS 2008	Total	-	-	-	-	-	-	-	-	-
	Benin	2006	DHS 2006	Total	56	-	25	47	-	20	-	-	20
		2006	DHS 2006	Urban	66	-	29	55	-	25	-	-	25
		2006	DHS 2006	Rural	50	-	21	42	-	18	-	-	17
	Burkina Faso	2006	MICS 2006	Total	52	-	23	18	-	10	-	-	-
		2006	MICS 2006	Urban	65	-	45	33	-	24	-	-	-
		2006	MICS 2006	Rural	47	-	15	14	-	6	-	-	-
	Cameroon	2006	MICS 2006	Total	32	-	20	27	-	13	-	-	-
		2006	MICS 2006	Urban	33	-	20	32	-	14	-	-	-
		2006	MICS 2006	Rural	30	-	20	22	-	12	-	-	-
	Central African Republic	2006	MICS 2006	Total	36	-	17	33	-	15	-	-	-
		2006	MICS 2006	Urban	54	-	27	52	-	24	-	-	-
		2006	MICS 2006	Rural	26	-	12	22	-	10	-	-	-
	Côte d'Ivoire	2006	MICS 2006	Total	27	-	6	17	-	6	-	-	-
		2006	MICS 2006	Urban	22	-	6	16	-	8	-	-	-
		2006	MICS 2006	Rural	31	-	6	18	-	4	-	-	-
	Democratic Republic of the Congo	2007	DHS 2007	Total	-	-	9	-	-	6	-	-	-
		2007	DHS 2007	Rural	-	-	-	-	-	-	-	-	-
	Equatorial Guinea	2007	Other Nat.	Total	-	54	26	-	-	42	-	-	-
		2008	Other Nat.	Total	-	64	-	-	-	-	-	-	-
	Ethiopia	2007	MIS 2007	Total	56	-	53	35	33	33	37	35	35
		2007	MIS 2007[a]	Total	69	-	65	41	37	42	37	34	43
		2007	MIS 2007	Urban	41	40	40	34	37	36	37	34	34
		2007	MIS 2007	Rural	59	57	56	34	33	33	37	36	34
	Gambia	2006	MICS 2006	Total	59	-	50	63	-	49	-	-	-
		2006	MICS 2006	Urban	49	-	13	55	-	38	-	-	-
		2006	MICS 2006	Rural	70	-	38	68	-	55	-	-	-
	Ghana	2006	MICS 2006	Total	30	-	19	33	-	22	-	-	-
		2006	MICS 2006	Urban	21	-	15	22	-	16	-	-	-
		2006	MICS 2006	Rural	37	-	22	38	-	25	-	-	-
		2008	DHS 2008	Total	-	-	33	-	-	28	-	-	-
	Guinea-Bissau	2006	MICS 2006	Total	79	-	44	73	-	39	-	-	-
		2006	MICS 2006	Urban	82	-	35	80	-	32	-	-	-
		2006	MICS 2006	Rural	78	-	49	71	-	42	-	-	-
	Kenya	2007	MIS 2007	Total	-	-	48	-	-	39	-	-	-
		2007	MIS 2007	Rural	-	-	-	-	-	-	-	-	-
		2008	DHS 2008	Total	-	-	48	-	-	39	-	-	-
		2008	DHS 2008	Rural	-	-	-	-	-	-	-	-	-
	Liberia	2007	DHS 2007	Total	-	-	-	-	-	-	-	-	-
	Madagascar	2008	Other Nat.	Total	-	-	59	-	-	60	-	-	-
	Malawi	2006	MICS 2006	Total	50	-	36	29	-	25	-	-	-
		2006	MICS 2006	Urban	72	-	56	52	-	43	-	-	-
		2006	MICS 2006	Rural	47	-	34	26	-	21	-	-	-

Annex 6.A – Household surveys of mosquito nets ownership and usage, 2006–2008 (continued)

WHO region/subregion	Country/area	Year	Source	Subgroup	% of HH with ≥1 any net	% of HH with ≥1 ever treated net	% of HH with ≥1 ITN	% of children <5 years who slept under any net	% of children <5 years who slept under ever treated net	% of children <5 years who slept under an ITN	% of pregnant women who slept under any net	% of pregnant women who slept under ever treated net	% of pregnant women who slept under an ITN
Africa	Mali	2006	DHS 2006	Total	69	-	50	41	-	27	-	-	29
		2006	DHS 2006	Urban	72	-	54	41	-	29	-	-	22
		2006	DHS 2006	Rural	68	-	48	41	-	26	-	-	31
	Mauritania	2006	MICS 2006	Total	-	-	3	-	-	-	-	-	-
		2007	MICS 2007	Total	-	-	-	-	-	-	-	-	-
	Mozambique	2007	MIS 2007	Total	-	-	16	-	-	7	-	-	-
		2007	MIS 2007	Rural	-	-	-	-	-	-	-	-	-
		2008	MICS 2008	Total	-	-	-	-	-	-	-	-	-
	Niger	2006	CDC-MMP National Survey	Total	-	-	65	-	-	56	-	-	48
		2006	DHS 2006	Total	69	69	43	15	15	7	13	13	7
		2006	DHS 2006	Urban	76	75	37	32	32	15	30	30	15
		2006	DHS 2006	Rural	68	67	44	12	12	6	11	11	5
	Nigeria	2007	MICS 2007	Total	-	-	8	-	-	6	-	-	-
		2008	DHS 2008	Total	-	-	-	-	-	-	-	-	-
		2008	DHS 2008	Rural	-	-	-	-	-	-	-	-	-
	Rwanda	2007	MIS 2007	Total	-	-	50	-	-	56	-	-	-
		2008	DHS 2008	Total	-	-	56	-	-	24	-	-	-
		2008	DHS 2008	Rural	-	-	-	-	-	-	-	-	-
	Sao Tome and Principe	2006	MICS 2006	Total	49	-	36	53	-	42	-	-	-
		2006	MICS 2006	Urban	58	-	44	62	-	51	-	-	-
		2006	MICS 2006	Rural	37	-	25	41	-	29	-	-	-
		2007	MOH 2007	Total	-	-	78	-	-	54	-	-	-
	Senegal	2006	MIS 2006	Total	57	-	36	28	-	16	-	-	17
		2006	MIS 2006	Urban	47	-	34	23	-	15	-	-	12
		2006	MIS 2006	Rural	65	-	38	30	-	17	-	-	20
		2008	MIS 2008	Total	-	-	63	-	-	31	-	-	-
	Sierra Leone	2007	MIS 2007	Total	-	-	59	-	-	56	-	-	-
		2008	DHS 2008	Total	-	-	37	-	-	26	-	-	-
	Togo	2006	MICS 2006	Total	46	-	40	41	-	38	-	-	-
		2006	MICS 2006	Urban	44	-	37	39	-	36	-	-	-
		2006	MICS 2006	Rural	47	-	42	42	-	40	-	-	-
		2008	CDC-MoH	Total	-	-	56	-	-	35	-	-	-
	Uganda	2006	DHS 2006	Total	34	21	16	22	13	9	24	13	10
		2006	DHS 2006	Urban	61	36	26	49	29	21	49	27	23
		2006	DHS 2006	Rural	29	19	14	18	11	8	22	12	9
	United Republic of Tanzania (Zanzibar)	2008	AIS/MIS 2008	Total	-	-	72	-	-	59	-	-	-
		2008	AIS/MIS 2008	Rural	-	-	-	-	-	-	-	-	-
	Zambia	2006	MIS 2006	Total	50	-	44	27	-	23	-	-	24
		2006	MICS 2006	Urban	51	-	45	31	-	26	-	-	18
		2006	MICS 2006	Rural	50	-	44	24	-	21	-	-	27
		2007	DHS 2007	Total	-	-	53	-	-	28	-	-	-
		2007	DHS 2007	Rural	-	-	-	-	-	-	-	-	-
		2008	MIS 2008	Total	-	-	62	-	-	41	-	-	-
		2008	MIS 2008	Rural	-	-	-	-	-	-	-	-	-
Eastern Mediterranean	Afghanistan	2008	NMLCP	Total	42	-	31	-	-	6	-	-	10
	Djibouti	2006	MICS 2006	Total	26	-	18	9	-	1	-	-	-
		2006	MICS 2006	Urban	26	-	18	9	-	1	-	-	-
		2006	MICS 2006	Rural	22	-	12	8	-	1	-	-	-
	Pakistan	2007	DHS 2007	Total	6	-	1	-	-	0	-	-	2

WHO region/subregion	Country/area	Year	Source	Subgroup	% of HH with ≥1 any net	% of HH with ≥1 ever treated net	% of HH with ≥1 ITN	% of children <5 years who slept under any net	% of children <5 years who slept under ever treated net	% of children <5 years who slept under an ITN	% of pregnant women who slept under any net	% of pregnant women who slept under ever treated net	% of pregnant women who slept under an ITN
Eastern Mediterranean	Somalia	2006	MICS 2006	Total	22	-	12	18	-	9	-	-	-
		2006	MICS 2006	Urban	27	-	16	25	-	15	-	-	-
		2006	MICS 2006	Rural	20	-	10	14	-	6	-	-	-
	Sudan (North)	2006	Sudan Household Health Survey	Total	37	-	18	-	-	28	-	-	-
South-East Asia	Indonesia	2007	DHS 2007	Total	32	4	3	31	4	3	23	2	2
		2007	DHS 2003 (National report)	Urban	18	2	1	19	2	2	11	1	1
		2007	DHS 2007	Urban	-	-	-	-	-	-	-	-	-
		2007	DHS 2007	Rural	42	5	4	40	6	5	33	4	3
Western Pacific	Cambodia	2007	CMS 2007	Rural	95	-	36	-	-	28	-	-	28
	Lao People's Democratic Republic	2008	IndoChina research / CMPE	Rural	97	-	56	-	-	43	-	-	50
	Viet Nam	2006	MICS 2006	Total	97	-	19	94	-	5	-	-	-
		2006	MICS 2006	Urban	92	-	5	88	-	12	-	-	-
		2006	MICS 2006	Rural	99	-	23	95	-	3	-	-	-

*Data updated by DHS since the original publication.

^aPercentages calculated using the population at risk.

AIS = AIDS Indicator Survey.

CDC-MMP = Centers for Disease Control and Prevention - Malaria Measles Partnership.

DHS = Demographic and Health Survey.

MICS = Multiple Indicator Cluster Survey.

MIS = Malaria Indicator Survey.

Annex 6.B – Household surveys of antimalarial treatment, 2006–2008

WHO region	Country/area	Year	Source	Subgroup	% of children < 5 with fever who took SP/Fansidar same or next day	% of children < 5 with fever who took chloroquine same or next day	% of children < 5 with fever who took ACT same or next day	% of children < 5 with fever who took any antimalarial drugs same or next day	% of children < 5 with fever who took SP/Fansidar	% of children < 5 with fever who took chloroquine	% of children < 5 with fever who took ACT	% of children < 5 with fever who took any antimalarial drugs	% of pregnant women who took at least 2 doses SP/Fansidar
Africa	Angola	2006	MIS 2006-07	Total	-	-	-	18	0	14	2	29	3
		2006	MIS 2006-07	Urban	-	-	-	27	-	-	-	38	4
		2006	MIS 2006-07	Rural	-	-	-	12	-	-	-	23	1
		2007	MIS 2007	Total	-	-	-	13	0	14	3	28	3
		2007	MIS 2007	Rural	-	-	-	-	-	-	-	-	-
		2008	MICS 2008	Total	-	-	-	-	-	-	-	-	-
	Benin	2006	DHS 2006	Total	-	-	-	42	1	49	0	54	3
		2006	DHS 2006	Urban	-	-	-	48	-	-	-	57	3
		2006	DHS 2006	Rural	-	-	-	39	-	-	-	53	3
	Burkina Faso	2006	MICS 2006	Total	-	-	-	41	0	46	0	48	1
		2006	MICS 2006	Urban	-	-	-	61	-	-	-	70	2
		2006	MICS 2006	Rural	-	-	-	36	-	-	-	42	1
	Cameroon	2006	MICS 2006	Total	-	-	-	38	2	8	2	58	6
		2006	MICS 2006	Urban	-	-	-	53	-	-	-	69	8
		2006	MICS 2006	Rural	-	-	-	29	-	-	-	50	4
	Central African Republic	2006	MICS 2006	Total	-	-	-	42	4	29	3	57	9
		2006	MICS 2006	Urban	-	-	-	48	-	-	-	68	15
		2006	MICS 2006	Rural	-	-	-	36	-	-	-	47	5
	Côte d'Ivoire	2006	MICS 2006	Total	-	-	-	26	2	31	3	36	8
		2006	MICS 2006	Urban	-	-	-	32	-	-	-	45	10
		2006	MICS 2006	Rural	-	-	-	23	-	-	-	32	7
	Democratic Republic of the Congo	2007	DHS 2007	Total	-	-	-	17	3	6	1	30	5
		2007	DHS 2007	Rural	-	-	-	-	-	-	-	-	-
	Equatorial Guinea	2007	Other Nat.	Total	-	-	-	-	-	-	-	-	-
		2008	Other Nat.	Total	-	-	-	-	-	-	3	16	-
	Ethiopia	2007	MIS 2007	Total	-	-	-	4	-	-	4	10	-
		2007	MIS 2007	Urban	-	-	-	4	-	-	-	13	-
		2007	MIS 2007	Rural	-	-	-	4	-	-	-	9	-
		2007	MICS 2007a	Total	-	-	-	5	-	-	-	-	-
	Gambia	2006	MICS 2006	Total	-	-	-	52	13	58	0	63	33
		2006	MICS 2006	Urban	-	-	-	54	-	-	-	59	31
		2006	MICS 2006	Rural	-	-	-	52	-	-	-	65	34
	Ghana	2006	MICS 2006	Total	-	-	-	48	1	42	4	61	27
		2006	MICS 2006	Urban	-	-	-	58	-	-	-	69	35
		2006	MICS 2006	Rural	-	-	-	44	-	-	-	57	24
		2008	DHS 2008	Total	-	-	-	-	-	-	12	24	-
	Guinea-Bissau	2006	MICS 2006	Total	-	-	-	27	2	41	2	46	7
		2006	MICS 2006	Urban	-	-	-	47	-	-	-	60	9
		2006	MICS 2006	Rural	-	-	-	18	-	-	-	39	7
	Kenya	2007	MIS 2007	Total	-	-	-	15	-	-	8	24	13
		2007	MIS 2007	Urban	-	-	-	-	-	-	-	-	-
		2008	DHS 2008	Total	-	-	-	-	-	-	-	24	-
		2008	DHS 2008	Rural	-	-	-	-	-	-	-	-	-
	Liberia	2007	DHS 2007	Total	-	-	-	26	3	43	9	59	12
	Madagascar	2008	Other Nat.	Total	-	-	-	-	-	-	-	-	-
	Malawi	2006	MICS 2006	Total	-	-	-	20	20	1	0	24	45
		2006	MICS 2006	Urban	-	-	-	24	-	-	-	30	52
		2006	MICS 2006	Rural	-	-	-	20	-	-	-	23	44
	Mali	2006	DHS 2006	Total	-	-	-	15	2	22	-	32	4
		2006	DHS 2006	Urban	-	-	-	16	-	-	-	35	10
		2006	DHS 2006	Rural	-	-	-	14	-	-	-	31	2

Annex 6.B – Household surveys of antimalarial treatment, 2006–2008 (continued)

WHO region	Country/area	Year	Source	Subgroup	% of children < 5 with fever who took SP/ Fansidar same or next day	% of children < 5 with fever who took chloroquine same or next day	% of children < 5 with fever who took ACT same or next day	% of children < 5 years with fever who took any antimalarial drugs same or next day	% of children < 5 years with fever who took SP/ Fansidar	% of children < 5 years with fever who took chloroquine	% of children < 5 years with fever who took ACT	% of children < 5 years with fever who took any antimalarial drugs	% of pregnant women who took at least 2 doses SP/Fansidar
Africa	Mauritania	2006	MICS 2006	Total	-	-	-	10	3	6	1	21	-
		2007	MICS 2007	Total	-	-	-	-	-	-	-	-	-
	Mozambique	2007	MIS 2007	Total	-	-	-	18	-	-	-	23	16
		2007	MIS 2007	Rural	-	-	-	-	-	-	-	-	-
		2008	MICS 2008	Total	-	-	-	-	-	-	-	-	-
	Niger	2006	CDC-MMP National Survey	Total	-	-	-	-	-	-	-	-	-
		2006	DHS 2006	Total	0	22	-	25	1	29	-	33	0
		2006	DHS 2006	Urban	2	29	-	34	2	38	-	45	1
		2006	DHS 2006	Rural	0	20	-	23	0	27	-	31	0
	Nigeria	2007	MICS 2007	Total	-	-	-	15	-	-	-	33	7
		2008	DHS 2008	Total	-	-	-	-	-	-	-	-	-
		2008	DHS 2008	Rural	-	-	-	-	-	-	-	-	-
	Rwanda	2007	MIS 2007	Total	-	-	-	0	-	-	5	6	17
		2008	DHS 2008	Total	-	-	-	-	-	-	-	-	-
		2008	DHS 2008	Rural	-	-	-	-	-	-	-	-	-
	Sao Tome and Principe	2006	MICS 2006	Total	-	-	-	17	1	2	6	25	-
		2006	MICS 2006	Urban	-	-	-	17	-	-	-	22	-
		2006	MICS 2006	Rural	-	-	-	16	-	-	-	28	-
		2007	MOH 2007	Total	-	-	-	-	-	-	-	-	-
	Senegal	2006	MIS 2006	Total	-	-	-	9	0	7	6	22	49
		2006	MIS 2006	Urban	-	-	-	12	-	-	-	19	55
		2006	MIS 2006	Rural	-	-	-	10	-	-	-	24	46
		2008	MIS 2008	Total	-	-	-	-	-	-	-	-	-
	Sierra Leone	2007	MIS 2007	Total	-	-	-	-	-	-	-	30	-
		2008	DHS 2008	Total	-	-	-	-	-	-	-	-	-
	Togo	2006	MICS 2006	Total	-	-	-	38	3	32	1	48	18
		2006	MICS 2006	Urban	-	-	-	49	-	-	-	57	18
		2006	MICS 2006	Rural	-	-	-	32	-	-	-	43	18
		2008	CDC-MoH	Total	-	-	-	-	-	-	11	37	-
	Uganda	2006	DHS 2006	Total	10	20	1	29	19	41	3	61	16
		2006	DHS 2006	Urban	2	10	0	27	6	24	4	58	17
		2006	DHS 2006	Rural	3	13	1	29	6	28	3	62	16
	United Republic of Tanzania (Zanzibar)	2008	AIS/MIS 2008	Total	-	-	-	37	-	-	10	38	52
		2008	AIS/MIS 2008	Rural	-	-	-	-	-	-	-	-	-
	Zambia	2006	MIS 2006	Total	-	-	-	37	33	-	13	58	61
		2006	MIS 2006	Urban	-	-	-	49	-	-	-	74	71
		2006	MIS 2006	Rural	-	-	-	35	-	-	-	55	56
		2007	DHS 2007	Total	-	-	-	21	23	1	11	38	63
		2007	DHS 2007	Rural	-	-	-	-	-	-	-	-	-
		2008	MIS 2008	Total	-	-	-	29	21	-	13	43	60
		2008	MIS 2008	Rural	-	-	-	-	-	-	-	-	-
Eastern Mediterranean	Afghanistan	2008	NMLCP	Total	-	-	-	-	-	-	-	8	-
	Djibouti	2006	MICS 2006	Total	-	-	-	3	4	5	0	10	-
		2006	MICS 2006	Urban	-	-	-	3	-	-	-	10	-
		2006	MICS 2006	Rural	-	-	-	0	-	-	-	0	-
	Pakistan	2007	DHS 2007	Total	-	-	0	3	-	-	0	3	0
	Somalia	2006	MICS 2006	Total	-	-	-	3	2	6	1	8	1
		2006	MICS 2006	Urban	-	-	-	7	-	-	-	14	1
		2006	MICS 2006	Rural	-	-	-	1	-	-	-	6	1
	Sudan (North)	2006	Sudan Household Health Survey Total		-	-	-	3	-	-	4	54	-

Annex 6.B – Household surveys of antimalarial treatment, 2006–2008 (continued)

WHO region	Country/area	Year	Source	Subgroup	% of children < 5 with fever who took SP/ Fansidar same or next day	% of children < 5 with fever who took chloroquine same or next day	% of children < 5 years with fever who took ACT same or next day	% of children < 5 years with fever who took any antimalarial drugs same or next day	% of children < 5 years with fever who took SP/ Fansidar	% of children < 5 years with fever who took chloroquine	% of children < 5 years with fever who took ACT	% of children < 5 years with fever who took any antimalarial drugs	% of pregnant women who took at least 2 doses SP/Fansidar
South-East Asia	Indonesia	2007	DHS 2003 (National report)	Urban	-	-	-	-	-	-	-	-	-
		2007	DHS 2007	Total	-	-	-	-	-	-	-	-	-
		2007	DHS 2007	Urban	-	-	-	-	-	-	-	1	-
		2007	DHS 2007	Rural	-	-	-	-	-	-	-	1	-
Western Pacific	Cambodia	2007	CMS 2007	Rural	-	-	-	-	-	-	-	-	0
	Lao People's Democratic Republic	2008	IndoChina research / CMPE	Rural	-	-	-	-	-	-	2	7	-
	Viet Nam	2006	MICS 2006	Total	-	-	-	2	2	0	0	3	-
		2006	MICS 2006	Urban	-	-	-	2	-	-	-	2	-
		2006	MICS 2006	Rural	-	-	-	2	-	-	-	3	-

[1] Data updated by DHS since the original publication.
[2] Percentages calculated using the population at risk.

AIS = AIDS Indicator Survey.

CDC-MMP = Centers for Disease Control and Prevention - Malaria Measles Partnership.

DHS = Demographic and Health Survey.

MICS = Multiple Indicator Cluster Survey.

MIS = Malaria Indicator Survey.

Other Nat. = Other national survey

Annex 7 – Funding for malaria control, 2008

WHO Region/Sub-region	Country	Year	Global Fund[a]	PMI[b]	The World Bank[c]	Government	Global Fund	The World Bank	bilaterals	UN Agencies	European Union	Other
Africa	Angola	2008	9,872,558	–	–	17,568,587	–	–	–	–	–	–
	Benin	2008	6,345,919	–	–	–	–	4,606,000	–	–	–	–
	Botswana	2008	–	–	–	1,000,000	–	–	–	–	–	–
	Burkina Faso	2008	7,283,872	–	–	58,662	406,699,675	–	–	–	–	–
	Burundi	2008	9,623,263	–	–	46,000,000	4,683,029	–	–	–	–	–
	Cameroon	2008	6,046,764	–	–	15,023,247	11,506,022	–	–	–	–	–
	Central African Republic	2008	2,294,055	–	–	19,000	3,992,312	600,000	–	–	–	–
	Comoros	2008	264,709	–	–	–	264,708	–	–	–	–	–
	Congo	2008	–	–	4,500,000	–	–	–	–	–	–	–
	Democratic Republic of the Congo	2008	18,188,352	–	–	2,000,000	4,071,981	43,000,000	–	–	–	–
	Equatorial Guinea	2008	6,305,881	–	–	776,600	8,245,229	–	–	–	–	–
	Eritrea	2008	4,754,718	–	–	–	4,792,642	300,000	–	–	–	–
	Ethiopia	2008	3,138,583	–	–	–	–	–	–	–	–	–
	Gabon	2008	1,338,162	–	–	1,276,856	450,693	–	–	–	–	–
	Gambia	2008	5,683,473	–	–	–	5,683,474	–	–	–	–	–
	Ghana	2008	10,544,980	–	–	–	16,206,474	–	–	–	–	–
	Guinea	2008	1,002,592	–	–	–	17,339,248	1,181,250	–	–	–	–
	Guinea-Bissau	2008	1,526,060	–	–	–	1,545,699	–	–	–	–	–
	Kenya	2008	18,964,849	–	–	32,566	37,543,798	–	–	–	–	–
	Liberia	2008	8,863,680	–	–	60,118	6,347,301	–	–	–	–	–
	Madagascar	2008	15,103,081	–	–	19,387	5,814,063	–	–	–	–	–
	Malawi	2008	14,961,664	–	–	24,000,000	–	–	–	–	–	–
	Mali	2008	4,233,040	–	–	–	6,703,715	1,749,540	–	–	–	–
	Mauritania	2008	1,342,027	–	–	–	–	–	–	–	–	–
	Mozambique	2008	11,625,136	–	–	–	–	–	–	–	–	–
	Namibia	2008	412,016	–	–	1,692,308	–	–	–	–	–	–
	Niger	2008	12,345,165	–	–	–	–	–	–	–	–	–
	Nigeria	2008	16,273,780	–	–	14,324,952	15,353,110	52,358,702	–	–	–	–
	Rwanda	2008	19,260,378	–	–	500,000	12,884,983	3,083,332	–	–	–	–
	Sao Tome and Principe	2008	2,424,782	–	–	115,990	535,989	40,000	–	–	–	–
	Senegal	2008	5,839,346	–	–	176,000	–	–	–	–	–	–
	Sierra Leone	2008	4,840,240	–	–	318,966	–	–	–	–	–	–
	Swaziland	2008	294,218	–	–	65,892	–	–	–	–	–	–
	Togo	2008	5,026,694	–	–	–	2,442,924	–	–	–	–	–
	Uganda	2008	6,335,768	–	–	19,445,544	–	–	–	–	–	–
	United Republic of Tanzania	2008	58,667,840	–	–	2,000,000	–	–	–	–	–	–
	Zambia	2008	15,423,129	–	8,000,000	2,000,000	–	–	–	–	–	–
	Zimbabwe	2008	–	–	–	1,675,435	1,100,000	–	–	–	–	–

Annex 7 – Funding for malaria control, 2008 (continued)

WHO Region/Sub-region	Country	Year	Global Fund[a]	PMI[b]	The World Bank[c]	Government	Global Fund	The World Bank	bilaterals	UN Agencies	European Union	Other
Americas	Bolivia (Plurinational State of)	2008	-	-	-	106,000,000	-	-	-	-	70,000	-
	Brazil	2008	-	-	-	6,720,000	-	-	-	-	-	-
	Costa Rica	2008	3,325,400	-	-	-	-	-	-	-	-	-
	Guatemala	2008	141,763	-	-	-	-	-	-	-	-	-
	Guyana	2008	3,322,684	-	-	560,600	337,620	-	-	-	14,000	-
	Haiti	2008	968,258	-	-	-	2,085,000	-	-	-	-	-
	Honduras	2008	793,799	-	-	-	-	-	-	-	-	-
	Nicaragua	2008	875,248	-	-	-	-	-	-	-	-	-
	Suriname	2008	-	-	-	-	-	-	-	-	-	-
Eastern Mediterranean	Afghanistan	2008	8,141,152	-	-	332,259	7,785,080	-	-	-	-	-
	Djibouti	2008	1,244,752	-	-	-	-	-	-	-	-	-
	Iran (Islamic Republic of)	2008	2,797,683	-	-	7,500,000	664,575	-	-	-	-	-
	Pakistan	2008	1,642,417	-	-	-	2,500,000	-	-	-	-	-
	Saudi Arabia	2008	-	-	-	27,345,844	-	-	-	-	-	-
	Somalia	2008	3,784,480	-	-	-	-	-	-	-	-	-
	Sudan*	2008	34,517,515	-	-	13,325,129	3,700,680	41,360	-	-	-	-
	Yemen	2008	5,044,737	-	-	2,465,870	4,185,533	-	-	-	-	-
Europe	Azerbaijan	2008	1,295,872	-	-	-	-	-	-	-	-	-
	Georgia	2008	705,430	-	-	47,904	603,680	-	-	-	-	-
	Kyrgyzstan	2008	-	-	-	68,500	647,245	-	-	-	-	-
	Tajikistan	2008	1,822,811	-	-	-	1,464,503	-	-	-	-	-
	Turkey	2008	-	-	-	40,850,967	-	-	-	-	-	-
	Uzbekistan	2008	509,704	-	-	120,813	320,146	-	-	-	-	-
South-East Asia	Bangladesh	2008	8,370,698	-	-	528,209	9,580,687	700,000	-	-	-	-
	Bhutan	2008	1,059,849	-	-	0	1	-	-	-	-	-
	Democratic Republic of Timor-Leste	2008	-	-	-	719,632	-	-	-	-	-	-
	India	2008	34,286,405	-	-	73,943,830	13,863,557	28,619,974	-	-	-	-
	Indonesia	2008	20,841,603	-	-	1,664,912	13,199,217	-	-	-	-	-
	Nepal	2008	4,480,142	-	-	961,457	924,791	-	-	-	-	-
	Sri Lanka	2008	3,929,226	-	-	4,144,123	157,300	-	-	-	-	-
	Thailand	2008	5,977,700	-	-	2,827,000	3,513,961	-	-	-	-	-
Western Pacific	Cambodia	2008	10,598,785	-	-	1,508,603	4,327,529	-	-	-	-	-
	China	2008	5,473,763	-	-	-	9,133,011	-	-	-	-	-
	Lao People's Democratic Republic	2008	7,840,252	-	-	594,912	7,242,608	-	-	-	-	-
	Papua New Guinea	2008	6,385,835	-	-	-	6,385,835	-	-	-	-	-
	Philippines	2008	5,310,226	-	-	1,600,000	-	-	-	-	-	-
	Republic of Korea	2008	-	-	-	792,000	-	-	-	-	-	-
	Solomon Islands	2008	-	-	-	3,613,227	483,416	-	-	-	-	-
	Vanuatu	2008	-	-	-	-	264,300	-	-	-	-	-
	Viet Nam	2008	8,395,846	-	-	4,599,534	3,178,551	-	-	-	-	-

[a] Source: The Global Fund web site (Malaria specific grants, Integrated and Health Systems Strengthening grants are not included)

[b] Source: PMI web site

[c] Source: The World Bank web site, funds for 3 years

* Data reported by Sudan represents only the northern states.